A

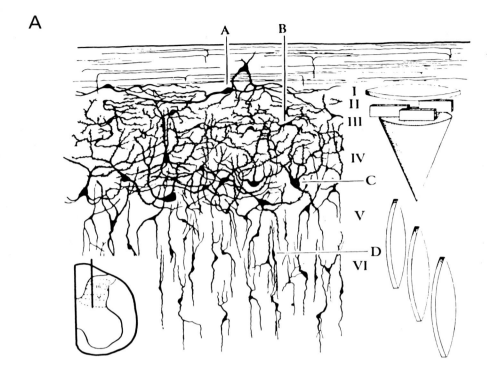

B

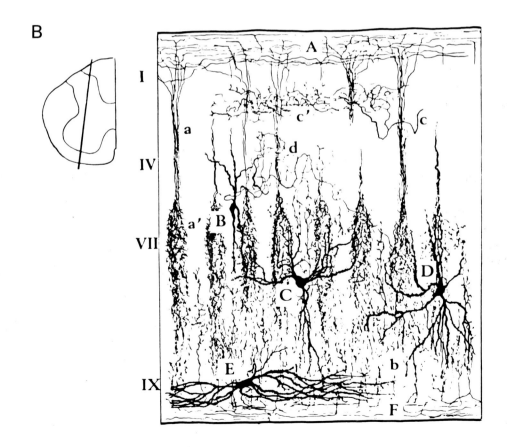

lamina. As will be seen (see Chapters 6–9), this is an oversimplification, but neurones with their somata in lamina IV have well-developed dorsally directed dendrites. Lamina IV neurones send axon collaterals to laminae III–V or VI but not into II (Matsushita 1969).

In laminae V–VIII the dendritic trees are organized transversely (Fig. 1.2A, B). This observation of the Scheibels has been confirmed by Matsushita (1969), Mannen (1975) and Proshansky and Egger (1977). Primary afferent collaterals are also organized in the transverse plane, running dorso-ventrally (Fig. 1.2B) and also arborizing widely across the cord (Sprague and Ha 1964; Sterling and Kuypers 1967a; Scheibel and Scheibel 1968, 1969; Réthelyi and Szentágothai 1973). In the central part of lamina VI there is an extensive terminal field of primary afferent fibres (Sprague & Ha 1964; Réthelyi and Szentágothai 1973). This area, often called the intermediate zone, is dorsal to the position of Ramon y Cajal's intermediate grey nucleus and the suggestion of Sprague and Ha that it be referred to simply as lamina VI has much to recommend it, except that the terminal field obviously extends into parts of adjacent laminae.

The motoneurones of lamina IX have well-developed longitudinally running dendrites (Sterling and Kuypers 1967b; Scheibel and Scheibel 1969) (Fig. 1.2B). But motoneuronal dendrites are not contained within the motor cell columns. Recent experiments involving the injection of horseradish peroxidase into motoneurones have revealed that their dendrites extend enormous distances, dorsally as far as lamina VI and also out into the white matter of the lateral and ventral columns (Cullheim and Kellerth 1976; see also Chapter 14).

Recent studies have shown, therefore, that there is very good agreement between Rexed's cytoarchitectonic scheme and the dendritic and synaptological organization in the dorsal horn, particularly in laminae I–IV. The motor cell columns are also quite clear. These two parts have been called the sensory and motor appendages respectively by Réthelyi and Szentágothai (1973). They consider that between these two appendages the 'real interneurone system' exists as a central core of double-cylindrical structure (double across the mid-line). This concept arose out of a consideration of the neurogenesis of the cord (Szentágothai 1967b) and was strengthened by a study of the dendritic architecture (Golgi–Kopsch) of *adult* feline cords (Réthelyi 1976).

The ideas of Réthelyi and Szentágothai can be traced back to earlier reports. Several attempts have been made at classifying neurones on the basis of their dendritic tree morphology as seen in Golgi preparations. Of relevance to the present discussion are the papers of Ramon-Moliner (1962), Ramon-Moliner and Nauta (1966) and Leontovich and Zhukova (1963). The 'isodendritic' neurones of Ramon-Moliner and Nauta (1966), which are essentially the 'radiate' neurones of the earlier paper by Ramon-Moliner (1962), are considered to be 'primitive' and typical of the reticular core of the brain stem. These neurones correspond with the reticular type of Leontovich and Zhukova (1963), who concluded that they formed a reticular formation in the cord, specifically in 'the whole of the zona intermedia, including the lateral horn . . . out to the ventral horn, penetrating between the motor nuclei . . . [up] to the dorsal horn, reaching the layer of large cells . . . at the ventral border of Rolando's substance'. The similarities between this description of the 'reticular formation' of the spinal cord and the central core of Réthelyi and Szentágothai (1973) are striking. In addition to the dendritic organization of the cord (Réthelyi 1976), Réthelyi and Szentágothai (1973) also consider the synaptic arrangements.

The central core concept is an interesting idea and merits serious consideration. Here, however, the system of Rexed will be used to describe the location of nerve cells, dendrites, axonal arborizations, etc. in the cord. The system has become so universally used that it would seem advisable to do this; where necessary the laminar descriptions will be qualified.

C. Physiological classifications of dorsal horn neurones

Electrophysiological experiments on the spinal cord seem to fall into two categories: on the one hand, those where neurones are identified quite precisely, and on the other, those where—often of necessity—identification is at best vague. The earliest microelectrode experiments, on motoneurones, set the standards for the first category. Motoneurones may be easily identified by antidromic excitation from the ventral root or peripheral nerve, and recently the identification has been developed to include the contractile properties of the motor unit (Burke et al. 1971a, 1973, 1974). The first category also includes experiments identifying, by antidromic excitation, neurones of various ascending pathways and two sorts of short-axoned interneurones in the ventral horn: the Renshaw cells and the Ia inhibitory interneurones (see Sect. D.II.2.b). Most of the second category deals with neurones for which identifications have not been provided. The neurones are situated in the dorsal horn and they have been the subject of a number of proposed classification systems. Some of the earliest attempts were made by Kolmodin (1957) and Kolmodin and Skoglund (1960), and Eccles et al. (1960). Many reports have also described certain cell types observed during the course of electrophysiological experiments in which the search stimuli would have limited the population of recordable neurones (such as the neurones recorded by Gray and his co-workers Armett et al. 1961, 1962; Gray and Lal 1965; Fuller and Gray 1966] and the neurones activated from cutaneous afferent units described by Tapper and his collaborators [Tapper et al. 1973; P. B. Brown et al. 1973]).

Perhaps the most influential scheme has been that of Wall (1967), which utilizes the laminar terminology of Rexed (1952, 1954). According to Wall, neurones in lamina 4 are excited by light tactile stimulation and have no surround or lateral inhibitory fields. Lamina 5 cells respond, in addition, to more intense mechanical stimulation and to visceral input (Pomeranz et al. 1968); they also have surrounding inhibitory fields. In lamina 6, neurones receive, in addition, excitatory input from muscle and joint receptors. Wall (1967) was careful to point out that his technique of using rather coarse microelectrodes preferentially selected the largest cells and that the laminae discerned by him should be regarded as zones of concentration of particular cell types rather than separate laminae of distinct specialization. It is, therefore, perhaps unfortunate that he called his layers laminae 4, 5 and 6, as it appears that many workers have Rexed's laminae IV–VI and Wall's laminae 4–6 inextricably mixed in their concepts of dorsal horn organization. Thus, if a cell has

certain *physiological* properties it is labelled a lamina IV, V or VI neurone. That is, its physiological properties as observed (and any fine differences between cells in their inputs, axonal projections, etc. are ignored) are used to determine its *anatomical* location in a cytoarchitectonic scheme. In some reports this has gone to the extent of ignoring the location of the cell: the position of the microelectrode tip is not specified (beyond its being somewhere in the dorsal horn), but the neurones are called lamina IV cells, etc.

An assumption in much current work is that all neurones in a certain lamina are similar from a functional point of view. But this is manifestly not so; it will be shown in Chapter 6, for example, that many neurones of the spinocervical tract with cell bodies in the dorsal half of Rexed's lamina IV respond to hair movement (light tactile input), heavy pressure and pinch and to muscle nerve stimulation. Undoubtedly, the *gradient* of cell properties described by Wall (1967) exists, but the division of neurones in Rexed's laminae IV–VI into defined physiological layers corresponding to the cytoarchitectonic laminae is arbitrary and has been much abused.

Recently another classification of dorsal horn neurones, based on their responses to mechanical and noxious stimulation of the skin, has been proposed (Iggo 1974; Handwerker et al. 1975; see also the earlier attempt by Gregor and Zimmermann 1972). The classification is: *Class 1*, neurones excited by sensitive cutaneous mechanoreceptors; *Class 2*, neurones excited by sensitive cutaneous mechanoreceptors and by nociceptors; *Class 3*, neurones excited only by nociceptors. This classification has been used in subsequent reports (Cervero et al. 1976, 1977).

The Class 1–3 system has been extended. Menétrey et al. (1977) have subdivided Classes 1 and 2 and added Class 4 in their study of dorsal horn neurones in the rat. Class 1A neurones are excited by hair movement and/or touch, Class 1B by hair movement and/or touch and pressure or pressure only. Class 2A neurones are excited by hair movement and/or touch, pressure, pinch and/or pin-prick, Class 2B by pressure, pinch and/or pin-prick. Class 4 neurones respond to joint movement or pressure on deep tissues. Cervero and Iggo (1978) and Cervero et al. (1979b) have added 'inverse classes' to the original categories, that is Classes $\bar{1}$, $\bar{2}$ and $\bar{3}$. The neurones of these classes are located in the substantia gelatinosa (lamina II) and are inhibited by peripheral stimuli as follows: Class $\bar{1}$, inhibited by sensitive cutaneous mechanoreceptors; Class $\bar{2}$, inhibited by sensitive cutaneous mechanoreceptors and by nociceptors; Class $\bar{3}$, inhibited by nociceptors.

The Class 1–3, etc. system cuts across other schemes. Thus, Class 1 cells appear similar to Wall's (1967) lamina 4 neurones and Class 2 to his lamina 5 and 6 neurones, but they are not limited to Rexed's (1952, 1954) laminae IV, V and VI. Many Class 3 cells are located in lamina I and are probably the marginal cells shown by Christensen and Perl (1970) to receive only noxious input. As mentioned above, the $\bar{1}$, $\bar{2}$ and $\bar{3}$ categories are located in lamina II; they are of particular interest because of their relevance to the 'gate theory' of Melzack and Wall (1965). Cells of the spino-cervical tract are also fitted into the scheme and include Class 1, 2 and 3 neurones (Cervero et al. 1977).

This classification, like that of Wall, does not take into consideration the identity of the neurones in terms of either their axonal projections or their responses to stimulation of known receptor types (different sorts of hair follicle receptors, Types I and II receptors, Pacinian corpuscles, joint and muscle receptors, etc.). The assumption is made that all Class 1 neurones etc. (cf. Wall's lamina 4 etc. cells) form a functionally homogeneous group. This is manifestly not so.

Obviously it is necessary, for communication of results and ideas, to group together units having similar physiological responses, but the schemes of Wall and Iggo should be considered no more than temporary means to aid that communication. It is the present writer's opinion that the anatomical and physiological classifications should be kept clearly differentiated. Ideally, a neurone should be identified as far as possible by means of its axonal projections and/or the characteristics of its input and response properties. If possible, it should be stained by intracellular dye deposition. Its anatomical location should then be described in terms of Rexed's scheme. This dual physiological and anatomical approach would, at the very least, avoid the unfortunate use of anatomical terminology to describe physiological response properties (such as 'lamina 4 type neurone'), and ought to lead, eventually, to a much more precise description of spinal cord organization. It has always been a tenet of the present writer that such an approach is not only

advisable but obligatory in any microelectrode experiments on the central nervous system.

D. Résumé of spinal cord anatomy

The remainder of this chapter is a brief résumé of the structure of the lumbosacral spinal cord (cat) as revealed by anatomical and physiological techniques up to the introduction of the technique of intracellular injection of the enzyme horseradish peroxidase (Cullheim and Kellerth 1976; Jankowska et al. 1976; Snow et al. 1976). The remainder of the book presents results obtained by that method. The literature up to 1971 was excellently reviewed by Réthelyi and Szentágothai (1973) and the following account draws heavily on that article.

I. Primary afferent fibres

1. Entrance into the spinal cord

The vast majority of primary afferent fibres from receptors in skin, subcutaneous tissue, muscle, fascia, joint capsules and viscera enters the central nervous system through the dorsal roots (or the corresponding divisions of the trigeminal system). The recently rediscovered afferent fibres that enter the spinal cord through the ventral roots (Coggeshall et al. 1973, 1974; Applebaum et al. 1976) are mainly non-myelinated and innervate visceral and, to a lesser degree, cutaneous receptors (Clifton et al. 1974, 1976). Their course and mode of termination within the spinal grey matter are unknown at present.

The concept that the lateral division of the dorsal root contains fibres of small diameter (Ranson 1913a) is, according to Szentágothai (1964), still acceptable, although he suggests that the small axons are concentrated at the periphery of the rootlets. In any event many of these small axons enter Lissauer's tract where they form the most medial component (Ranson 1913a, 1914a; Ranson and Hess 1915; Ranson and Billingsley 1916).

Upon entering the cord, the primary afferent fibres bifurcate and give rise to ascending and descending branches from which collaterals arise. According to Réthelyi and Szentágothai (1973) there is no evidence for the existence of non-bifurcating primary afferent fibres (nor for any fibres that enter the grey matter directly). Non-bifurcating fibres do occur, however, and they commonly innervate hair follicle receptors (see Chapter 2), although most other types of primary afferent fibres are represented in the non-bifurcating category.

2. Collaterals

The collaterals given off the ascending and descending branches of primary afferent fibres enter the grey matter through any part of its border with the dorsal columns. Since the ascending and descending branches of the primary afferent fibres move medially in their ascent and descent (Kahler 1882), then collaterals enter the dorsal horn laterally when they arise from the parent fibre close to its entry into the cord, and more and more medially as they are given off farther and farther away from the point of entry. The position of the terminal arborization of a collateral is not, however, governed by the position of entry of the collateral into the grey matter but by the location of its receptors. The somatotopic organization of the terminations of primary afferent fibres in the cord has been discussed by Réthelyi and Szentágothai (1973); it will be considered in several of the following chapters.

There is a wealth of descriptive material on the morphology of the different types of primary afferent fibre collaterals in the cord. Unfortunately, anatomical methods, by their very nature, are unable to provide identification of the collaterals in terms of their receptor types. At best, only tentative identifications may be made with the help of other, often electrophysiological, evidence. Alternatively, the anatomical evidence per se, such as the diameter of the parent axons, may be used to consider a particular group of axons, for example the small fibres and their collaterals to the substantia gelatinosa.

Anatomical methods have shown that fibres of small diameter give rise to terminal arborizations that run longitudinally in lamina II. According to Réthelyi (1977) the only primary afferent fibres to terminate within lamina II are the non-myelinated (C) fibres. It remains to be seen whether this is the case, but as will be shown in the following chapters very few, if any, myelinated primary afferent axons have terminal arborizations within lamina II. Fine fibres are also distributed to lamina I (Szentágothai 1964; Sterling and Kuypers, 1967a). The substantia gelatinosa (lamina II) has long been assumed to play a role in nociception, and more recently the marginal cells of lamina I have also been considered in this light (Christensen and Perl 1970). The non-myelinated fibres are known to include a considerable number, particularly in cat, that respond only to noxious stimulation. The pieces of evidence fit together nicely and it may be assumed that laminae I and II receive input from the small-diameter primary afferent fibres. However, the final identification of the fine-calibre axons entering laminae I and II has not been made. It is known that many axons in Lissauer's tract are propriospinal in nature (Szentágothai 1964).

Collaterals arising from large myelinated fibres of known primary afferent origin have been described. Among the best known are the recurving collaterals that, having descended through the dorsal horn, turn and ascend back into laminae IV and III where they break up into the 'flame-shaped arbors' of Scheibel and Scheibel (1968). They were described by Ramon y Cajal (1909), but it was Sterling and Kuypers (1967a) and the Scheibels (1968) who realized that the 'flames' were the end-on views of longitudinally running columns or sheets of terminals. These arborizations were assumed to arise from cutaneous afferent fibres because the field potentials evoked by stimulation of low-threshold cutaneous axons are maximal in laminae III and IV (see, for example, Coombs et al. 1956; Willis et al. 1973). The 'flame-shaped arbors' are now known to arise from axons innervating hair follicle receptors (Brown et al. 1977c; see Chapter 2).

Large-diameter collaterals descending directly to the motor nuclei have been assumed to belong solely to the primary (Ia) afferent fibres from muscle spindles, because of the well-known monosynaptic connexion between such axons and the motoneurones. Undoubtedly Ia afferent fibres do have collaterals of this type (see Chapter 11), but the observation that Group II muscle afferent fibres from the secondary spindle endings also have monosynaptic excitatory connexions to motoneurones (Kirkwood and Sears 1974; Stauffer et al. 1976) throws doubt on this as an exclusive identification (but see Chapter 13).

Few other collaterals have been given even tentative identifications on the basis of separate anatomical and physiological experiments

(Réthelyi and Szentágothai 1973). One such tentative identification that has been shown to be correct is that of relatively large-fibre collaterals that arborize in laminae VI and VII but which do not reach the motor nuclei. Réthelyi and Szentágothai (1973) thought these were from Golgi tendon organs (Ib fibres) and this is now known to be so (Brown and Fyffe 1978b, 1979; Hongo et al. 1978; see Chapter 12).

II. Identified neurones in the spinal cord

New and very powerful techniques have been developed in recent years that have been used to identify neurones in the central nervous system with little margin of error. These methods, particularly orthograde and retrograde transport techniques and the intraneuronal injection of a variety of markers, have revolutionized the study of nervous tissue. It is, of course, the main purpose of this book to present the information provided by one of these techniques (intracellular injection of the enzyme horseradish peroxidase) in detail. In this section the location of identified spinal cord neurones will be described. Figure 1.3 shows the locations of these neurones in terms of the cytoarchitectonic scheme of Rexed (1952, 1954).

1. Cells of origin of ascending pathways

a) *Spinocervical tract* (see Chapter 6). The cells of origin of this somatosensory pathway have been shown by electrophysiological methods (Eccles et al. 1960; Hongo et al. 1968; Bryan et al. 1973; Brown et al. 1976, 1977b, 1980b) and by retrograde horseradish peroxidase tracing (Craig 1976, 1978; Brown et al. 1980a) to be in laminae III, IV and V (Fig. 1.3A). Very few cells are located outside of these laminae. The axons of the tract ascend the cord in the ipsilateral dorsolateral funiculus (Morin 1955; Lundberg and Oscarsson 1961).

b) *Post-synaptic dorsal column pathway* (see Chapter 8). In 1968 Uddenberg described second-order axons within the fasciculus cuneatus (Uddenberg 1968a, b). They were presumably travelling to the cuneate nucleus. It has subsequently been shown that input to the dorsal column nuclei from the cord is not restricted to primary afferent fibres ascending the dorsal columns, but also includes fibres from post-synaptic neurones. These fibres travel both through the

dorsal columns (Angaut-Petit 1975a,b; Rustioni 1973, 1974) and the ipsilateral dorso-lateral funiculus (Gordon and Grant 1972; Dart and Gordon 1973; Rustioni 1973, 1974; Rustioni and Molenaar 1975), and projections to nucleus Z have been described (Rustioni 1973). Rustioni and Kaufman (1977) have concluded that most of the neurones that give rise to axons projecting to the dorsal column nuclei are situated in lamina IV and the medial part of lamina V (Fig. 1.3A), together with the medial part of lamina VI in the upper cervical cord, on the ipsilateral side. To

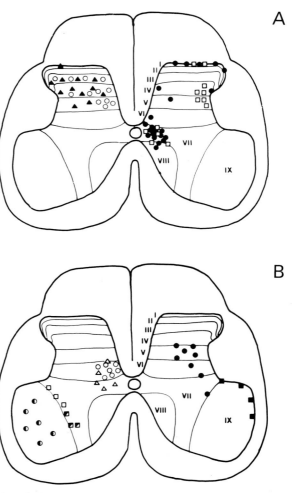

Fig. 1.3. Summary diagrams of the locations of some identified neurone systems. **A** ▲, spinocervical tract (cat); ○, neurones with axons ascending the dorsal columns (the postsynaptic dorsal column system); ●, spinothalamic tract (cat); □, spinothalamic tract (monkey). **B** ○, dorsal spinocerebellar tract (from Clarke's column); △, neurones projecting to cerebellum (Aoyama et al. 1973); ●, ■, ventral spinocerebellar tract; □, Ia inhibitory interneurones; ◪, Renshaw cells; ◖, motoneurones.

some extent, therefore, the post-synaptic dorsal column path and the spinocervical tract take origin from overlapping parts of the dorsal horn (lamina IV mainly). It is not known whether a single neurone can project both to the lateral cervical nucleus (spinocervical tract) and to the dorsal column nuclei (post-synaptic dorsal column path).

c) *Spinothalamic tract.* At the time Réthelyi and Szentágothai (1973) wrote their review, the location of spinothalamic tract cells was uncertain. Since then there has been considerable research, especially using electrophysiological methods (Dilly et al. 1968; Trevino et al. 1972, 1973, 1974; Willis et al. 1974; Albe-Fessard et al. 1974a, b; Carstens and Trevino 1978b), that has shown in both cats and primates the presence of spinothalamic projections and recorded the locations of the cell bodies. The retrograde horseradish peroxidase tracing technique has been used by Trevino and Carstens (1975) and Carstens and Trevino (1978a) to determine the location of spinothalamic tract neurones in cats and monkeys. Their results have confirmed and extended the localization data provided by electrophysiological experiments. There are species differences. In the cat (Fig. 1.3A) the cells are mainly in lamina I, medial lamina VII and dorsal lamina VIII contralateral to the site of injection; ipsilaterally labelled cells are found in medial lamina VII and dorsal lamina VIII. There are few cells elsewhere. When injections are limited to the nucleus ventralis posterior lateralis no cord cells are labelled. In the monkey labelled cells are located almost entirely on the side of the cord contralateral to the site of injection and are situated laterally in the neck of the dorsal horn (corresponding with lateral laminae IV and V in the cat, although the cytoarchitectonic organization of the primate cord has not been studied in detail). Other cells are found in the marginal layer (lamina I) and in positions corresponding with laminae VII and VIII.

d) *Dorsal spinocerebellar tract.* This tract, as has been known for many years, originates in the dorsal nucleus of Clarke (Clarke's column) (Fig. 1.3B). Clarke's column terminates caudally at about L-4. It has been studied in detail at both light and electron microscope levels (Réthelyi 1968, 1970). The identities of the different neurone types in Clarke's column are well worked out: the large cells are the tract neurones and the smaller border cells are interneurones, probably inhibitory interneurones (Réthelyi and Szentágothai 1973).

e) *Ventral spinocerebellar tract.* The most direct evidence on the location of ventral spinocerebellar tract neurones comes from intracellular dye injection experiments (Jankowska and Lindström 1970). The tract arises (Fig. 1.3B) from spinal border cells (Cooper and Sherrington 1940), as predicted by Burke et al. (1971b). These cells are also found within the motor nuclei. The tract also arises from cells situated more dorsally and medially in the lateral parts of laminae V, VI and VII as recorded by Eccles et al. (1961b) and Hubbard and Oscarsson (1962) (see also Ha and Liu 1968). The axons of ventral spinocerebellar tract neurones cross the mid-line in the ventral commissure to ascend the contralateral ventral column.

f) *Other ascending tracts.* Very little is known about the identity of the cells of origin of other ascending pathways. It seems highly likely that the marginal cells of lamina I project to targets in addition to various thalamic nuclei (Trevino and Carstens 1975). Thus, they seem to project to the lateral cervical nucleus (Craig 1976; see Chapter 6) and to the hind brain (Kumazawa et al. 1975; Molenaar and Kuypers 1978).

Much remains to be discovered about the locations of the cells of origin of many ascending pathways. Especially outstanding are the cells of the various indirect pathways to the cerebellum. In this connexion the recent observation (Aoyama et al. 1973) of neurones situated medially in laminae V, VI and VIII (Fig. 1.3B) that are excited monosynaptically by Group I muscle afferent fibres from the hind limb is of particular interest. Some of these neurones project as far as the cerebellum (direct pathway) and were observed as far caudally as L-6.

2. Identified interneurones with short axons

a) *Renshaw cells.* These neurones, intercalated on the recurrent inhibitory path from motoneurone to motoneurone (Eccles et al. 1954b), were the first inhibitory neurones to be characterized by intracellular dye injection (Jankowska and Lindström 1971). Renshaw cells are located (Fig. 1.3B) at the medio-ventral border of the motor nuclei, and even with the limitations imposed by Procion Yellow injection Jankowska and Lindström could trace Renshaw cell axons into the ventro-medial funiculus, showing that they are funicular neurones, as suggested earlier on the basis of Golgi studies by Scheibel and Scheibel (1966a). It is of historical interest that Renshaw cells were successfully injected with Fast Green dye as long ago as 1965 (Thomas and Wilson; see also Erulkar et al. 1968).

b) *Ia inhibitory interneurones*. The identification of the Ia inhibitory interneurones is one of the most fascinating stories in spinal cord research. After an initial (and logical) suggestion that they were located in laminae VI and VII (Eccles et al. 1954c, 1956, 1960) it was subsequently found that they were deeper in the cord, in the ventral part of lamina VII just dorsal and medial to the motor nuclei (Hultborn et al. 1971a, b, c) (Fig. 1.3B). The use of sophisticated electrophysiological techniques (Jankowska and Roberts 1972a, b) indicated that these neurones had axons passing into the ventro-lateral funiculus and that their cell bodies were in the same segment as the entering Ia fibres and not in the segment of the antagonist motoneurones, as sug-

gested by Eccles et al. (1954c). Finally, intracellular injection of Procion Yellow (Jankowska and Lindström 1972) provided ultimate proof of their location in lamina VII just dorsal and medial to the motor nuclei.

3. Motoneurones

The location of motoneurones in the motor nuclei (Fig. 1.3B) and their appearance in sections stained with silver techniques are so well known that repetition here is unwarranted. Because of their size and the general interest in α-motoneurones as 'model' or 'standard' vertebrate nerve cells they were among the first cells to be injected intracellularly with dyes (Procion Yellow, Barrett and Graubard 1970; Barrett and Crill 1971, 1974a, b; radioactive amino acids, Lux et al. 1970: horseradish peroxidase, Cullheim and Kellerth 1976, 1978; Cullheim et al. 1977). The smaller γ-motoneurones have also been injected with horseradish peroxidase (Westbury, 1979). For completeness, the locations of motoneurones are included in Figure 1.3B.

2   Axons innervating hair follicle receptors

The hairy skin of mammals is richly endowed with receptors that respond to movement of the hairs. Hairs project from the surface of the skin and therefore extend the sensory surface outwards, so that the hair follicle receptors can act as 'short-distance receptors'. The receptors in the hair follicles are innervated by myelinated axons with conduction velocities that cover nearly all the myelinated fibre range, from the fastest (Aα) to the slowest (Aδ). Only the slowest myelinated axons, the post-δ group of Koll et al. (1961), appear not to innervate hair follicles. Each hair follicle usually receives innervation from a number of afferent nerve fibres, and each axon supplies several hair follicles, the number depending on the type of hair follicle afferent unit (see below).

Adrian (1931), in the first electrophysiological study of cutaneous receptors in mammals, recorded from the largest Aα axons innervating hair follicle receptors and noted that the responses to hair movements were rapidly adapting. This conclusion was supported by the early work in Japan by Maruhashi et al. (reported in 1952). Soon after Adrian's observations, Zotterman (1939) noted that both large and small action potentials could be evoked in fine branches of the cat's saphenous nerve upon stroking the fur. Zotterman concluded that the axons with smaller action potentials (axons with smaller diameter) innervated receptors with a higher sensitivity than those innervated by the axons with larger action potentials (larger-diameter fibres). This result was later confirmed by Hunt and McIntyre (1960c).

In addition to the rapidly adapting hair follicle receptors on the head, body, limbs and tail there are some slowly adapting hair follicle receptors. The vibrissae and other special facial hairs (Fitzgerald 1940; Iggo 1968; Gottschaldt et al. 1973) and the carpal tactile hairs on the cat's foreleg (Nilsson and Skoglund 1965) respond during maintained displacement of the hair in addition to responding during movement. Only the rapidly adapting hair follicle units will be considered in this book.

A. Physiology of hair follicle afferent units

I. Classification

Recent studies of the rapidly adapting hair follicle receptors in cats and other mammals have employed well-controlled mechanical stimulation of the hairs. Quantitative stimulus–response relations have been determined and a number of different types of hair follicle afferent unit recognized. Two independent studies on single units have each divided hair follicle afferent fibres into three categories (Brown and Iggo 1967; Burgess et al. 1968). Unfortunately, the two classifications agree on only one of the categories.

Brown and Iggo (1967) used both morphological and electrophysiological criteria to classify the hair follicle afferent units. Three types of hairs were recognized when the animal's coat was examined with an operating microscope. (1) The down hairs (Danforth 1925) were wavy, unpigmented and the shortest and finest of the hairs; they emerged in groups of two to four from a common orifice. (2) The guard hairs (Danforth 1925) were straight, often pigmented and longer and thicker; they emerged singly from a follicle. (3) The tylotrichs of Straile (1958, 1960, 1961) were similar to the guard hairs but were the longest hairs of the coat and usually the thickest, and with a vascular follicle often associated with a Type I receptor (see Chapter 4). Three types of physiological responses were observed, each associated with a particular class of hair: (1) Type D, in response to movement of down hairs, had a very high sensitivity to hair movement and was carried by Aδ axons; (2) Type G, in response to movement of guard hairs, included both sensitive and very insensitive responses and was carried by axons conducting faster than the Aδ wave; (3) Type T, in response to movement of the tylotrichs, usually had a high sensitivity to hair movement and was carried by axons with a higher mean conduction velocity than the Type G response.

Burgess et al. (1968) used essentially physiological means to classify the hair follicle afferent fibres. Their Type D units correspond exactly with the Type D units of Brown & Iggo (1967). Burgess et al. did not recognize the Type T category (or the tylotrich hairs) and they divided the remaining units into G_1 and G_2 categories. G_1 hair units were the least sensitive of all the hair follicle types, had axons with the highest conduction velocities and were responsive to moving the longest hairs. G_2 hair units were much more sensitive than the G_1 units and, like the D units, responded with a stream of impulses to hair movement; their axons had conduction velocities slower than the G_1 units and they responded equally well to moving both long and short guard hairs. Burgess et al. (1968) also described another category, the 'insensitive hair receptors', which did not fit into their D, G_1, G_2 classification. Subsequently, the G classes have been further subdivided by the addition of an 'intermediate' (G_I) category (Burgess and Perl 1973; Burgess et al. 1974; Whitehorn et al. 1974; Horch et al. 1977).

The two classifications obviously require some discussion. We (Brown and Iggo) recognized the Type T units first in the rabbit, where tylotrichs are very obvious. In the rabbit, tylotrichs emerge from follicles that contain, on their lip, a Type I receptor (*Haarscheibe* of Pinkus 1904). Indeed, occasionally the tylotrich emerges through the Type I receptor. In the cat, the association with Type I receptors is not so tight, but many (perhaps the majority) of tylotrichs emerge very close to a Type I receptor and the tylotrich follicle is very vascular.

The present writer has difficulty in sorting out the different G categories in the work of Burgess and his collaborators. This difficulty is compoun-

ded by the addition of two more classes, the field receptors F_1 and F_2 (Burgess et al. 1968, 1974; Perl 1968; Burgess and Perl 1973; Whitehorn et al. 1974). According to Burgess and Perl (1973) field receptors are not excited by movement of single hairs but may be excited when a number of hairs are moved together. In the cat, field receptors are said to be most numerous in the hairy skin that surrounds the foot and toe pads, an area of skin where it is particularly difficult to sort out receptor types. This skin contains many tylotrichs and Type I receptors and the close proximity of Pacinian corpuscles and sensitive rapidly adapting mechanoreceptors in the glabrous skin complicates matters enormously.

At the very least, the classification of Brown and Iggo (1967) has the merit of simplicity. But it seems to the present writer to be a more useful system. Type G and T hair follicle units make different connexions onto spinal cord neurones and onto neurones (probably in the dorsal column nuclei) with axons in the medial lemniscus (Brown and Franz 1969; Brown 1971; Brown et al. 1974; but see P. B. Brown et al. 1975). The T, G, D classification will be used in this book.

II. Responses to hair movement

The sensitivities of hair follicle receptors to movement of hairs vary widely. The Type D units form a clear-cut group. They are exquisitely sensitive to movement of the down hairs and respond with a regular discharge of impulses to movement of the hair at constant velocity (Fig. 2.1A), the rate of discharge increasing with increasing velocity of displacement. Types G and T units have a wide range of sensitivities. At one extreme, many (particularly Type T) behave like Type D units and carry a stream of impulses during hair movement (Fig. 2.1B, C). This discharge is regular and there is a logarithmic relation between the rate of discharge and the velocity of hair movement (Fig. 2.1B, C–F). The sensitive hair units code the rate of hair movement precisely and the stimulus–response relation is maintained within the central nervous system, at least across one set of synapses (Brown and Franz 1969; Brown et al. 1974). At the opposite extreme many Type G and some Type T units are insensitive (Fig. 2.1D). These insensitive units respond only with one or two impulses upon movement of a single hair and

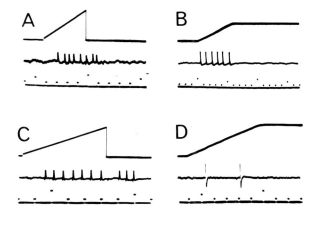

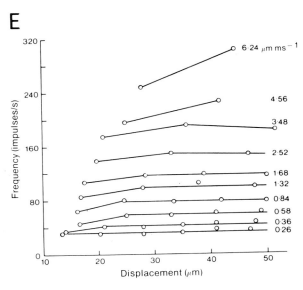

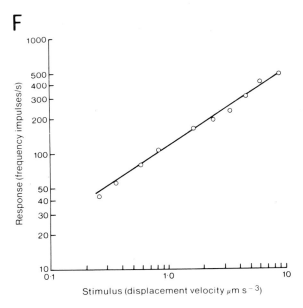

require a number of hairs to be moved simultaneously for a stream of impulses to be evoked.

III. Receptive fields

The receptive field organization of hair follicle units differs according to the type of unit. On the hind limb, forelimb and tail the fields are approximately circular or oval with the long axis in the long axis of the limb or tail. For Type D units it is likely that all down hairs within the perimeter of the receptive field contribute to the unit, although the extreme sensitivity of the Type D units makes this difficult to investigate. Many fewer hairs activate Type G (10–20 hairs per unit on the leg) and Type T units (2–7 hairs per unit on the leg), so that the perimeters of their receptive fields encompass hairs that do not contribute to the unit. There is considerable overlap of Type G and T receptive fields.

The size of a hair follicle receptive field depends on its position on the body. Fields are smallest on the toes (about 0.5 cm^2 or less) and increase in size on more proximal parts of the limb (Fig. 2.2). Fields are largest on the thorax and abdomen (50–75 cm^2). In general, the smaller the area of the receptive field the fewer the number of hairs whose movement activates the unit. Thus, Type T units with fields on the toes frequently have only two or three hairs in the field contributing to the unit, although these hairs may not be adjacent to one another.

Fig. 2.1. Responses of hair follicle afferent units to the movement of single hairs. **A–D** show responses recorded from single axons evoked by constant-velocity displacement of the hair as indicated in the upper trace of each set of records. **A** Type D unit; **B** Type T unit; **C** and **D** Type G units. The time marks are at millisecond intervals. **E** Graph of the responses of a Type T hair follicle unit to displacements of a single hair at constant velocity (μm ms^{-1}) as indicated at the right-hand end of each *curve*. Each *point* represents the average of ten impulse intervals from consecutive records, the frequency being calculated from the reciprocal of the impulse intervals. The results show both the relative uniformity of the impulse intervals at any given velocity of displacement and the greater number of impulses discharged (for the same final displacement) at lower velocities. **F** Graph, on logarithmic coordinates, of the responses of the unit shown in **E** to constant-velocity displacement of a single hair. The slope of the *straight line* through the *points* is 0.62. (From Brown and Iggo 1967.)

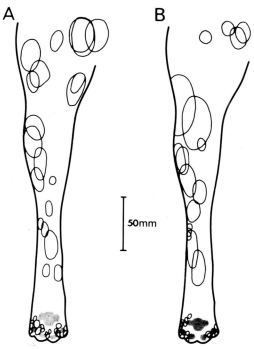

Fig. 2.2. Receptive fields of hair follicle afferent units on the hind limb. **A** Type G units; **B** Type T units. In general the fields are very small on the toes and become larger on more proximal parts of the limb. (From Brown 1968.)

B. Central projections of hair follicle afferent fibres

Many spinal cord neurones respond to hair movement, but the details of the projections of the different types of hair unit have not been worked out. The vast majority of Type G and T units have axons that ascend the dorsal columns to the dorsal column nuclei: the axons of Type D units do not (Petit and Burgess 1968; Brown 1973).

All the ascending somatosensory pathways have some neurones that respond to hair movement. The majority of spinocervical tract cells receive monosynaptic excitation from hair follicle afferents (Brown and Franz 1969; Brown 1971; Brown et al. 1973, 1975) and many neurones of the post-synaptic dorsal column pathway respond to hair movement too (Uddenberg 1968b; Angaut-Petit 1975b). In the primate, spinothalamic tract neurones may also respond to hair movement (Willis et al. 1974). In addition to the neurones giving rise to long ascending axons,

many dorsal horn cells also respond to hair movement and some of their responses are monosynaptically evoked (see Tapper et al. 1973; P. B. Brown et al. 1975). Some of these interneurones should be on the pathways responsible for primary afferent depolarization (Jänig et al. 1968b). It is to be expected, therefore, that hair follicle afferent fibres will distribute their collaterals to those parts of the cord containing the above neurones, that is to laminae III, IV and V, and possibly deeper.

The exteroceptive component of the dorsal spinocerebellar tract receives monosynaptic input from cutaneous axons, including hair follicle afferent fibres (Lundberg and Oscarsson 1960; Mann 1971). According to Lindström and Takata (1971), the cell bodies of these dorsal spinocerebellar tract neurones are in Clarke's column and it would therefore be expected that hair follicle afferent fibres would send collaterals to the column. Not all the exteroceptive neurones projecting from the lumbosacral cord to the cerebellum (whether or not they should be called dorsal spinocerebellar tract neurones is debatable) are in Clarke's column (Aoyama et al. 1973; Tapper et al. 1975). It is not known whether they receive monosynaptic excitation from hair follicle afferent fibres.

C. Morphology of axons innervating hair follicle receptors

The following account of the morphology of hair follicle afferent fibres is limited to axons belonging to Type G and T units. Type D units have smaller-diameter axons (Aδ) of about 2–4 μm which are not easily accessible for the long-term intra-axonal microelectrode penetrations necessary for the injection of horseradish peroxidase. However, Light and Perl (1979b) have recently achieved intra-axonal staining of Type D hair follicle afferents; these have the same morphology as the larger hair follicle axons.

No obvious differences have been observed between axons of Type G and T units. They will, therefore, be described together, as they were in our original report (Brown et al. 1977c).

I. Entry of axons into the spinal cord, branching and collateral distribution

The vast majority of dorsal root axons divides soon after entering the spinal cord, usually within at most a few hundred micrometres of leaving the root. According to Réthelyi and Szentágothai (1973) no convincing evidence for non-bifurcating axons has ever been reported. But hair follicle afferent fibres form an exception to this rule. The majority of hair follicle axons do not divide after entering the cord but turn towards the brain and, moving medially over the dorsal horn, ascend the cord in the dorsal columns, giving off collaterals as they do so.

Figure 2.3 shows, in schematic fashion, the branching pattern of a sample of 14 hair follicle afferent fibres injected with horseradish peroxidase. Twelve of these could be traced into the dorsal roots and nine did not bifurcate after leaving the root. Although axons innervating other cutaneous or muscle receptors occasionally do not divide upon entering the cord, only hair follicle afferent units have such a large proportion (about two-thirds) that do not.

The interest of this observation is not so much that hair follicle afferent fibres behave differently from other axons (though that raises some questions) but resides in the fact that, given the non-bifurcating nature of most hair follicle afferent fibres, information from their receptors is fed into the cord at the level of and rostral to the point of entry of the axon. Information from other cutaneous receptors is distributed both rostrally and caudally of the point of entry of the axon. A problem therefore arises concerning the somatotopic organization of the dorsal horn. Is the input from hair follicle receptors out of register with that from other cutaneous receptors in hairy skin? This is possible unless: (1) there is a

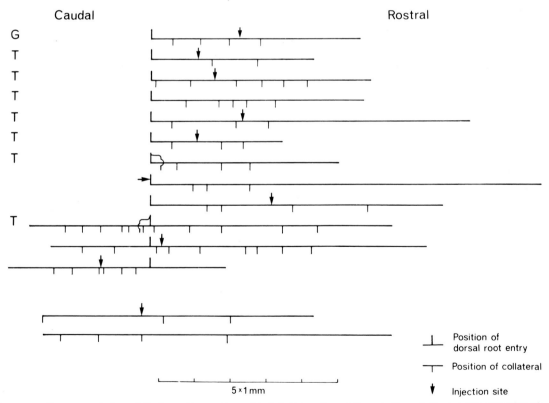

Fig. 2.3. Diagrammatic representation of the branching pattern of hair follicle afferent fibres in the spinal cord. The total length of each axon stained is shown, together with (where possible) the position of its entry into the cord through the dorsal root, the position of the origin of each stained collateral, and the site of injection of horseradish peroxidase. Axons identified as belonging to Type T or Type G units have been indicated on the left-hand side of the figure. The majority of axons that could be traced into the dorsal root did not bifurcate upon entering the cord but turned rostrally.

systematic shift in the position at which hair follicle afferent fibres enter the cord relative to other cutaneous afferents, particularly the slowly adapting Types I and II from hairy skin; (2) the minority of hair follicle axons that do bifurcate provide sufficient information to compensate for the preponderance of rostral projections. There is no evidence that receptive fields of dorsal horn neurones are out of register. No reports exist of neurones with a receptive field consisting of two separated parts, one excited by hair movement and the other by stimulating other receptors in *hairy* skin. Many dorsal horn neurones may be recorded close together with excitation from different receptor types within the same receptive field area (see P. B. Brown et al. 1975).

It seems most likely that there are sufficient caudally projecting branches of hair follicle afferent fibres to avoid the problem of the receptive fields being out of register. But hair follicle axons may, in general, enter the cord at a more caudal level than other afferent fibres whose receptive fields are in the same area of skin. Unfortunately, this latter suggestion will be very difficult to test experimentally. A satisfactory experiment would need to examine population responses. If a similar position exists in the rabbit as has been found in the cat, an answer might be found by examining the ingoing volley upon electrical stimulation of cutaneous nerves from hairy skin. In the rabbit, cutaneous axons with the lowest electrical threshold in the sural nerve belong to Type I units. The next most excitable group of axons, innervating Type T hair follicle receptors, have electrical thresholds of more than 1.4 times the threshold for the whole nerve (Brown and Hayden 1971). It might be possible to demonstrate different levels of entry for the two kinds of afferent fibres.

The lengths of axon stained by injected horseradish peroxidase in the sample of hair follicle afferent fibres shown in Fig. 2.3 ranged from 3.8 to 10.5 mm. Hair follicle units with peripheral axons conducting in the $A\alpha-\gamma$ range nearly all project to the dorsal column nuclei (Petit and Burgess 1968), a distance, in the adult cat, of some 200–300 mm from the lumbosacral enlargement. The amount of axon revealed by the injection of horseradish peroxidase is small indeed. Even when a caudally projecting branch was present it did not terminate in a collateral (see Fig. 2.3), so the method does not stain this

shorter branch in its entirety either. One of the axons in the stained sample did end caudally as a collateral. It was, presumably, part of a caudally directed branch, although it could not be traced into a dorsal root. It had a length of 7.6 mm. Wall and Werman (1976) have presented electrophysiological evidence showing that cutaneous axons entering the cord at the L-2 level may project caudally as far as S-1, for distances up to 73 mm. Imai and Kusama (1969) have shown, by means of the Nauta degeneration method, that axons entering the cord at L-4 may reach at least as far as S-1 (S-1 was the most caudal segment examined). Of course, the identity of the axons in terms of the receptors they innervated was not available to Imai and Kusama and it is not clear from the paper of Wall and Werman whether hair follicle afferents were included in those that projected such long distances in the caudal direction. Some hair follicle afferent fibres may project caudally for several segments.

Figure 2.3 also shows the distribution of collaterals from hair follicle afferent fibres. An assumption made in all the work described in this book is that for any axon injected with horseradish peroxidase all collaterals between the most caudal and most rostral ones stained are also revealed. In other words, the method does not stain collaterals in an all-or-none manner, staining some but missing others in between. The evidence for this is necessarily indirect. The intensity of staining along an axon varies steadily, being most intense at the site of injection and becoming fainter with distance from the injection site. This gradation in staining intensity applies also to the collaterals of an axon: there are no sudden changes in the density of staining. The most intensely stained collaterals are those near the injection site and they become fainter the further they are away from the injection site. Groups of better-stained collaterals separated by more faintly staining ones are not seen. Injection sites may usually be recognized by slight extra-axonal spillage at the most intensely stained part of an axon.

On the basis of the assumption that all collaterals between the most rostral and the most caudal ones stained on an axon are revealed by the method, some quantitative data on the density and distribution of collaterals may be obtained. Brown et al. (1977c) stained 13 axons of hair follicle units. These axons gave rise to a total of 63 collaterals over distances up to 7.4 mm (mean

3.6 mm). On average, therefore, a hair follicle axon gives off a collateral about every millimetre for the first centimetre or so after its entry into the cord. Occasionally a collateral arises from the axon within the dorsal root or very soon after it leaves the root. Obviously the method of intra-axonal staining provides no information on the total number of collaterals arising from a single axon, only a lower limit. In general, a more intensely stained axon is stained for a longer length and has more stained collaterals than a weakly stained axon.

The frequency with which collaterals arise from a hair follicle axon is determined by: (1) their proximity to the dorsal root entrance zone of the axon, and (2) the medio-lateral position of their terminal arborizations in the dorsal horn. Collaterals arise more frequently near the entrance of the axon into the cord than they do further away. Within about 2 mm of either side of the entrance point collaterals arise at intervals of 100–1300 μm; further than 2 mm from the dorsal root entrance they usually arise at intervals of more than 800 μm (see Fig. 2.3). Collaterals also arise more frequently if their terminal arborizations are situated in the medial part of the dorsal horn than if they are in the lateral part. All arborizations from a single axon are in the same general medio-lateral position; for example in the lateral third, the middle third, etc. (see below). The medio-lateral position of a collateral's terminal arborization is determined by the receptive field of the unit. For ten axons, with collaterals in the L-6–S-1 segments, 32 intercollateral distances were measured. Collaterals with terminals in the lateral half of the horn had a mean spacing of 1165 μm, whereas those with terminals in the medial half of the horn had a mean spacing of 718 μm: the difference of the means is significant at the 5% level (Student's t-test).

II. Morphology of collaterals and their arborizations

Collaterals arise from all parts of the parent axon or its major branches: in the dorsal root, as the axon moves across the dorsal horn from the dorsal root entrance to take up its position ascending the dorsal columns and, where there is a caudally directed branch, from along its length.

Collaterals are given off more or less at right angles from the parent axon. They do not drop vertically, however, but run rostrally as well as ventrally towards the dorsal horn so that their entry into the grey matter is rostral of their point of origin. This orientation, which is common to all collaterals of all primary afferent fibres, was overlooked in our earlier description (Brown et al 1977c). It was only when the more obvious rostral trajectory of Group Ia muscle afferent collaterals was noted (Brown and Fyffe 1978a) that the earlier cutaneous material was re-examined. The rostral trajectory is easily seen when sections cut in the sagittal plane are examined (see Fig. 2.9). Usually the collateral enters the dorsal horn about 100–300 μm rostral to its point of origin.

Hair follicle collaterals may also be directed laterally or medially, according to the relative positions of the parent axon and the terminal arborization (see Figs. 2.5–2.7). Collaterals enter the dorsal horn on any position on its dorsal or medial border: their entrance is not limited to the medial part of the substantia gelatinosa as has been suggested by Réthelyi and Szentágothai (1973). Usually, collaterals enter the dorsal horn at its dorsal border and descend through Rexed's laminae I–IV, sometimes dividing into branches on the way (Fig. 2.4), and continuing their rostro-ventral path.

Reconstructions of hair follicle afferent fibre collaterals made from serial transverse sections show that the collaterals have a striking and quite specific morphology (Figs. 2.5–2.7; see also Fig. 2.4). The collaterals descend through the first four or five laminae of the cord, and in lamina IV or V they make a U-shaped turn and ascend back into laminae IV and III where they undergo repeated subdivision and break up into terminal arborizations. They are, in fact, the 'flame-shaped arbors' of Scheibel and Scheibel (1968) and may be identified as the 'collaterales grosses et profondes de la substance de Rolando' described by Ramon y Cajal (1909). It should be noted, however, that in the adult cat these collaterals do not encroach to any great extent into the substantia gelatinosa (see below).

The flame-shaped arbor structure of hair follicle afferent collaterals is shared only with collaterals from rapidly adapting mechanoreceptors in glabrous skin (see Chapter 3). No other types of cutaneous or muscle afferent fibre collaterals have this morphology and these two differ in their sagittal organization. As will be seen from the

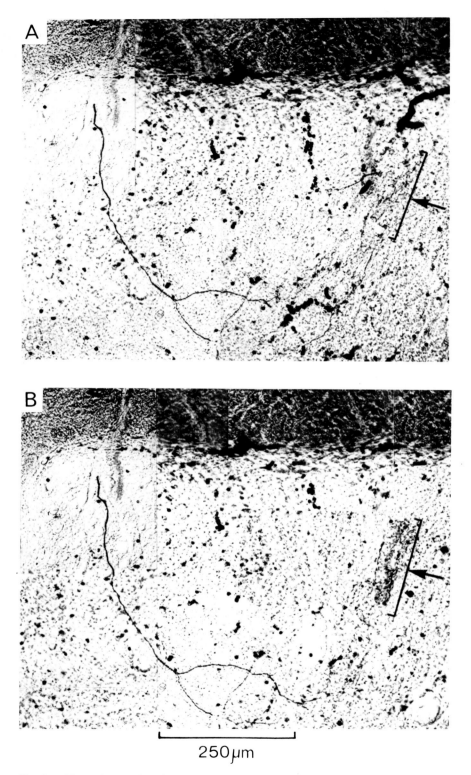

Fig. 2.4. Photomicrographs of a collateral from a Type T hair follicle unit. **A** and **B** are montages made from micrographs of adjacent 100-μm transverse sections of the spinal cord to show two different parts of the terminal arborization (indicated by the arrowed bracket). The boundary between the white matter of the dorsal column and the grey matter of the dorsal horn may be clearly seen towards the top of each figure. (From Brown et al. 1977c.)

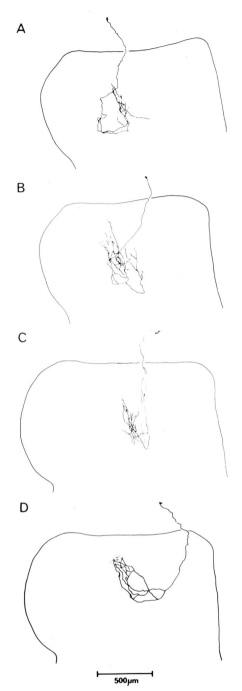

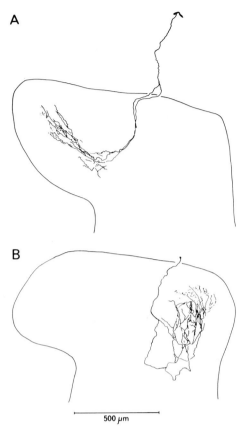

A

B

C

D

A

B

Fig. 2.5. Reconstructions, in the transverse plane, of four adjacent collaterals from an axon of a Type T hair follicle unit. **A** is the most caudal and **D** the most rostral of the four. From **A** to **D** the parent axon moves from a lateral to a medial position over the dorsal horn. Each collateral enters the dorsal horn at its dorsal border, descends (sometimes dividing as it does so) through the horn to lamina IV where it reverses direction and ascends to break up into the flame-shaped arbors of Scheibel and Scheibel (1968). The outline of the dorsal horn is shown; lateral border to the left, medial border to the right. (From Brown et al. 1977c.)

Fig. 2.6. Reconstructions, in the transverse plane, of hair follicle afferent fibre collaterals. **A** a collateral terminating in the lateral part of the horn; **B** a collateral, from a Type G unit, terminating in the medial part of the horn. Both collaterals show the characteristic flame-shaped terminal arborization. The positions of boutons are shown and they can be seen to be restricted almost entirely to lamina III. The outline of the dorsal horn is shown; lateral border to the left. (From Brown et al. 1977c.)

following chapters, each type of primary afferent fibre has collaterals with specific, and different, morphologies.

The terminal arborizations of hair follicle afferent collaterals, when viewed in the transverse plane, are elliptical or lozenge-shaped, centred on lamina III with only slight extension into the most dorsal part of lamina IV and, occasionally, minimal intrusion into lamina II (substantia gelatinosa). In the Scheibels' evocative description these 'Flame-shaped arbors . . . like successive positions of the large hand on a clock face, sweep over the dorso-lateral cord from ten o'clock to a virtually upright 'high noon' position against the dorso-medial white matter'. In other words, the arborizations are oriented so that their long axes are at right angles to the dorsal and dorso-lateral borders of the dorsal horn, or, more correctly, oriented at right angles to lamina II.

In adult cats the terminal arborizations of hair follicle collaterals measure 150–400 μm in width. Scheibel and Scheibel (1968) and Réthelyi and Szentágothai (1973) give values of 20–30 μm for the kitten. In all studies the width of the arborizations represents about one-tenth to one-seventh of the transverse width of the dorsal horn at the level of lamina III, about the same proportion as indicated by Ramon y Cajal (1909, in his Fig. 121) from the new-born kitten. There is, therefore, no change in relative width of the terminal arborization after birth. But there does seem to be a change in the dorso-ventral distribution. The illustrations in Ramon y Cajal (1909), Szentágothai (1964), Scheibel and Scheibel (1968) and Réthelyi and Szentágothai (1973) from kittens show the arborizations extending through lamina II (substantia gelatinosa). In our material from adult cats, only a few collaterals have terminals that enter even the most ventral parts of lamina II.

In a recent Golgi–Kopsch study in adult cats Réthelyi (1977) has presented results consistent with the observations we have made. Réthelyi has proposed that only non-myelinated afferent fibres terminate in lamina II and he is of the opinion that the recurving collaterals (now shown to be from hair follicle afferent fibres) do not enter lamina II but run longitudinally in laminae III and IV. This is essentially in agreement with Sterling and Kuypers (1967a), who studied the cat's brachial cord. The longitudinal organization of these arborizations will be discussed below.

The difference between new-born and adult animals indicates that some changes occur during post-natal growth. In the legend to their Fig. 9, Réthelyi and Szentágothai (1973) state: 'During later development the neuropil lobuli [these are the 'flame-shaped arbors'] become elongated in dorsoventral direction.' The authors do not elaborate further on this 'elongation'. It may represent growth in the dorso-ventral direction within lamina III, associated with either withdrawal of the dorsalmost extension of the arborization from lamina II or an increase in the thickness of lamina

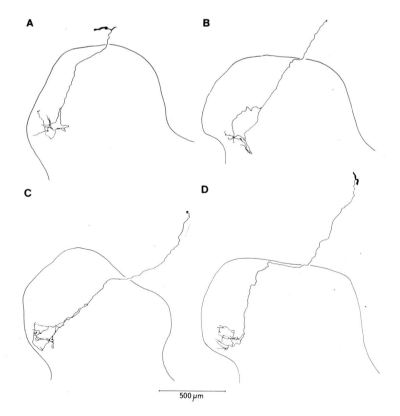

500 μm

Fig. 2.7. Reconstructions, in the transverse plane, of four adjacent collaterals from an axon of a Type T hair follicle afferent unit. **A** is the most caudal, **D** the most rostral. This axon innervated hairs on the base of the tail and its collaterals were in the S-2–S-3 segments. Presumably the caudal position is responsible for the somewhat atypical morphology of the collaterals, but the flame-shaped arbors may still be seen at right angles to the lateral edge of the horn. (From Brown et al. 1977c.)

II that is both absolute and relative to lamina III. The end result would be that lamina II becomes almost completely free of the endings of hair follicle afferent collaterals.

The situation at birth and the subsequent changes taking place during early post-natal development are not clear. Scheibel and Scheibel (1968) state that in the new-born rat and cat the arborizations are poorly differentiated, extending only part way up lamina III. By the 20th to 30th day of post-natal life maturation has taken place and the arborizations now occupy all of lamina III and part of II, with occasional extensions into lamina I.

In the adult the situation is clear. Our results and those of Sterling and Kuypers (1967a) and Réthelyi (1977) show that information from hair follicle receptors is, except for a most limited amount, denied direct access to lamina II. Obviously further work needs to be done to clarify the reasons for the differences between neonatal and adult animals.

The 'flame-shaped arbors' seen in transverse sections of the cord are the end-on views of longitudinally running columns, or sheets, of arborizations. This was first clearly described by Scheibel and Scheibel (1968), although Sterling and Kuypers (1967a) had pointed out the predominantly longitudinal orientation of the arborizations of dorsal root fibres. In the Scheibels' material from new-born kittens the longitudinal extent of 'single terminal afferents' (presumably single collaterals) ranged from 150 to 500 μm with a median value of 270 μm. One such terminal field tended 'to confluesce and overlap along the sagittal axis' with adjacent fields. Because of the nature of their material (rapid Golgi method) Scheibel and Scheibel were not able to determine whether the overlapping terminal fields arose from collaterals of the same or different axons. The horseradish peroxidase technique has clarified the situation in the adult cat.

It was apparent from serial transverse sections (Brown et al. 1977c; see Figs. 2.5, 2.7) that hair follicle afferent terminal arborizations are arranged in sagittally organized sheets. But sections cut in the sagittal plane show the arrangement more clearly (Figs. 2.8, 2.9). In well-stained axons the terminal arborizations of adjacent collaterals form a continuous sheet in the sagittal plane throughout the thickness of lamina III.

The sheet of terminal arborizations of the col-

laterals from a single hair follicle afferent fibre is continuous in the long axis of the cord. There are no sudden jumps in its medio-lateral position: if it is in the most lateral part of the dorsal horn caudally it remains lateral at more rostral levels, and if medial it remains medial. There is, however, a gradual medial shift of the sheets as they ascend the cord. The total extent of this shift is unknown owing to the limitations of the horseradish peroxidase method, and even within the stained portion it is difficult to estimate because of the changes in width and shape of the dorsal horn between and within segments. In Fig. 2.5 the dorsal horn increases in width from the most caudal collateral (A) to the most rostral (D) and the arborization moves from a position just lateral of the centre of the horn (A) to a position just medial to the centre (D). When whole dorsal roots are cut (Sterling and Kuypers, 1967a; Imai and Kusama 1969) degenerating fragments are seen to follow a similar pattern: that is, in segments rostral to the cut root they are medial to their position in the segment of the cut root, and caudal to the cut root they are lateral (see particularly Fig. 4 in Sterling and Kuypers, 1967a; Figs. 1 and 2 in Imai and Kusama 1969).

At this point it is necessary to stress that both the preceding and subsequent discussions refer to the organization of hair follicle collaterals at and near to the segmental level of entry of their parent axons (L-5–S-2). At more rostral levels it is to be expected that collaterals are given off from hair follicle afferent fibres to neurones in Clarke's column. We have not examined these collaterals.

None of the hair follicle afferent fibres examined so far has given rise to more than one sagittally oriented sheet of terminal arborizations. The possibility that a single collateral might divide to supply more than one sheet of terminals (as depicted in Fig. 6 of Scheibel and Scheibel 1968) has not been observed. In Golgi material it is difficult to be sure whether two arborizations arise from the same or different axons. With the intra-axonal injection of horseradish peroxidase into single fibres no such difficulty arises. It remains possible, however, that a single fibre might provide flame-shaped arbors to two different transversely separated sheets of terminals. But such a possibility must be slight because of the somatotopic organization of the dorsal horn (see below and Chapters 6 and 7): sagittal columns of neural elements representing the same or over-

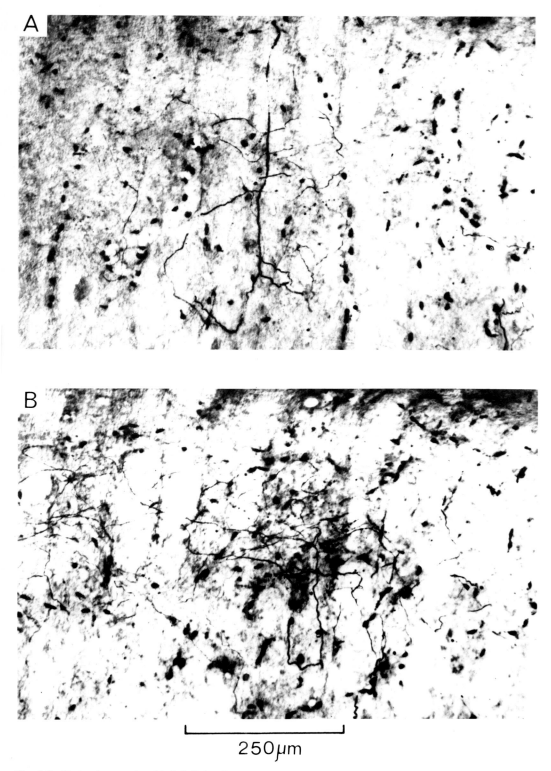

250μm

Fig. 2.8. Photomicrographs of hair follicle afferent fibre collaterals taken from adjacent serial longitudinal sections of spinal cord (100-μm thick sections). The sagittally oriented sheet of terminal arborizations is clearly seen, as is the main part of the collateral as it descends through the dorsal horn and recurves back into the more superficial layers before breaking up into numerous branches.

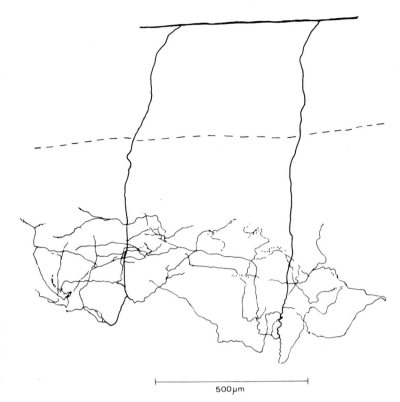

Fig. 2.9. Reconstruction, in the sagittal plane, of two adjacent collaterals from a hair follicle afferent fibre. The collaterals leave the parent axon and run rostrally as they descend to the dorsal horn. The recurving nature of the collaterals is apparent as they turn from their deepest points and ascend to break up into their terminal arborizations. The longitudinal organization of the arborization is clearly shown in this plane, as is the continuity of the arborizations from the two collaterals, forming the sagittal sheet of arborization typical of the hair follicle afferent fibres. The dorsal border of the dorsal horn is indicated by the dashed line. These reconstructions are from the same collaterals as those shown in Fig. 2.8.

500 μm

lapping parts of the skin are arranged so that in the transverse plane there is a very steep gradient of receptive fields with very little smearing. If single hair follicle afferents were prone to supply more than one such column—and the widths of the columns are similar to the widths of the sheets of terminal arborizations—then the steep transverse gradient in the somatotopic map across the dorsal horn could hardly be generated. Szentágothai (1964) also noted that there is probably no overlap in the transverse plane between neighbouring arborizations of these collaterals.

In the adult cat the length of the terminal arborization of a hair follicle collateral depends on its medio-lateral position in the dorsal horn. The longest arborizations (up to 1800 μm) are found in the lateral quarter of the horn; those in the medial part of the horn are usually 500–800 μm long. As would be expected these values for the adult are considerably greater than those for the kitten (270–500 μm: Scheibel and Scheibel 1968).

The observation that the sagittal spread of the terminal arborization of a single hair follicle collateral depends on its medio-lateral position in the dorsal horn gains in interest when it is realized

that there is a similar organization for the dendritic trees of some dorsal horn neurones. Thus, spinocervical tract neurones, which receive monosynaptic excitation from hair follicle afferent fibres, have dendritic trees whose sagittal extents are remarkably similar to those of the arborizations of hair follicle collaterals in the same part of the cord (see Chapters 6 and 7).

III. Synaptic boutons

1. Morphology

Synaptic boutons of hair follicle afferent fibre collaterals are shown in the photomicrographs of Fig. 2.10 and in the camera lucida drawings of Fig. 2.11. The commonest type of terminal axon carries boutons *en passant*, the last 30–75 μm of axon being less than 1 μm in diameter and carrying up to 12 boutons. Boutons are usually about 6 μm × 4 μm in size, although some are smaller (3 μm × 2 μm) and on occasion set off from the terminal axon on short, 1-μm stalks (Fig. 2.11C).

The arrangement of boutons *en passant* is shown particularly well when sections are cut in

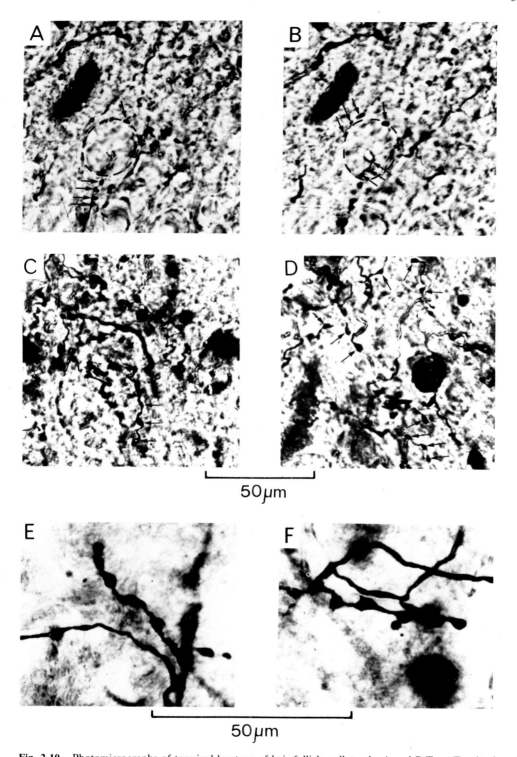

Fig. 2.10. Photomicrographs of terminal boutons of hair follicle collaterals. **A** and **B** Type T unit; the micrographs are of the same field of view taken at different focal planes in this 100-μm thick transverse section. The outlines of a cell body may be seen (indicated by dashed lines) and boutons appear to end in relation to it. This field of view is shown in the camera lucida drawings of Fig. 2.11. **C** and **D** boutons of a Type G unit seen in transverse sections. In **A–D** some boutons are indicated by *arrows*. (From Brown et al. 1977c.) **E** and **F** boutons of hair follicle collaterals as seen in sagittal sections. The longitudinal arrangement of the terminal axons is clearly seen. Note the greater magnification in **E** and **F**.

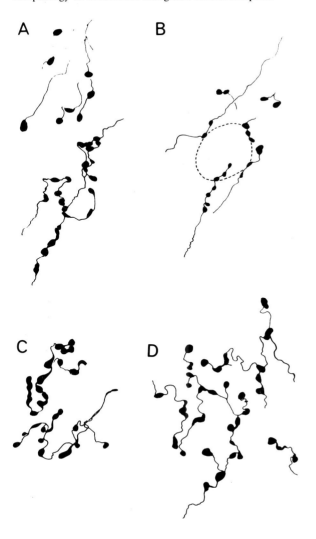

Fig. 2.11. Camera lucida drawings of synaptic boutons of hair follicle afferent fibre collaterals. **A–D** are from transverse sections: **A** and **B** from a Type T unit; **C** and **D** from a Type G unit. Most boutons are of the *en passant* type and in **B** the outline of a cell body is indicated that appears to receive boutons from four terminal branches of the same collateral. Photomicrographs of the field of view shown in **B** are illustrated in Fig. 2.10 A, B. (From Brown et al. 1977c.) **E** and **F** are from longitudinal sections and show clearly the organization of the terminal parts of the collaterals as they run in the sagittal plane (the label E is placed between two terminal axons). Each part of this figure (**A–F**) is from a separate field of view from different histological sections.

the sagittal plane (Fig. 2.10E, F; Fig. 2.11E, F). The longitudinal organization of the terminal axons is apparent. Terminal axons of hair follicle collaterals run in close association with the longitudinally oriented dendrites of many of the neurones with cell bodies in laminae III and IV; they are also seen to terminate on neuronal somata in lamina III (Fig. 2.10A, B and Fig. 2.11B).

Terminal axons end as a bouton *terminal* (Fig. 2.11). Frequently the last 20–60 μm of the axon branches, up to as many as five times, each branch carrying boutons *en passant* and ending as a bouton *terminal*.

2. Distribution

The vast majority of synaptic boutons of hair follicle afferent fibres is in lamina III. A few are in the dorsal 100 μm or so of lamina IV, although it is very difficult in unstained sections to determine the border between laminae III and IV, so that boutons assessed as being in lamina IV may really be in III. Only rarely are boutons found in lamina

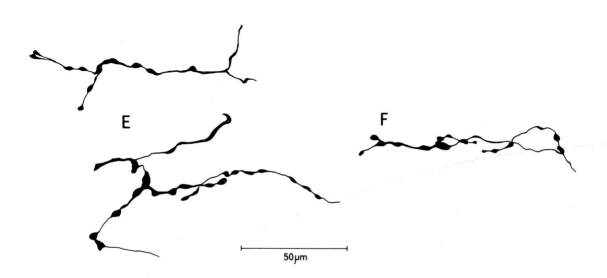

50μm

II and, when they are, they are always very close to the border with lamina III. This border is very obvious (Brown et al. 1976). There are occasional boutons in deeper parts of the dorsal horn.

The distribution of boutons is, of course, restricted to the area of distribution of the flame-shaped arbors. But it is more limited, particularly ventrally as the ventral parts of the 'flames' are made up of the ascending branches of the axon collaterals. Thus the boutons are more clearly confined to lamina III than are the flame-shaped arbors.

It is apparent that information from hair follicle receptors is distributed almost exclusively to a single lamina—lamina III. Except for axons from rapidly adapting mechanoreceptors in glabrous skin, myelinated cutaneous and muscle afferent fibres distribute their input to several laminae, and the restriction of the hair follicle receptor input to, essentially a single lamina is a striking feature. It means that only neurones with somata or dendrites in lamina III will receive direct excitation from hair follicle afferent fibres; those in more superficial or deeper parts of the cord will receive any excitation they obtain from hair follicle afferents through the mediation of interneurones. It should be remembered, however, that dorsal spinocerebellar tract neurones receive monosynaptic excitation from hair follicle afferent fibres (Lundberg and Oscarsson 1960; Mann 1971).

3. Density

The terminal arborizations of hair follicle afferent collaterals contain a very high density of synaptic boutons, a density greater than that for any other type of collateral from myelinated afferent fibres. Some idea of this density may be gained from the photomicrographs in Fig. 2.10.

In lamina III there are between 21 and 79 boutons per 100 μm^3 (45.7 $\pm$ 21.7, mean $\pm$ s.d.; $n = 12$). This is a much greater density than that for any other type of cutaneous or muscle afferent fibre that we have measured. It is presumably responsible, in part, for the powerful excitatory synaptic action that hair follicle afferent fibres have on their target neurones, such as neurones of the spinocervical tract. Because of the overlapping nature of the terminal arborizations of hair follicle collaterals and the differences in length of individual arbors it has not been possible to assess how many boutons might be carried by a single collateral.

IV. Organization of collaterals in the dorsal horn

1. Organization of collaterals from a single axon

An attempt is made in Fig. 2.12 to illustrate the salient points of the morphology and organization of hair follicle axons and their collaterals near the dorsal root entrance of the axon into the spinal cord. The figure also serves as a summary of much of the data presented in this chapter. It is drawn to scale and shows two hair follicle afferent fibres entering through different dorsal roots, one distributing its terminals to medial dorsal horn and the other to lateral horn.

Information from a hair follicle afferent unit is distributed to the spinal cord from a continuous sheet of terminal arborizations occupying the complete dorso-ventral extent of lamina III with little or no intrusion into adjacent laminae. Hair follicle afferent fibres are unique among the larger myelinated afferent fibres in that: (1) they have recurving collaterals that give rise to the flame-shaped arbors of the Scheibels (1968), and are identified as the 'collaterales grosses et profondes de la substance de Rolando' described by Ramon y Cajal (1909), except that the substantia gelatinosa (lamina II) does not receive a substantial input from them; (2) their input to the cord is restricted essentially to a single one of Rexed's laminae (lamina III); (3) they form a continuous sheet of terminals with no interruptions. This last point sets them apart from axons of rapidly adapting mechanoreceptors in glabrous skin (see Chapter 3).

Hair follicle afferent fibres also show a number of other unusual features. Most of them do not bifurcate upon entering the cord but turn rostrally and ascend. The majority of other afferent fibres bifurcate into ascending and descending branches. Collaterals arising from a single axon are closer together near the dorsal root entrance than farther away. Most injections of horseradish peroxidase have been made within about 2–3 mm of the dorsal root entrance of the axons. It is possible that for all types of afferent fibres, collaterals arise further apart the farther they are away from the entrance zone, but this tendency is pronounced in hair follicle axons (and also those of Pacinian corpuscle and tendon organ afferents).

The total length of the sheet of terminals, in lamina III, from a single hair follicle axon is unknown. The greatest stained length in our sample

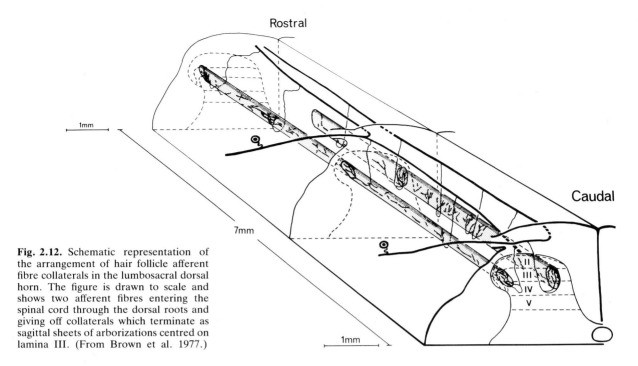

Fig. 2.12. Schematic representation of the arrangement of hair follicle afferent fibre collaterals in the lumbosacral dorsal horn. The figure is drawn to scale and shows two afferent fibres entering the spinal cord through the dorsal roots and giving off collaterals which terminate as sagittal sheets of arborizations centred on lamina III. (From Brown et al. 1977.)

has been 7.4 mm, which must be a lower limit to the range. The order of magnitude of the upper limit may be assessed by considering the somatotopic arrangement of the dorsal horn (see Chapter 6). Neurones of the spinocervical tract, which are monosynaptically excited by hair follicle afferents, are arranged in sagittally running columns with neurones in a column having overlapping receptive fields and, in all probability, common inputs. These longitudinal columns of neurones may be as long as 1.5–2.0 cm in the lumboscral cord, and the figures provide realistic estimates for the lengths of the sheets of hair follicle afferent terminals. Even these lengths may underestimate the true values. Certainly some primary afferents project caudally through many segments (Imai and Kusama 1969; Wall and Werman 1976).

Whatever the upper limit to the length of terminal sheets from hair follicle axons it is obvious that a single circular or oval skin area, which is the receptive field of a single hair follicle afferent unit, is represented in the dorsal horn as a sheet only some 150–400 μm thick but enormously elongated to many millimetres. In other words, a receptive field whose length is, at the most, about twice its width is transformed into a sheet with a length 100 or more times its width. From a number of these sheets, overlapping in the sagittal plane, neurones with somata and dendrites in lamina III sample the hair follicle input. Scheibel and Scheibel (1968) attempted to analyse the relation between the sheets of terminals and the dorsal horn neurones receiving input from them (see their Fig. 15). They considered the sheets of terminals to represent strip-shaped areas of skin running in the long axis of the limb. This is unlikely; the cutaneous areas are more likely to be a similar shape to the receptive fields of single hair follicle afferent fibres, but perhaps rather larger in size due to a certain amount of overlapping in the sagittal plane of individual sheets from single axons.

Scheibel and Scheibel (1968) also showed (their Fig. 15) a neurone with its cell body in lamina IV extending its dendrites into several (three) sets of sheets of terminals across about half the width of the dorsal horn. Similar illustrations had appeared earlier (see Fig. 121 in Ramon y Cajal 1909; Fig. 2 in Szentágothai 1964), also from neonatal material. In the adult cat, however, the width of a sheet of hair follicle terminals is about the same as the width of the dendritic tree of the vast majority of neurones with cell bodies in lamina IV (see Chapter 7). It is tempting to conclude that this similarity is no coincidence but that the widths of the sheets of terminals and the widths of the dendritic trees of the neurones are matched one to the other, as are the lengths of the arborizations of single collaterals and the lengths of the dendritic trees of many of the same neurones. It is as if the dendritic tree sampled from the terminal arbor of a single collateral. The situation cannot be as simple as this (see Chapter 7) but may approach it. The consensus of anatomical opinion would seem to be that the sheets of terminal arborizations do not overlap in the transverse plane. The evidence from our horseradish peroxidase experiments would not contradict this interpretation, but the crucial experiments of injecting with horseradish peroxidase a number of hair follicle afferents that have similar receptive fields have not been performed.

One firm conclusion may be drawn from a consideration of the arrangement of hair follicle afferent fibre collaterals in the dorsal horn: neurones in the dorsal horn that collect information from hair follicle afferent fibres should reflect, in their receptive field organization, the longitudinal organization of the terminal arborizations. As will be shown in Chapter 6, they do.

2. Somatotopic organization

When microelectrode recordings are made from neurones in the dorsal horn it is observed that a map of the hind limb is unfolded across the horn in lumbosacral segments. Distal and/or ventral skin is represented medially and proximal and/or dorsal skin in represented laterally (Wall 1960; Bryan et al. 1973; Brown and Fuchs 1975; Brown et al. 1980b). Details of the map are presented in Chapter 6. The gradient of the map in the transverse plane is very steep: in the L7 segment toes are represented medially and hip and outer thigh laterally, with leg and foot in between. These maps are recorded, for the most part, from neurones with cell bodies in or close to lamina IV. Such cells have many of their dendrites in lamina III, where they have ample opportunity for coming into contact with the boutons of hair follicle afferent fibres.

The primary central representation of the body surface in the spinal cord must be made by the terminal arborizations of cutaneous afferent fibres. The hair follicle afferents will play an important part in this representation as hairy skin covers nearly all the body surface. There should be a precise hind limb map formed by the hair

follicle afferent terminals across lamina III.

There is the possibility that the somatotopic information in the primary afferent fibres is 'scrambled' in the dorsal horn. The map recorded from dorsal horn neurones would then have to be generated by very selective synaptic contacts between the afferent fibres and the neurones. This seems unlikely, a priori, and, as will be shown below, the afferent terminal arborizations are arranged in a precise manner.

Obviously it is a relatively straightforward matter to record from the cells of the second-order map. It is not possible, however, to record from the terminal arborizations of hair follicle afferent fibres to determine the topography of the primary representation. But the position of single hair follicle afferent fibre arborizations is revealed by intra-axonal injection of horseradish peroxidase and the receptive field of the unit may be determined at the time of injection. Figure 2.13 shows the results of such an exercise for nine hair follicle afferent fibres. The representation of the body surface by the hair follicle afferent fibres is the same as the dorsal horn neurones receiving monosynaptic excitation from them (for example, neurones of the spinocervical tract as may be seen by comparing Fig. 2.13 with Figs. 6.13 and 6.14).

It is obvious that the neuronal receptive field maps are generated from the afferent fibre maps. Indeed, it is because the hair follicle terminal arborizations, and those of other types of cutaneous afferent unit, are arranged in longitudinally running sheets (or columns) that the neurones receiving input from them are also arranged in columns running up and down the cord, cells in any one column having overlapping receptive fields.

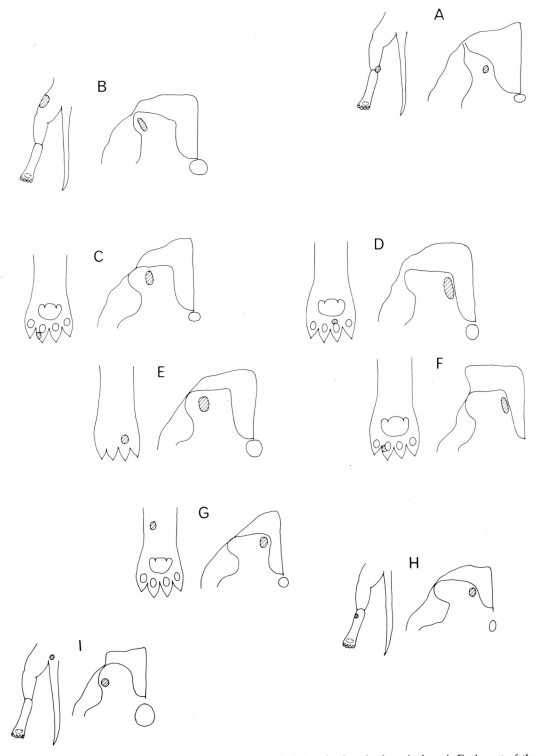

Fig. 2.13. Somatotopic organization of hair follicle afferent terminal arborizations in the spinal cord. Each part of the figure shows the receptive field of the afferent and the position of its terminal arborization in a transverse view of the dorsal horn. The figure is arranged so that rostral parts of the cord are at the top and caudal parts at the bottom; terminals in the lateral parts of the horn are to the left and those in the medial horn to the right. Proximal and dorsal parts of the hind limb are represented laterally, and distal and ventral parts medially.

3   Axons innervating rapidly adapting mechanoreceptors in glabrous skin

The axons of two receptor types will be considered in this chapter: the rapidly adapting mechanoreceptor in the dermis of the glabrous skin of the cat's foot and toe pads, and the Pacinian corpuscle, found in the subcutaneous tissue under and near to the glabrous skin of the foot and toe pads. By definition the rapidly adapting pad receptors are limited to the glabrous skin, and in fact the receptor organ, the Krause corpuscle or end bulb, is also limited to glabrous skin. Pacinian corpuscles are, of course, found in many places in addition to the subcutaneous tissue associated with the foot and toe pads. For example they are found in subcutaneous tissue in hairy regions of the body, in interosseous ligaments and in the mesentery. It is, therefore, somewhat arbitrary to include them in this chapter. However, clusters of Pacinian corpuscles are associated with the foot and toe pads and they may be very easily excited from the glabrous skin. It seems reasonable to assume that these corpuscles may have specialized reflex functions, as those associated with the carpal tactile hairs (Nilsson and Skoglund 1965; Nilsson 1969a,b) and the vibrissae (Gottschaldt et al. 1973) appear to have. Recently Jänig and Spilok (1978) have shown that excitation of Pacinian corpuscles in the central pad will lead to a very marked sudomotor response from the glabrous skin.

Another reason for treating these two receptor types together is that their close anatomical association has led to their being studied, and excited, together in many experiments. In fact until about 1970 they were not clearly differentiated in the literature but were thought to be a single class of rapidly adapting mechanoreceptor (e.g. the work of Gray and his colleagues: see below).

In view of the general interest in cutaneous receptors and the relation between their structure and function throughout the last 25 years or so, it is somewhat surprising that it was as late as 1968

that the first well-controlled electrophysiological study of the innervation of the cat's foot pad appeared (Jänig et al. 1968a). That there are both rapidly and slowly adapting mechanoreceptors which may be activated by displacement of the glabrous skin of the cat's foot has been known since the early report of Adrian and Zotterman (1926) and the work of Maruhashi et al. (1952). But the report of Jänig et al. (1968a) established that there are three types of sensitive mechanoreceptors that may be excited by pad displacement: a slowly adapting receptor now known to be of the Type I variety (see Chapter 4) and two rapidly adapting mechanoreceptors of which one has the properties of Pacinian corpuscle receptors. As will be described below, not only do the two types of rapidly adapting receptors have different end organs (Pacinian corpuscles and Krause corpuscles respectively) and different stimulus–response properties, but they are also innervated by axons whose central terminations differ and which have collaterals with distinctive morphologies.

A. Axons innervating Pacinian corpuscles

I. Pacinian corpuscles and their response properties

The structure and response properties of Pacinian corpuscles are too well known to require detailed presentation here. The Pacinian corpuscle and its smaller relatives, the paciniform corpuscles, have a distinctive morphology. The nerve terminal is surrounded by a many-layered capsule in which the layers (lamellae) are arranged in a typical 'onion skin' way. This accessory structure acts as a mechanical filter and prevents slow displacements from deforming the nerve ending at the centre of the 'onion' (Hubbard 1958; Loewenstein and Mendelson 1965; Ozeki and Sato 1965).

Typical Pacinian corpuscles are present in the subcutaneous tissue of the foot and toe pads (Adrian and Umrath 1929; Gray and Matthews 1951; Malinovsky 1966; Lynn 1969; Jänig 1971a), usually between 4 and 6 mm below the skin surface of the central pad. Jänig (1971a) counted between 15 and 30 corpuscles within and below the fat lobules associated with the central pad, a rather narrower range than the 11 to 43 counted by Lynn (1971). In addition there are other Pacinian corpuscles associated with the toe pads and on the digits between the tendons and the bones (Adrian and Umrath 1929; Malinovsky 1966; Lynn 1971). Obviously the distal parts of the hind limb contain a high concentration of these endings. Most, if not all, of these will be excited by mechanical displacement of the glabrous skin, if that displacement is abrupt enough (see below).

Pacinian corpuscles respond typically to vibration, and they are in fact tuned to frequencies in the range 150 to 300 or 400 Hz: that is, as long as the displacement is above a certain amplitude threshold (from less than 1 μm to 20–40 μm (Jänig et al. 1968a; Lynn 1971; Iggo and Ogawa 1977) for receptors in cat hind foot) the response follows the stimulus with one action potential for each sinusoid wave. Minimal amplitude thresholds are often difficult to determine because of the difficulties of finding the most sensitive spot on the skin, but once found the majority of Pacinian corpuscles will fire in response to indentations of 1 μm or less (Hunt 1961; Sato 1961; Lindblom and Lund 1966; Talbot et al. 1968; Nilsson 1969b; Merzenich and Harrington 1969).

Classically Pacinian corpuscles have been considered as vibration detectors, and certainly this interpretation is valid when one thinks of them in their natural environment. It has been pointed out however (see Burgess and Perl 1973) that they are really acceleration detectors—a valid point of view when one is considering their properties in the situation of an analytical experiment directed towards understanding their mechanisms of transduction. Operationally, of course, they behave as vibration detectors, except, perhaps, for those in the mesentery, which can act as acceleration detectors during jumping and the usually artificial or accidental situation of falling.

According to Jänig et al. (1968a) a displacement of the central pad of 20 μm in 1 ms will activate between 50 and 100 mechanoreceptors and by far the most of these will be Pacinian corpuscles. This is an important conclusion since it allows a retrospective identification of the receptor population studied by Gray and his colleagues in their quantitative analysis of receptors in the central foot pad (Armett and Hunsperger 1961; Armett et al. 1962). The receptors studied by these workers were, in all probability, Pacinian corpuscles. Unfortunately this identification means that the model of a population of receptors in the cat's central foot pad (Armett et al. 1962; Fuller and Gray 1966) is unrealistic with regard to both the spatial distribution of receptive fields and the variation of sensitivity within a field (see Lynn 1971).

Pacinian corpuscles in and around the foot and toe pads are innervated by axons conducting at about 45–65 m s^{-1} (Jänig et al. 1968a). Iggo and Ogawa (1977) give much lower values (23–34 m s^{-1}) but undoubtedly their figures are due to the use of electrical stimulation applied to the receptive field. The values given by Iggo and Ogawa are, therefore, misleading and those of Jänig et al., which were measured from the dorsal root to the plantar nerves about 15 mm cranial to the central foot pad, are accurate.

II. Central projections of afferent fibres innervating Pacinian corpuscles

Very little is known about the central projections of Pacinian corpuscle afferents in spite of their characteristic response properties. Indeed, since the afferent fibres innervating Pacinian corpuscles do not show much if any reduction in conduction velocity after entering the spinal cord (Jänig et al. 1968a; Brown 1968, 1973; Petit and Burgess 1968) Boivie and Perl (1975) hazard the suggestion that they may not have major branches at the segmental level. Branching is thought to lead to a reduction in diameter of the parent axon, although there is no a priori reason why absence of such a diameter reduction (conduction velocity decrease) should mean that no major branching has taken place. Indeed if it is accepted that Gray and his co-workers were studying Pacinian corpuscle input to the cord then there should be a population (or populations) of neurones in the medial part of the dorsal horn at lumbosacral level receiving such input (Armett et al. 1961, 1962).

Even if the cord neurones studied by Gray's group were not receiving Pacinian corpuscle excitation, and this seems most unlikely, Boivie and Perl's suggestion is too extreme. It was shown convincingly by Jänig et al. (1968b) that axons innervating Pacinian corpuscles, upon reaching the cord, activated interneurones responsible for the primary afferent depolarization of (mainly) axons innervating other rapidly adapting mechanoreceptors including the Pacinian corpuscle afferents themselves. At the very least, therefore, it is to be expected that neurones of the 'phasic' system producing primary afferent depolarization are excited via collaterals from Pacinian corpuscle afferent fibres. It remains to be seen whether the interneurones recorded by Gray's group and those on the pre-synaptic inhibitory pathway are one and the same population.

Of the three well-described somatosensory pathways originating in the spinal cord—the spinocervical, the spinothalamic and the postsynaptic dorsal column tracts or pathways—only the spinocervical tract would appear to have been examined properly for Pacinian corpuscle input. This does not receive excitation from any low-threshold receptor in glabrous skin and therefore does not receive input from Pacinian corpuscles (Brown and Franz 1969). Cells of the spinothalamic tract in the primate may respond at only the onset and termination of a mechanical stimulus (Willis et al. 1974). These neurones may, therefore, receive Pacinian corpuscle input, but the matter has not been examined rigorously. The position is similar for the post-synaptic dorsal column pathway. Angaut-Petit (1975b) described neurones of this system (in cat) with receptive fields that included glabrous skin and which responded with a rapidly adapting discharge to 'light tactile stimulation'. It will be shown in Chapter 8 that neurones sending axons into the dorsal columns may receive input from Pacinian corpuscles.

Direct evidence of Pacinian corpuscle input to neurones of the spinocerebellar tracts is also lacking. Mann (1971) examined input to the dorsal spinocerebellar tract mainly from hairy skin, but did show that some neurones received input from slowly adapting receptors in the foot and toe pads. No mention was made of any response that could have been due to Pacinian corpuscle activa-

tion in isolation. All ventral spinocerebellar tract neurones receive excitation from cutaneous nerves (see Oscarsson 1973) but analysis of the receptor types involved has not been carried out.

Undoubtedly the best-known central projection of Pacinian corpuscle afferent fibres is one that is really outside the scope of this book. This is the projection through the dorsal column–medial lemniscal–thalamic system to the cerebral cortex. At each 'relay station' in this pathway neurones have been recorded which have the characteristics to be expected if they were to receive information from Pacinian corpuscles (Poggio and Mountcastle 1960, 1963; Perl et al. 1962; Gordon and Jukes 1964; Mountcastle et al. 1969; Hyvärinen and Poranen 1978).

III. Morphology of axons innervating Pacinian corpuscles in the foot and toe pads

In our work (Brown et al. 1979, 1980a) afferent fibres innervating Pacinian corpuscles associated with the foot pad and toe pads of the cat's hind limb have been identified during electrophysiological experiments as follows. They had diffuse, poorly localized receptive fields limited to one pad. They were exquisitely sensitive to mechanical stimulation, usually responding with one or two impulses to tapping on the frame holding the hind limb. They followed, in a one-to-one fashion, the vibrations of a tuning fork (500 Hz) placed on the pad containing the receptive field, and sometimes followed in the same way when the fork was placed on the frame that held the animal. There is no reason to suspect that any receptor other than the Pacinian corpuscle was innervated by the axons recorded from. Indeed the later morphological analysis of the central parts of the axon indicated a class of unit different from any other studied. The axons had conduction velocities of 57–75 m s^{-1}.

1. Entry of axons into the spinal cord, branching and collateral distribution

In contrast to the great majority of hair follicle afferent fibres (see Chapter 2) but in line with the usual pattern for primary afferent fibres entering the cord, the axons of Pacinian corpuscle units usually bifurcate into rostral and caudal branches shortly after entering the cord. Both the rostral and caudal branches then run medially as they ascend or descend over the dorsal horn to lie in the dorsal columns medial to the dorsal horn (Figs. 3.1, 3.2).

The collaterals of Pacinian afferent fibres arise closer together from the descending branch of the axon than they do from the ascending branch, as do those of Golgi tendon organ afferents. On the descending branch collaterals arise on average about every 330 μm, whereas on the ascending branch they arise about every 880 μm. The mean spacing of collaterals from axons of Pacinian afferent is 688 ± 469 μm (means ± s.d.), a value very similar to those for other cutaneous axons that, like the axons of Pacinian corpuscle units with receptors in the foot and toe pads, distribute their collaterals to the medial parts of the dorsal horn (for example, axons of Type I slowly adapting receptors in glabrous skin [Chapter 4], Type II slowly adapting receptors near the claw bases [Chapter 5], and hair follicle receptors on the distal foot and toes [Chapter 2]. As will be discussed in Chapter 10, it seems to be a general rule of the organization of cutaneous collaterals that on average they arise closer together if they distribute their terminals to the medial parts of the dorsal horn.

2. Morphology of collaterals and their arborizations

In line with the general principles that have emerged from intra-axonal staining with horse-radish peroxidase, collaterals of Pacinian corpuscle afferent fibres have a morphology that is quite distinctive and characteristic of the unit type. Reconstructions of these collaterals are shown in Figs. 3.1 and 3.2 (reconstructions in the transverse plane) and Fig. 3.3 (reconstruction in the sagittal plane).

The axons from Pacinian corpuscles of the foot and toe pads distribute their collaterals to the medial third or less of the dorsal horn (Figs. 3.1, 3.2), entering the horn at its dorsal or medial border. If entering from the former they descend through laminae I and II, sometimes dividing on the way, and enter lamina III where they soon undergo repeated subdivision. When entering from the medial border the collaterals may enter lamina III directly. Like all primary afferent fibre collaterals they usually have a rostral trajectory as they descend from the parent axon towards their main branching site (Fig. 3.3).

Like most primary afferent fibre collaterals, those of axons from Pacinian corpuscles have not been described in detail in reports in which classical anatomical methods have been used. But their morphology is distinctive and characteristic. Each collateral provides terminal arborizations to two main areas of the dorsal horn. There is a main termination dorsally in laminae III and IV and a lesser area of termination ventrally in laminae V and VI. These two areas may nearly always be clearly seen in reconstructions of single collaterals, with an obvious gap, containing no terminal axons, between the two areas in the vicinity of the IV–V border or in dorsal lamina V. The two areas are connected by a few (two to four) fairly thick branches of the collateral.

Within the two areas of arborization the branches of the collaterals tend to run in different directions. As seen in the reconstructions from sagittal sections (Fig. 3.3) or photomicrographs of such sections (Fig. 3.4A–C), in the dorsal termination area the axons run in the plane of the section in the longitudinal axis of the cord, whereas in the ventral area the axons run in the transverse plane in a dorso-ventral direction (Fig. 3.5).

The total arborizations from individual collaterals have a dorso-ventral depth of some 700–800 μm. This is much greater than that of hair follicle afferent fibre collaterals which have *terminal* arborizations limited mainly to lamina III even though branches of the collateral are deeper than this. In fact, along with the Type II slowly adapting units, Pacinian corpuscle units have collaterals with the largest dorso-ventral distribution of any large myelinated axon running in cutaneous nerves.

The collateral arborization is less extensive in the transverse plane, the medio-lateral measurement usually being 170–350 μm and rarely up to 500 μm. In the rostro-caudal direction the arborization is much longer dorsally than ventrally. The dorsal region of termination is about 400–750 μm and the dorsal regions of adjacent collaterals frequently overlap with one another (Fig. 3.3). There is overlap between adjacent ventral terminal arborizations only rarely.

3. Synaptic boutons

a) *Morphology and distribution.* Photomicrographs of the bouton-carrying parts of Pacinian corpuscle axon collaterals are shown in Fig. 3.4A–C and Fig. 3.5. There are distinct differences

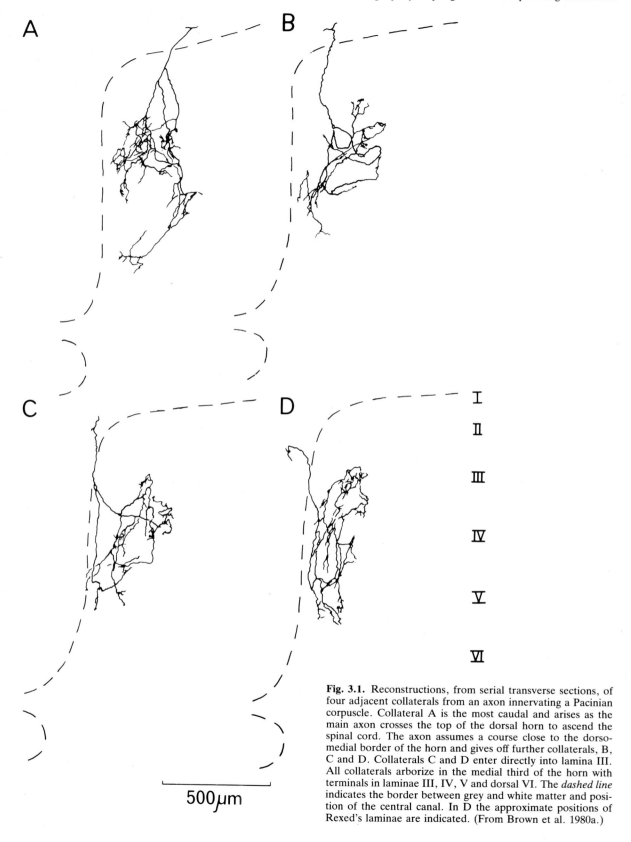

Fig. 3.1. Reconstructions, from serial transverse sections, of four adjacent collaterals from an axon innervating a Pacinian corpuscle. Collateral A is the most caudal and arises as the main axon crosses the top of the dorsal horn to ascend the spinal cord. The axon assumes a course close to the dorso-medial border of the horn and gives off further collaterals, B, C and D. Collaterals C and D enter directly into lamina III. All collaterals arborize in the medial third of the horn with terminals in laminae III, IV, V and dorsal VI. The *dashed line* indicates the border between grey and white matter and position of the central canal. In D the approximate positions of Rexed's laminae are indicated. (From Brown et al. 1980a.)

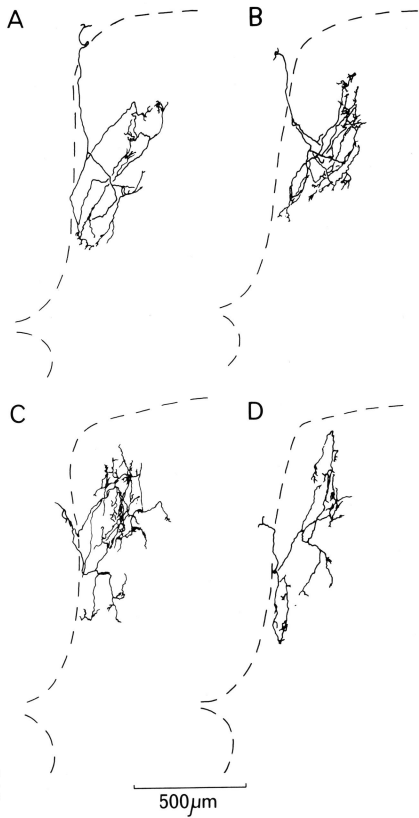

Fig. 3.2. Reconstructions, in the transverse plane, of four adjacent collaterals from a Pacinian corpuscle axon. (From Brown et al. 1980a.)

500µm

in the arrangement of the boutons in the two termination regions.

In the dorsal region the terminal axons run predominantly in the longitudinal axis of the cord and carry many boutons *de passage*. Up to 12 or 14 boutons may be strung out along the last 50 μm of the axon, although six to ten are more common numbers. The longitudinal organization of the terminal axons in the dorsal region is more marked in lamina III than in lamina IV.

In the ventral region (laminae V and VI) the terminal axons run dorso-ventrally and are contained within the transverse plane. Boutons *en passant* are present in this region (Fig. 3.5B) but are uncommon in comparison with those in laminae III and IV. The usual arrangement in the ventral region is for a terminal axon to branch several times (two to four), the branches being close together and each terminating in a bouton,

perhaps having one bouton *de passage* before the bouton *terminal*. This leads to the arrangement of boutons in small clusters of about three to six boutons close together. In counterstained sections these clusters may be seen ordered around neuronal somata (Fig. 3.5C). The clustering has not been seen in lamina III and only occasionally in lamina IV.

The boutons on Pacinian corpuscle axon collaterals vary widely in size. The smallest are 1.0 μm × 1.0 μm while the largest may be 5.5 μm × 2.5 μm. These very large boutons are considerably bigger than any other boutons of primary afferent fibres (cutaneous or muscle) that we have seen. In counterstained sections the large boutons are not in close proximity to neuronal somata and are presumably, therefore, contacting dendrites.

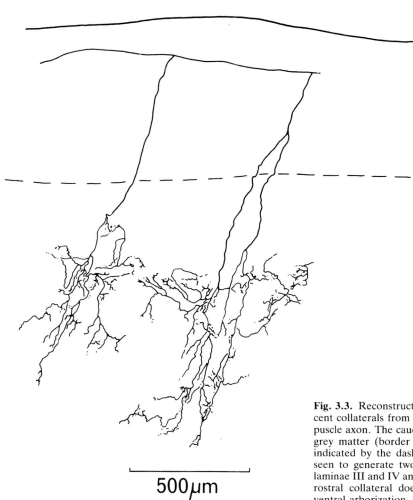

500 μm

Fig. 3.3. Reconstruction, from sagittal sections, of two adjacent collaterals from the ascending branch of a Pacinian corpuscle axon. The caudal collateral divides before it enters the grey matter (border between the grey and white matter is indicated by the dashed line). The caudal collateral can be seen to generate two sets of arborizations, one dorsally in laminae III and IV and one ventrally in laminae V and VI; the rostral collateral does not generate such a well-developed ventral arborization. (From Brown et al. 1980a.)

b) *Density*. Single collaterals of Pacinian corpuscle afferent fibres carry between 47 and 367 boutons (170 ± 94, mean ± s.d.; n = 19). Because of the greater development of the terminal arborization in laminae III and IV most boutons are in this region.

4. Organization of collaterals in the dorsal horn

The organization of Pacinian corpuscle collaterals is summarized in Fig. 3.6, which should be compared with the similar figures in this and other chapters on primary afferent fibres (see also Chapter 10).

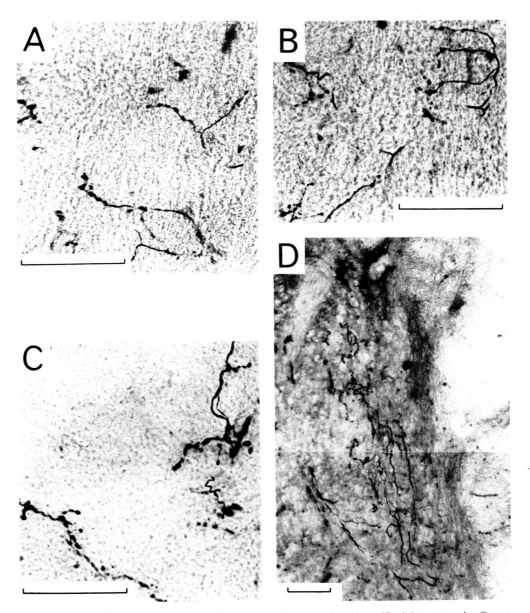

Fig. 3.4. A–C Photomicrographs, from 100-μm sagittal sections of spinal cord, of terminal branches of Pacinian corpuscle afferent fibre collaterals. Each example shows boutons in laminae III–IV. The terminal axons are oriented within the plane of these sagittal sections. Dorsal is at the top, rostral to the left.

D Photomicrograph, from a single 100-μm thick transverse section of cord, showing part of a collateral from an axon innervating a rapidly adapting mechanoreceptor in glabrous skin. The medial and dorsal borders of the dorsal horn can be seen. Although the collateral branches penetrate deep into lamina IV they change direction and recurve dorsally to terminate within lamina III.

The scale bars all represent 100 μm. (From Brown et al. 1980a.)

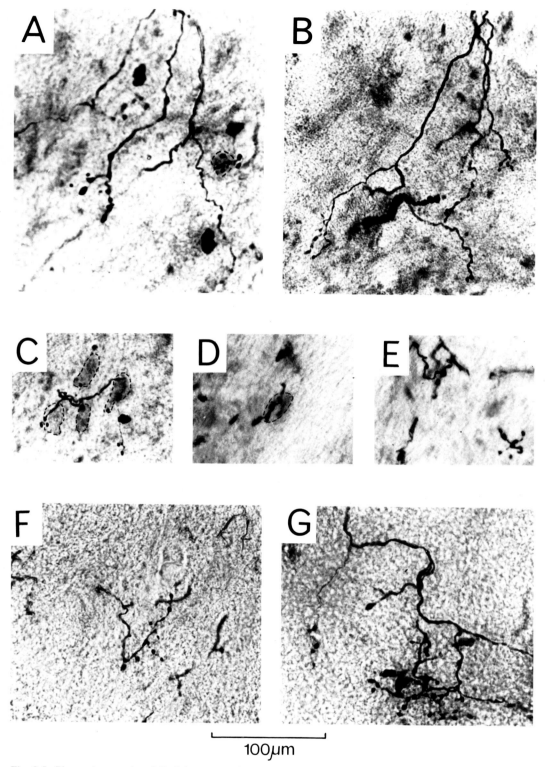

100μm

Fig. 3.5. Photomicrographs of Pacinian corpuscle axon collateral branches in laminae V and VI. All are from 100-μm thick sections: **A–C** from transverse sections, **D–G** from sagittal sections. In counterstained sections (**A, C, D**) neurones apparently contacted by boutons are outlined with *dashed lines*. Many of the fine terminal branches carry only one or two boutons and distribute these in small clusters. (From Brown et al. 1980a.)

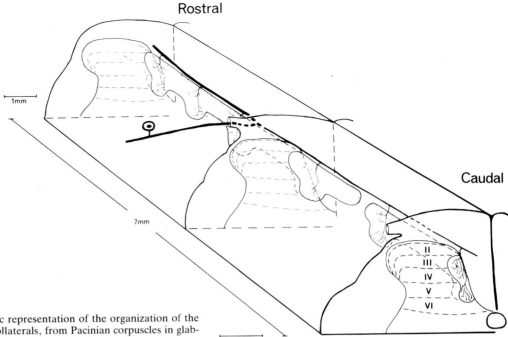

Fig. 3.6. Schematic representation of the organization of the axons, and their collaterals, from Pacinian corpuscles in glabrous skin. (From Brown et al. 1980a.)

Axons from Pacinian corpuscle units usually bifurcate into ascending and descending branches shortly after entering the cord and each branch gives off numerous collaterals, certainly as many as any other cutaneous axon. Therefore, as expected, the suggestion of Boivie and Perl (1975) that Pacinian corpuscle axons might have no major branches at the segmental level is refuted. Furthermore the present findings show that the degree of branching of an axon is not necessarily reflected by the degree of reduction of its conduction velocity. Axons of Pacinian corpuscles branch as much as other cutaneous axons at the segmental level and yet their conduction velocities change much less (Jänig et al. 1968a; Brown 1968, 1973, and unpublished observations).

Pacinian corpuscle afferent collaterals have a characteristic morphology that has not apparently been described prior to our reports (Brown et al. 1979, 1980a and the present volume). As befits the position of the receptors in the tissue beneath the glabrous skin of the foot and toe pads, the collaterals distribute their terminations to the most medial parts of the dorsal horn in laminae III–VI. Along with all other large myelinated afferent fibres they do not send terminals to laminae I or II.

Pacinian corpuscle afferent collaterals distribute their information to two distinct regions of the dorsal horn: a major region in laminae III and IV and a minor region in laminae V and VI. There are characteristic differences in both terminal axon orientation and bouton density in the two regions that indicate a high likelihood that at least two different populations of neurones are being influenced.

In the dorsal region, especially in lamina III, the axons run in the longitudinal axis of the cord and carry many boutons *en passant*. In this respect they are similar to the terminal axons of the hair follicle afferent fibre collaterals (Chapter 2). Many dendrites in lamina III also run in the longitudinal axis of the cord (Scheibel and Scheibel 1968) and the terminal axons of Pacinian corpuscle afferent fibres with their boutons *de passage* are ideally suited to contact these, although it should be noted that there is no evidence that they contact the dendrites of spinocervical tract neurones that run in this lamina (see Chapter 6).

In the ventral region (laminae V and VI) the terminal axons are oriented mainly within the transverse plane of the cord and run dorsoventrally. This orientation reflects that of many dendrites in the region (Scheibel and Scheibel

1968; Proshansky and Egger 1977; see also Chapter 9), although counterstained sections reveal that many of the clusters of boutons on Pacinian corpuscle collaterals are arranged around neuronal cell bodies.

In both the dorsal and ventral regions, the organization of boutons in *en passant* and cluster formations, together with the large size of many boutons, suggests very tight coupling between the afferent fibres and the neurones they contact.

B. Axons innervating rapidly adapting mechanoreceptors in glabrous skin

I. The receptor and its response properties

As mentioned above it was only recently (Jänig et al. 1968a) that the responses of rapidly adapting mechanoreceptors and of Pacinian corpuscles of the foot and toe pads were clearly differentiated from one another in electrophysiological experiments on single units. The differences were soon confirmed (Lynn 1969). Attempts were then made to identify the receptors morphologically, the Pacinian corpuscle being the first to be recognized (Lynn 1969). Jänig (1971a) combined electrophysiological and histological methods and demonstrated that the rapidly adapting mechanoreceptors were, in all probability, encapsulated endings of the Krause corpuscle type.

The most complete combined electrophysiological and histological study is that of Iggo and Ogawa (1977), who carried the structural study to the level of the electron microscope. As pointed out by these authors, combined studies of this type on receptors in or below the thick glabrous skin of the cat's pads are less easy to interpret than similar studies on the thin skin of hairy-regions. But both Jänig (1971a) and Iggo and Ogawa (1977) conclude that the responsible receptor is the Krause corpuscle and there can be little doubt that this is a correct identification.

In point of fact Iggo and Ogawa conclude that the receptor is the cylindrical type of corpuscle (*cylindrische Endkolben*) of Krause (1860). Its

morphology has been well described at both light and electron microscope levels (Krause 1860; Winkelmann 1958; Malinovsky 1966; Ormea and Goglia 1969; Polacek and Halata 1970; Munger and Pubols 1972; Iggo and Ogawa 1977). The corpuscles are located in the dermis within about 2 mm of the surface of the pads, within the dermal papillae. In the foot pad they are 5–40 μm in transverse diameter (Iggo and Ogawa 1977) and 30–125 μm in length. Most corpuscles (about 40% according to Malinovsky 1966) have a single nerve terminal; the remainder have two or three. The terminal (neurite) is surrounded by 10–12 concentric lamellae, with desmosomes between adjacent lamellae.

In contrast with the Pacinian corpuscles the rapidly adapting mechanoreceptors have small well-localized receptive fields of less than 1 mm^2 to about 20 mm^2, and usually show two or more sensitive spots in the field (Jänig et al. 1968a; Lynn 1969; Iggo and Ogawa 1977). Tuning curves may be found for the rapidly adapting receptors but their best frequencies (10–200 Hz: Iggo and Ogawa 1977) are lower than those for Pacinian corpuscles in the pads (100–300 Hz: Jänig et al. 1968a; Iggo and Ogawa 1977). It is generally thought that the indentation threshold for rapidly adapting mechanoreceptors is less than that for the Pacinian corpuscles (Jänig et al. 1968a; Lynn 1969)—but see Iggo and Ogawa (1977). According to Iggo and Ogawa (1977) the rapidly adapting receptors encode stimulus indentation velocity (in a similar way to the hair follicle receptors (Brown and Iggo 1967); see Chapter 2) rather than stimulus indentation amplitude.

The rapidly adapting mechanoreceptors in the dermis of the foot and toe pads are innervated by axons conducting at about 45–75 m s^{-1} (see Fig. 7 in Jänig et al. 1968a). As with the values for Pacinian corpuscle afferent nerve fibres, the values given by Iggo and Ogawa (1977) for the conduction velocities of fibres innervating these receptors (24–48 m s^{-1}) are misleading due to the method of measurement used.

II. Central projections of afferent fibres innervating rapidly adapting mechanoreceptors in the foot and toe pads

The position with regard to the central projections of afferent fibres innervating rapidly adapting mechanoreceptors in the foot and toe pads is essentially the same as that for the Pacinian afferent—almost nothing is known of them. Near the level of entry of the axons into the spinal cord there should be a population of interneurones receiving input from them. These interneurones are on the same pathway as that responsible for primary afferent depolarization of other cutaneous afferent fibres, particularly those innervating rapidly adapting receptors of the hair follicles and Pacinian corpuscles (Jänig et al. 1968b). Whether or not any of the interneurones recorded by Armett et al. (1961, 1962) and Gray and Lal (1965) receive excitation from the rapidly adapting mechanoreceptors of the pads is not known.

Afferent fibres from rapidly adapting mechanoreceptors in glabrous skin do not excite the cells of origin of the spinocervical tract (Brown and Franz 1969). The spinocervical tract, therefore, does not receive input from either the Pacinian corpuscles or the Krause corpuscles. As will be described later, it does not receive excitation from the Type I slowly adapting receptors of the glabrous skin either. With regard to the spinothalamic tract and the post-synaptic dorsal column pathway there may be input from the rapidly adapting mechanoreceptors of the pads, since cells of these systems may respond at the onset and termination of mechanical stimulation (Willis et al. 1974; Angaut-Petit 1975b; see Chapter 8). But the position is not clear; the responses may be due to input from other receptors. Obviously a detailed receptor-oriented study is needed for these latter two systems. The situation for the spinocerebellar tracts is similarly unclear.

It seems reasonable to assume that axons of some of the rapidly adapting pad units ascend the dorsal columns to the dorsal column nuclei, because rapidly adapting responses to glabrous skin stimulation have been recorded (Perl et al. 1962; Gordon and Jukes 1964). Some axons of the medial lemniscus certainly have properties that would be expected if their neurones were to receive a convergent input from these receptors (Brown et al. 1974).

III. Morphology of axons innervating rapidly adapting mechanoreceptors

Identification of the rapidly adapting mechanoreceptors in the glabrous skin of the foot and toe pads is relatively straightforward. They are innervated by myelinated axons (conducting at $54–60$ m s^{-1} in our sample), have small well-localized receptive fields and do not follow the vibrations of a tuning fork in a one-to-one manner. All of the sample of axons identified as innervating Krause corpuscles satisfied these criteria. In addition the morphological characteristics of their collaterals were quite distinctive and indicated that a separate population of afferent units was being studied. Although only three axons of this type have been stained successfully with horseradish peroxidase we are quite confident that they represent this class of unit (Brown et al. 1980a).

1. Entry of axons into the spinal cord, branching and collateral distribution

All three axons in the sample could be traced into the dorsal root and two of them bifurcated shortly after leaving the root and entering the cord. Fifteen collaterals arose from the stained axons at an average spacing of 783 ± 338 μm (mean $\pm$ s.d.) with a range of $400–1500$ μm. These spacings are similar to those of other cutaneous afferent fibre collaterals that, like those of the rapidly adaptiing mechanoreceptors, distribute their terminal arborization to the medial parts of the lumbosacral dorsal horn (see Chapter 10).

2. Morphology of collaterals and their arborizations

The collaterals from axons innervating the rapidly adapting mechanoreceptors in glabrous skin have a distinctive morphology, as shown in Figs. 3.7 and 3.8 for collaterals reconstructed from transverse sections of the cord (see also Fig. 3.4D). The collaterals are distributed to the most medial parts of the dorsal horn, sometimes to the medial quarter or less.

When examined in single transverse sections or in reconstructions from serial transverse sections some collaterals bear a resemblance to the flame-shaped arbors of hair follicle afferent fibre collaterals (see Chapter 2), and in a casual examination the two types may be confused. The resemblance lies in the general morphology as seen in the transverse plane and also in the distribution of the terminal arborizations: both hair follicle collaterals and those from the rapidly adapting receptors in glabrous skin send their information almost exclusively to lamina III. Careful examination, however, reveals a number of differences. The major difference between the two types is that hair follicle collaterals form a continuous longitudinal column or sheet of arborizations running up and down the cord for many millimetres, with arborizations from adjacent collaterals overlapping, while those of the rapidly adapting mechanoreceptors are restricted in the longitudinal axis. This restriction is to between 400 and 600 μm in our material and there are

gaps between adjacent collaterals of 100–700 μm. Usually, each collateral terminates in its own private volume of cord measuring 400–600 μm in the longitudinal direction, 50–300 μm in the transverse axis and about 300 μm dorso-ventrally. Some collaterals (Fig. 3.8A, C) have a greater development dorso-ventrally, with boutons in lamina IV.

3. Synaptic boutons

The bouton-carrying terminal axons of collaterals from rapidly adapting mechanoreceptors are mainly limited to lamina III; on some collaterals there are boutons in lamina IV. In the former respect these collaterals are similar to those from hair follicle afferent fibres. However, the orientation of the terminal axons, although running mainly in the longitudinal axis of the cord, is not as strictly confined to the rostro-caudal direction

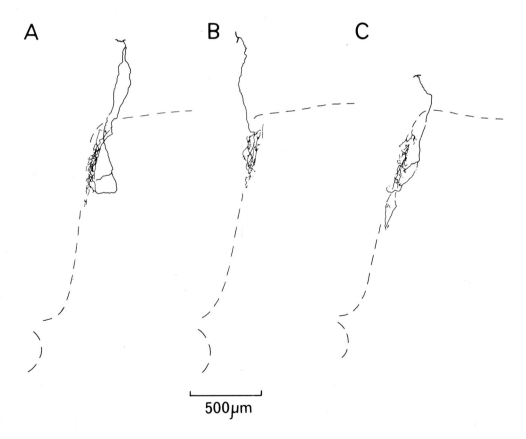

500 μm

Fig. 3.7. Reconstructions, from serial transverse sections, of three adjacent collaterals from an axon innervating rapidly adapting mechanoreceptors in glabrous skin. **C** is the most rostral. The resemblance to the transverse view of hair follicle afferent collaterals is clear (see Figs. 2.5, 2.6). Most of the boutons of these collaterals are distributed to lamina III close to its medial border. (From Brown et al. 1980a.)

as that of the hair follicle collateral terminal arborizations or as that of Pacinian corpuscle afferent fibres in the same part of the dorsal horn.

Many of the boutons carried by collaterals from Krause corpuscle axons are of the *en passant* variety but small groups or clusters may also be observed. In comparison with the boutons of hair follicle afferent fibre collaterals, therefore, those from rapidly adapting mechanoreceptors are more heterogeneous in their arrangement.

4. Organization of collaterals in the spinal cord

Figure 3.9 summarizes the organization of collaterals from axons innervating Krause corpuscles, and should be compared with the other similar figures in this (Fig. 3.6) and other chapters (see also Chapter 10). These collaterals have a distinctive morphology which, although similar in some respects to that of collaterals from hair follicle afferent fibres, differs from that of any other

collaterals from large myelinated cutaneous or muscle axons.

The superficial resemblance between collaterals from Krause corpuscles and hair follicle receptors is interesting. Both are rapidly adapting mechanoreceptors with rather similar stimulus–response properties (Brown and Iggo 1967; Iggo and Ogawa 1977). Both have central axon collaterals with flame-shaped arbors when viewed in transverse sections, and these arborizations, in addition to having very similar morphologies, are situated in the same dorsal horn laminae. There are important differences, however, in both their morphology and their post-synaptic target neurones. Morphologically the most obvious differences are: (1) hair follicle axon collateral arborizations form continuous columns from adjacent collaterals along the length of the dorsal horn that run for many millimetres, whereas rapidly adapting mechanoreceptor axon collater-

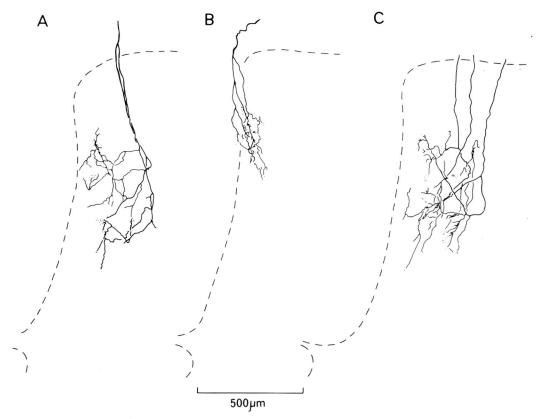

Fig. 3.8. Reconstructions, in the transverse plane, of five adjacent collaterals from an axon innervating rapidly adapting mechanoreceptors in glabrous skin. The collaterals in **A** and **C** send more branches into lamina IV than those shown in **B** and Fig. 3.7. (From Brown et al. 1980a).

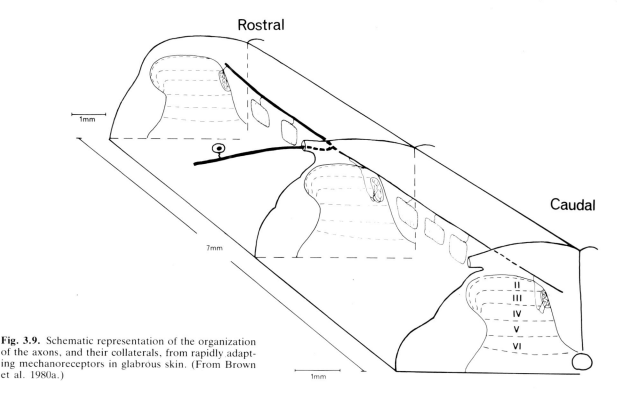

Fig. 3.9. Schematic representation of the organization of the axons, and their collaterals, from rapidly adapting mechanoreceptors in glabrous skin. (From Brown et al. 1980a.)

als are limited to their own private volume of cord, and (2) the arrangements of the synaptic boutons. With regard to the target neurones of the two types it is known that hair follicle afferent fibres excite many neurones of the spinocervical tract whereas axons from the rapidly adapting mechanoreceptors in glabrous skin do not (see Chapter 6). Therefore, it is not reasonable to assume that the two types of afferent unit perform identical functions for hairy and glabrous skin respectively: the central processing of informa-

tion from these two types of receptors obviously differs. Finally, the observation that there are two quite different types of collaterals from axons innervating glabrous skin, and that the two types are never found on the same axon, provides quite independent confirmation that glabrous skin does indeed contain two types of rapidly adapting mechanoreceptors—the Pacinian and the Krause corpuscles—with each having characteristic response properties.

4   Axons innervating slowly adapting Type I mechanoreceptors

The skin of mammals contains two types of slowly adapting sensitive mechanoreceptors. The distinction into two classes was first made clearly by Iggo (1963b), on the basis of the electrophysiological responses recorded from nerves innervating hairy skin. Iggo originally called the two types of receptors 'touch spots' and 'touch fields'. The designations were later changed to Type I and Type II receptors or afferent units (Iggo 1966; Chambers and Iggo 1967; Brown and Iggo 1967). Type I responses had been described earlier by a number of workers but, unfortunately, up to the mid 1960s no clear distinction was made between the Type I and II responses (Hunt and McIntyre 1960b; Werner and Mountcastle 1965).

The first clear description of Type I units was given by Frankenhaeuser (1949). He made the important observation that (in the rabbit) there were obvious structures, visible on the skin surface, at the points of highest sensitivity. The discovery that Type I responses come from a distinct kind of receptor organ was also made independently by Iggo (1963a) and Tapper (1963, 1964, 1965) in the cat. Subsequent studies have shown that the receptors are present in other mammals: rabbit (Brown and Iggo 1967; Brown and Hayden 1971) and primates including man (Lindblom and Tapper 1967; Iggo 1963b; Perl 1968; Harrington and Merzenich 1970; Knibestöl and Vallbo 1970). Type I discharges have also been recorded in non-mammalian vertebrates (reptiles: Kenton et al. 1971).

Type I responses have been recorded too from the glabrous skin of mammals, by Jänig et al. (1968a), and it has been shown (Jänig 1971a, b) that collections of tactile (Merkel) cells are present at the epidermo-dermal junction under the positions of the sensitive spots of the afferent units. Since Merkel cells are a feature of the receptors in hairy skin (see below) it is reasonable to conclude that the Type I responses recorded from glabrous skin and hairy skin both originate from the same receptor type, even though the two receptors have somewhat different morphologies.

A. Morphology of the Type I receptor

The recognition by Iggo (1963a) and Tapper (1963) that a particular type of electrophysiological response was always associated with displacement of distinctive structures visible in hairy skin was a landmark in the history of somatosensory physiology. It crystallized the discussion about specificity of cutaneous receptors and the relationships between structure and function. The arguments are now dead and outside the scope of this book. But from the early 1960s onwards the evidence has been accumulating that shows, without doubt, that all cutaneous receptors are specific in that they only respond to one type of (adequate) stimulus. Wherever it has been possible to determine the structure of the receptor then that has been specific too.

I. In hairy skin

The structure of the Type I receptor as it appears in light and electron microscope preparations from the skin of the cat is shown (diagrammatically) in Fig. 4.1. The receptor is a dome-shaped structure some 100–400 μm in diameter that projects from the surface of the skin. Under the light microscope (Fig. 4.1A) it can be seen that it contains a thickened epidermis. On the epidermal side of the basement membrane is a single layer of cells associated with the expanded terminals of the myelinated axon that innervates the receptor. These cells are the *Tastzellen* originally described by Merkel (1875). In the dermis there are many bundles of collagen fibres together with blood vessels. The light microscope appearance of the receptor was originally described by Pinkus (1904).

Under the electron microscope the Merkel cell is seen (Fig. 4.1B) to be invaginated, deep to the nucleus, by the plate-like expansion of the nerve terminal. The tactile cells are attached to the overlying epidermal cells by desmosomes and there are cylindrical cytoplasmic expansions from the tactile cells that indent the epidermal cells. There is a close relationship between the tactile cell and the expanded nerve ending. They are always separated by a gap of about 15 nm, but structures similar to synapses are present and there are accumulations of dense-cored vesicles in the cytoplasm of the tactile cells that overlie the 'synapses'. Treatment with reserpine did not affect these osmiophilic granules (Iggo and Muir 1969).

In the rabbit and in rodents (Straile 1960; Smith 1967) the receptor has a similar structure to that in primates, although in the latter it protrudes less from the skin (Smith 1970).

II. In glabrous skin

The structure of the Type I receptors in the glabrous skin of the cat's foot pad, as seen under the light microscope, has been described by Jänig (1971a, b). There is no dome-shaped touch corpuscle as there is in hairy skin. Instead, in the epithelial pegs there are clusters of Merkel cells at the epidermo-dermal junction. The characteristic electrophysiological responses recorded in the afferent fibre from Type I receptors (see below) are presumably due to the properties of the tactile cells.

B. Physiology of Type I units

I. From hairy skin

Each Type I receptor is innervated by a single myelinated axon with a conduction velocity of between 33 and 95 m s^{-1} (Brown and Iggo 1967). Burgess et al. (1968) give values of about 45–85 m s^{-1} (see their Fig. 7A). Both sets of results are from cat.

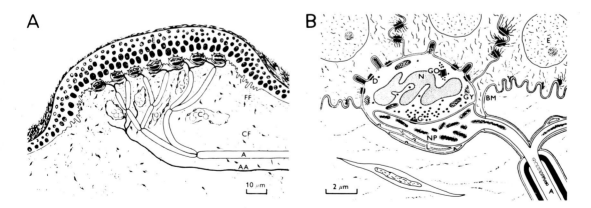

Fig. 4.1. The structure of the slowly adapting Type I receptor.
   A shows the structure as seen in light microscope sections. A, single myelinated axon; AA, non-myelinated axon; BM, basement membrane; C, capillary; E, thickened epidermis; FF and CF, fine and coarse bundles of collagen fibres; I, indentations of the epidermis at the periphery of the corpuscle; T, tactile (Merkel) cell with its associated nerve plate.
   B shows the structure of a tactile cell and its nerve plate as seen in electron microscope preparations. A, myelinated axon; D, desmosome; E, epidermal cell nucleus; G, granular vesicles in the tactile cell near a junction with the nerve plate (NP); GO, Golgi apparatus; GY, glycogen; L, lamellae underlying the nerve plate; N, multilobulated nucleus of tactile cell; P, cytoplasmic process from the tactile cell. (Modified From Iggo and Muir 1969.)

Between one and five Type I receptors are innervated by a single afferent fibre (Burgess et al. 1968; Iggo and Muir 1969); Tapper (1965) gives a range of one to seven endings per axon. Most axons innervate one to three receptors (see also Hunt and McIntyre 1960b).

According to Tapper (1965) the receptive fields of Type I units are non-intersecting. That is, within the skin area surrounded by the perimeter of the receptive field of a single Type I unit there are no touch corpuscles that do not belong to that unit. The sensitive part of the receptive field of a Type I unit is strictly limited to the receptors; the field is 'spotty', and the receptors have to be displaced in order for a response to be elicited. Type I receptors, unlike Type II receptors, are not responsive to the skin being stretched but require displacement in a direction at, or close to, right angles to the skin surface. The dense collagenous core of the receptor probably provides mechanical insulation from skin displacement occurring at a distance.

Type I units rarely show any background (spontaneous, resting) activity. This property further differentiates them from Type II units, which nearly always display a background discharge upon isolation.

Type I units show both a phasic and a tonic response to mechanical stimulation: a phasic response during movement and a tonic response during a maintained displacement (Tapper 1965; Burgess et al. 1968; Iggo and Muir 1969; Harrington and Merzenich 1970). The phasic response is dependent on both the velocity and the amplitude of the displacement (Fig. 4.2) and has the very low threshold of less than 1 mg weight (Iggo 1963a) or 1–5 μm displacement (Iggo and Muir 1969). The tonic response shows an initial fairly rapid adaptation during the first second or so of a maintained displacement, then a period of more slow adaptation for some tens of seconds; finally there may be a non-adapting phase if the mean impulse rate is greater than about 10 s^{-1} (Burgess et al. 1968; Iggo and Muir 1969). A characteristic feature of the tonic response is its marked irregularity, in contrast to that of Type II units. The

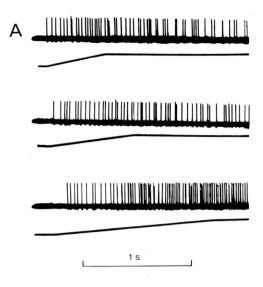

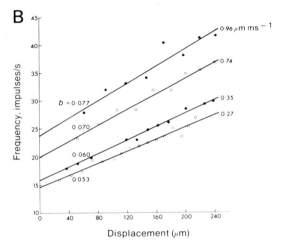

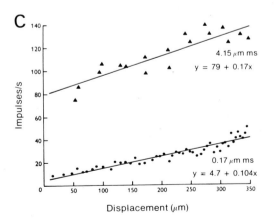

Fig. 4.2. Responses of Type I units to skin indentation. **A** Responses recorded from a single unit (*upper trace*) to displacement of the receptor (*lower trace*). In each set of records the final displacement was 250 μm. The irregularity of the discharge is characteristic. **B** The dynamic response during constant-velocity displacement at the indicated velocities. The values of the regression coefficients of the fitted lines (*b*) are indicated on each graph. **C** Dynamic responses at two velocities (final displacement, 300 μm). Each *point* is the mean of 16 responses. (From Iggo and Muir 1969.)

general features of the Type I tonic response are shown in Fig. 4.3. For a detailed discussion of the responses of Type I units the reader is referred to the excellent review by Burgess and Perl (1973).

Perhaps the most important point about Type I units for anyone wishing to examine their central projections is that they may be recognized with certainty during an electrophysiological experiment. This is because the receptors can be seen in hairy skin with the aid of an operating microscope and their discharge characteristics and receptive field properties are unique.

II. From glabrous skin

Responses of Type I receptors in glabrous skin, in both cat and monkey, are essentially similar to those in hairy skin (Iggo 1963b; Jänig et al. 1968a; Jänig 1971b). There is no surface indication of the presence of Type I receptors in glabrous skin. Type I discharges may be recorded, however, from cutaneous nerves innervating glabrous skin and Jänig (1971b) has provided the evidence to link these Type I discharges with Merkel cells at the epidermo-dermal junction.

C. Central projections of Type I afferent fibres

In view of the interest in Type I receptors, which have been well studied at the primary afferent fibre and structural levels, and the fact that they are so easily recognized in hairy skin, it is most surprising that so little is known about their central connexions. Of the ascending systems that arise in the spinal cord (see Chapter 1) only two have been shown to receive excitatory input from Type I units. These are the dorsal spinocerebellar tract (Mann 1971; Mann et al. 1971) and the post-synaptic dorsal column pathway (Angaut-Petit 1975b). Type I afferent fibres do not excite spinocervical tract neurones (Brown and Franz 1969) and nor do they project directly to the gracile nucleus through the dorsal columns from the hind limb (Petit and Burgess 1968), although they do appear to project to the cuneate nucleus through the cuneate fascicle from the forelimb (Uddenberg 1968a; Brown et al. 1974). Whether or not they project to any other ascending system is at present not known.

There are neurones in the dorsal horn that respond to mechanical stimulation of Type I receptors. Tapper et al. (1973) and P. B. Brown et al. (1973) have described dorsal horn neurones receiving an exclusive excitatory input from Type I receptors and also other neurones receiving a convergent input from various mechanoreceptors including those of Type I (see also Mann et al. 1971). Some of these dorsal horn neurones may send their axons through the dorsal columns as part of the post-synaptic dorsal column pathway.

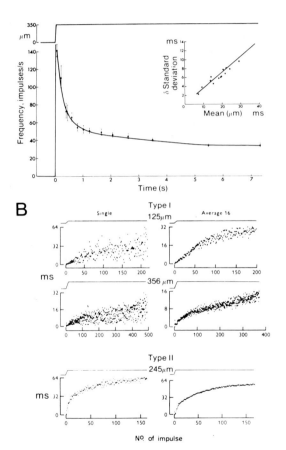

Fig. 4.3. Responses of Type I units to skin indentation. **A** Time course of the discharge in response to a 350-μm indentation (*top trace*). Each *point* is the mean of 16 responses. The *inset* shows the relation between the mean and standard deviation for each set of values. **B** Variability of the responses. The interspike intervals are plotted against the sequential interval number. On the left are shown responses to single-stimulus presentations and on the right the averaged responses to 16 stimuli. The lowest pair of records is from a Type II unit for comparison, to demonstrate the regularity of the Type II responses. (From Iggo and Muir 1969.)

Others have been shown to send their axons into the dorso-lateral funiculus (Mann et al. 1971), but their destination is unknown. The plantar cushion reflex (Egger and Wall 1971) is evoked by light pressure on the glabrous skin of the foot pad and it seems likely that the receptors involved are Type I receptors.

D. Morphology of axons innervating Type I receptors

Type I receptors occur in both hairy and glabrous skin. The first question that arises, therefore, is whether the axons from the two skin types are morphologically similar after they enter the spinal cord. The axons from the two types of skin are of similar size range (Brown and Iggo 1967; Burgess et al. 1968; Jänig 1971a). Collaterals from axons innervating Type I receptors in the foot and toe pads would be expected to be distributed to the medial part of the dorsal horn because of the somatotopic organization in the horn (see Chapters 2, 6 and 10).

In fact the branching patterns and collateral morphologies of the two types are essentially the same, and they will be treated as a single group in the following account. The only observed differences between the two relate to the intercollateral spacings and the morphology and density of the boutons (Brown et al. 1978). These differences will be described in the appropriate sections below.

I. Entry of axons into the spinal cord, branching and collateral distribution

Figure 4.4 shows the branching patterns of 13 axons of Type I units, nine from hairy skin and

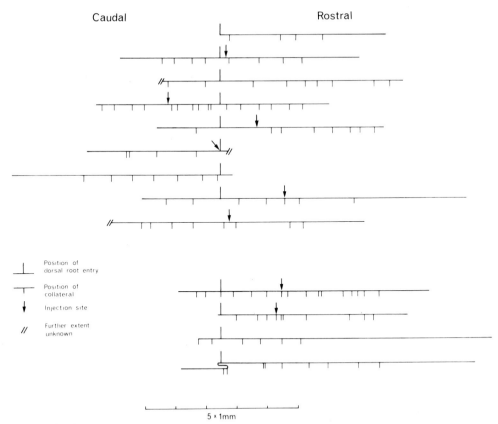

Fig. 4.4. Diagrammatic representation of the branching patterns of axons of Type I units in the spinal cord; the upper nine are from hairy skin, the lower four from glabrous skin. The total length of each axon stained is shown together with (where possible) the position of its entry into the cord through the dorsal root, the position of origin of each stained collateral and the site of injection of horseradish peroxidase. (From Brown et al. 1978.)

four from glabrous skin. Twelve of the axons could be traced back into the dorsal root, thus allowing examination of their behaviour at and near their entrance point to the spinal cord. Eleven axons bifurcated into rostral and caudal branches within a few hundred micrometres of leaving the root. Type I axons are, therefore, similar to the vast majority of cutaneous and muscle afferent fibres in that they nearly all bifurcate upon entering the cord.

The rostral and caudal branches of Type I axons move medially across the cord as they ascend and descend respectively. This behaviour is common to all axons we have stained. Type I axons often come to lie deep in the dorsal columns medial to the deeper laminae of the dorsal horn (Fig. 4.9), the caudal branch being particularly liable to take up this position.

The limitations of the horseradish peroxidase injection method restrict staining of axons to a maximum of about 10 mm. Even for Type I axons that appear to be distributed only to segments near the level of entry (see above) this restriction leads to only a part of the axon being revealed. None of the rostral or caudal branches in our material has ended as a collateral. Caudal branches were stained for up to 6.8 mm, which is thus a lower limit to the true length.

Between four and 16 collaterals arose from the stained Type I axons (mean 8.6) over rostrocaudal distances of 2300–7300 μm. These values also provide lower limits to the numbers of collaterals arising from Type I axons. The average intercollateral distance for Type I axons from hairy skin is greater than that for axons from glabrous skin. For 62 intercollateral distances in axons from hairy skin the mean value was 720 μm (±403, s.d.), whereas for 37 collateral spacings in axons from glabrous skin it was 531 μm (±363, s.d.). The difference between the means is significant at the 1% level (Student's t-test). This is one of the differences that has been observed between Type I axons from the two types of skin. Whether it reflects a true difference in kind between the two sorts of afferent units, it is not possible to say. In general, collaterals destined for the medial third of the dorsal horn arise closer together than those destined for the lateral third. This has been shown most convincingly for the hair follicle afferents (Chapter 2). Type I axons from the glabrous skin of the foot and toe pads all send their collaterals to the medial third of the

dorsal horn (see below). The difference in collateral spacing may, therefore, be simply a reflexion of the medio-lateral distribution of the collaterals.

II. Morphology of collaterals and their arborizations

Like all afferent fibres, Type I collaterals have a distinctive morphology. They do not appear to have been described in anatomical investigations using silver staining methods. Fig. 4.5A and B shows montages made from photomicrographs of two adjacent collaterals from a Type I axon from hairy skin, and Fig. 4.5C shows montages of different parts of the same collateral from a Type I axon that innervated glabrous skin. The morphology of the collaterals is more clearly seen in reconstructions made from camera lucida drawings of transverse sections of the cord, as shown in Figs. 4.6–4.10, and sagittal sections.

Collaterals from Type I axons follow the general pattern and run rostrally as they descend from their point of origin towards the grey matter, entering the grey matter usually some 100–300 μm rostral to their origin. Within about 1–3 mm of either side of the dorsal root entrance of the parent axons the collaterals enter the dorsal horn through it dorsal border (Figs. 4.6, 4.7, 4.8). More rostrally and caudally the collaterals enter the dorsal horn through its medial border (Fig. 4.9).

The collateral morphology is most distinctive for collaterals from axons innervating hairy skin and which enter the dorsal horn through its dorsal border. The collaterals descend through the most dorsal four or five laminae, sometimes dividing on the way. At the level of lamina IV or V the collaterals pursue a broad C-shaped path. The curve of the C is convex laterally in all collaterals from our sample. From this basic C shape, further loops arise as the collateral divides and subdivides. Finally the branches of the collateral turn

Fig. 4.5. A and **B** Photomicrographs of two adjacent collaterals of an axon from a Type I unit from hairy skin. The montages were made from micrographs of 100-μm transverse sections of the cord. The dorsal border of the dorsal horn may be seen near the top of each montage. **C** Montages from different parts of the same Type I collateral from an axon innervating glabrous skin. (From Brown et al. 1978.)

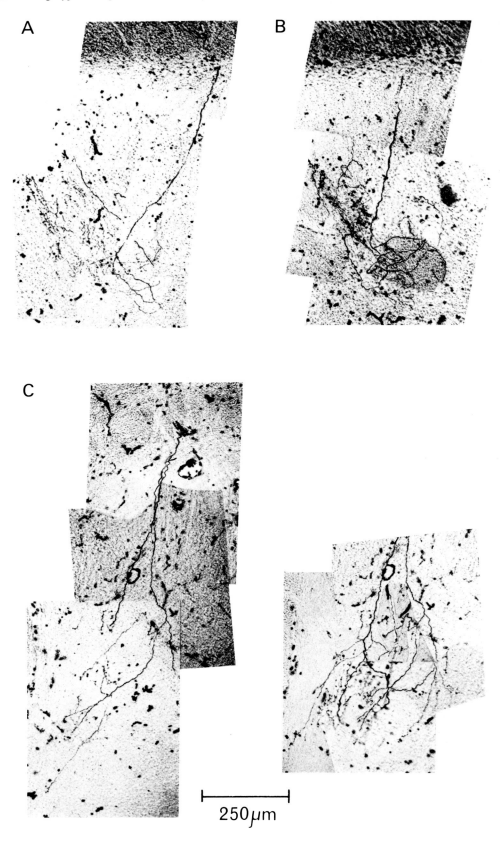

250µm

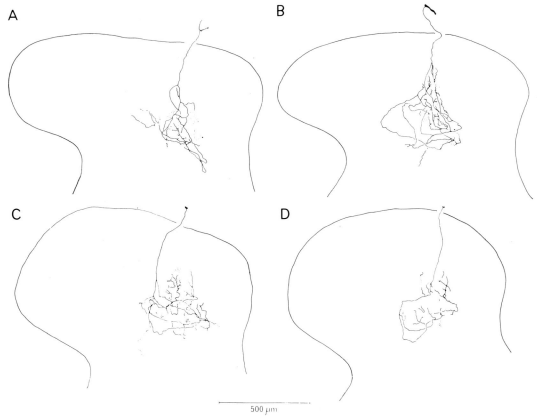

Fig. 4.6. Reconstructions, from transverse sections, of four adjacent collaterals of an axon from a single Type I unit from hairy skin. A is the most caudal and D the most rostral. The outline of the dorsal horn is shown, lateral border to the left. (From Brown et al. 1978.)

and ascend back through the horn, often from as deep as lamina VI, as a spray of fibres in laminae V, IV and III.

Collaterals from axons innervating glabrous skin have essentially the same morphology (Fig. 4.8). The C-shaped trajectory, however, is not so well marked and is often flattened to an L-shape (Fig. 4.8). The C or L is again convex laterally, but it often gives rise to branches that run horizontally to the termination area in the medial part of the dorsal horn (Fig. 4.8C).

Where collaterals arise from axons deep in the dorsal columns they enter the dorsal horn through its medial border. They do not have the broad C- or L-shaped trajectory shown by collaterals entering through the dorsal border and instead run laterally towards their termination sites, sometimes fairly straight across the horn but often in a U-shaped loop convex ventrally. Collaterals entering through the medial border of

the dorsal horn are shown in Fig. 4.9.

The terminal arborizations of Type I collaterals are contained within laminae III, IV and V. Collaterals from axons from hairy skin usually have their lamina V terminals restricted to its dorsal part, whereas collaterals from axons innervating glabrous skin often have terminals throughout lamina V. In the vast majority of collaterals of both types, however, the arborizations are superficial to the most ventral parts of the collateral, which often reach lamina VI and, less frequently, lamina VII.

In reconstructions from transverse sections of the cord the terminal arborization areas (those areas containing synaptic boutons) are elliptical or disc-shaped. They measure 250–500 µm at their widest part in the transverse plane, and from 250 to 650 µm in the dorso-ventral direction. In the transverse plane, therefore, Type I collateral terminal arborizations are wider and deeper than

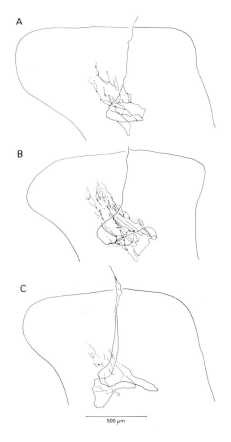

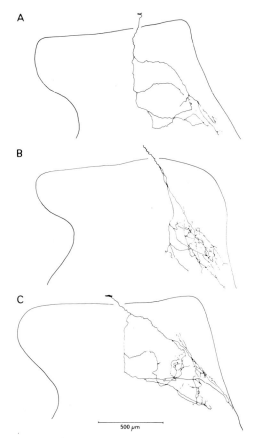

Fig. 4.7. Reconstructions, from transverse sections, of three adjacent collaterals of an axon from a Type I unit from hairy skin. **A** is the most caudal and **C** the most rostral. Note the similarity with the collaterals in Fig. 4.6. (From Brown et al: 1978.)

Fig. 4.8. Reconstructions, from transverse sections, of three adjacent collaterals of an axon from a Type I unit from glabrous skin. For further description see the legend to Fig. 4.6. (From Brown et al. 1978.)

those of hair follicle collaterals (Chapter 2) and those of rapidly adapting mechanoreceptors (Chapter 3), but not as wide or as deep as those of Type II collaterals (Chapter 5).

In the sagittal plane of the cord the terminal arborizations of Type I collaterals extend for between 100 and 700 μm (mean of 13 collaterals that were particularly well stained; 400 μm ± 158, mean ± s.d.). They are less extensive than those of hair follicle afferent fibres but more extensive than those of Type II afferent fibres (Chapters 2 and 5). Like the terminal arborizations of other primary afferent fibres in the dorsal horn, those of Type I collaterals from a single axon are in line with one another in the sagittal plane, as can be seen from Figs. 4.6–4.9.

There are gaps between adjacent terminal arborizations from the same axon. That is, in the sagittal plane the terminal arborizations of adjacent collaterals from the same axon are usually separated from one another by cord containing no terminals from that axon. The gaps are between 100 and 500 μm in the long axis of the cord. Only rarely do the terminals of one collateral intermingle with those of an adjacent one. This is in marked contrast to hair follicle afferent fibre collaterals, which form a continuous sagittal column of terminals (Chapter 2), but is more in line with other types of cutaneous afferent fibre collaterals.

III. Synaptic boutons

Type I afferent fibres from hairy skin and from glabrous skin differ in the morphology, the distribution and the density of their synaptic boutons.

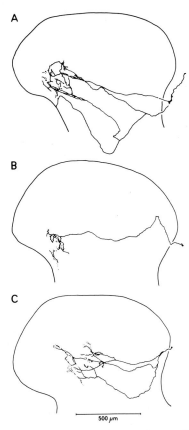

Fig. 4.9. As Fig. 4.7, but to show collaterals entering the dorsal horn from deep in the dorsal columns. The axon innervated hairy skin. (From Brown et al. 1978.)

1. Morphology

Synaptic boutons of Type I afferent collaterals are shown in the camera lucida drawings of Fig. 4.10 and the photomicrographs of Fig. 4.11. Type I afferent fibres innervating hairy skin have terminal arborizations that carry mainly boutons of the *en passant* variety. Up to 9 or even 12 boutons may be strung out on the last 30–50 μm of axon, which is usually 1 μm or less in diameter and ends as a bouton *terminal*. Most boutons on these axons are about 6 μm × 4 μm, although some are smaller (3 μm × 2 μm), and frequently set off from the terminal axon on short, 1-μm stalks (Fig. 4.10A). In sagittal sections it can be seen that the bouton-carrying terminal axons do not run so predominantly in either the longitudinal or transverse axes as do those of hair follicle afferents and Type II afferents respectively, although there is a slight tendency towards a longitudinal orientation.

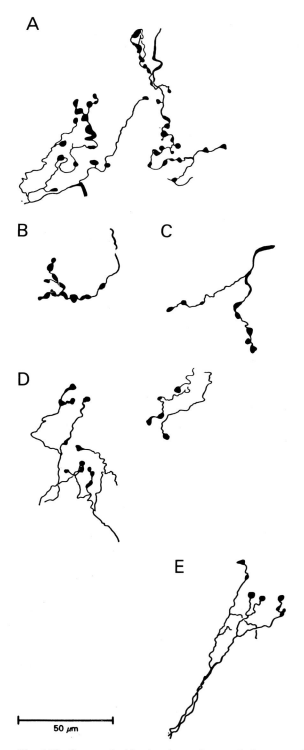

Fig. 4.10. Camera lucida drawings of synaptic boutons of Type I units, from transverse sections of spinal cord. Note the well-developed boutons *en passant* in the examples from hairy skin (**A–C**) and the predominance of boutons *terminaux* in the examples from glabrous skin (**D** and **E**). (From Brown et al. 1978.)

Type I afferent fibres that innervate glabrous skin give rise to very few boutons of the *en passant* type (Fig. 4.10D, E; Fig. 4.11C, D). Instead, these collaterals end in a bouton *terminal* with just one or two boutons *de passage* within 20 μm or so of the bouton *terminal*. The boutons are similar in size to those of Type I afferents from hairy skin. In sagittal sections it may be seen that there is no obvious preferred direction for the terminal axons.

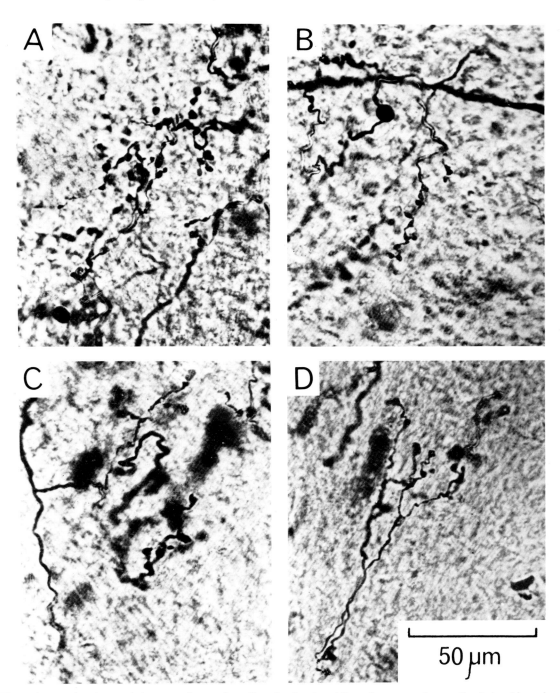

Fig. 4.11. Photomicrographs of synaptic boutons of axons from Type I units. **A** and **B** are from axons innervating hairy skin and show many boutons *en passant*. **C** and **D** are from axons innervating glabrous skin and have fewer boutons *en passant* but relatively more boutons *terminaux*. All photomicrographs are of 100 μm thick transverse sections. (From Brown *et al.*, 1978.)

2. Distribution

The synaptic boutons of Type I afferent fibres are found in laminae III, IV and V (near the level of entry of the axons into the spinal cord). The distribution of boutons from axons innervating hairy skin is somewhat more restricted than that from axons innervating glabrous skin. Axons from hairy skin distribute to laminae III, IV and the dorsal part of V, whereas those from glabrous skin have boutons in III, IV and nearly all of V.

Neurones receiving monosynaptic excitation from Type I units will need to have their somata or dendrites in laminae III–V. Neurones excited by Type I units have been found in laminae III–VI by Tapper et al. (1973) and some of these excitatory inputs are monosynaptic (P. B. Brown et al. 1973, 1975). Obviously the neurones in laminae III–V are ideally placed to receive the input, while neurones in lamina VI will have to send their dendrites dorsally into lamina V in order to receive monosynaptic connexions; this is ccertainly possible (see the illustrations in Scheibel and Scheibel 1968; and Chapter 9). Neurones receiving monosynaptic excitation from the plantar cushion have their somata in the medial part of lamina IV and are ideally placed to receive Type I input (Egger and Wall 1971), as are many cells sending their axons into the dorsal columns (Chapter 8).

Type I afferent fibres also give collaterals to the dorsal spinocerebellar tract, presumably to cells in Clarke's columns (see Mann 1971; Lindström and Takata 1971). The present account refers only to the organization and distribution of collaterals at and near the level of entry of the axons into the spinal cord.

3. Density

The density of boutons in the terminal arborizations of the two varieties of Type I afferent fibres differs, axons from hairy skin have a much higher density of boutons than those from glabrous skin.

The numbers of boutons have been counted in cubes of tissue of side 100 μm. There were between 16 and 46 boutons in 100 μm^3 for Type I axons innervating hairy skin (mean 24.2 boutons; $n=13$ arborizations). There were between 9 and 26 boutons (mean 15.3) in 100 μm^3 for 6 arborizations from Type I axons innervating glabrous skin. These values are considerably less than those for both hair follicle afferent fibres and axons from Pacinian corpuscles (see Chapters 2 and 3).

IV. Organization of collaterals in the dorsal horn

Figure 4.12 summarizes the morphology of Type I axons and their collaterals near the dorsal root entrance of the axon into the spinal cord. It should be compared with the other similar diagrams for cutaneous and muscle afferent fibres.

Information from Type I afferent fibres is distributed to the spinal cord from an interrupted cylinder of terminal arborizations that occupies laminae III, IV and V (dorsal part of V for axons from hairy skin, most of V for axons from glabrous skin). Each collateral from a single axon usually supplies its own private volume of cord; there is rarely any overlap between terminal arborizations of adjacent collaterals from the same axon. The interrupted cylinder of terminal arborizations (more correctly a series of flattened spheres) from a single axon runs in the longitudinal axis of the cord. The general principle that single cutaneous axons distribute their input into longitudinally running columns (sheets, etc.) in the dorsal part of the spinal grey matter is maintained (see Chapter 10).

Individual collaterals from Type I axons have a characteristic morphology, best seen in reconstructions from transverse sections and for collaterals from axons innervating hairy skin. Collaterals pursue a broad C-shaped curve as they descend through the dorsal horn, giving off branches as they do so, finally turning to produce ascending branches to laminae III to V. The convexity of the C is nearly always towards the lateral surface of the cord. Collaterals from axons innervating glabrous skin are distributed to the medial third of the dorsal horn and their C-shaped trajectory is not so well marked, often being flattened to an L. Even so the morphology of Type I collaterals is characteristic.

No other type of cutaneous or muscle afferent has collaterals with the specific morphology of Type I axons; the C- or L-shaped path taken by the collaterals is distinctive. Furthermore, the 'flattened sphere' type of terminal arborization in laminae III–V is also characteristic of Type I collaterals. Examination of the classical and recent anatomical literature has failed to reveal illustrations that could without any doubt be of these collaterals. This is surprising in view of their obvious appearance. The only other type of primary afferent collaterals that are at all similar to the

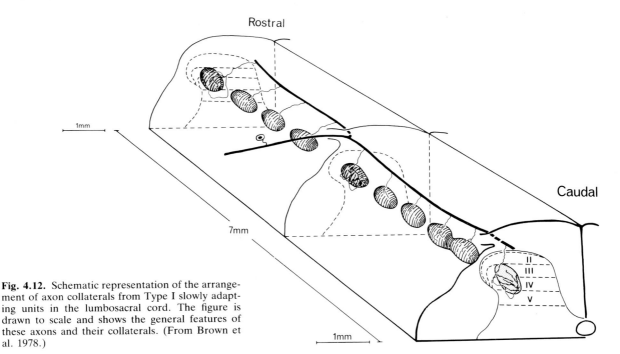

Fig. 4.12. Schematic representation of the arrangement of axon collaterals from Type I slowly adapting units in the lumbosacral cord. The figure is drawn to scale and shows the general features of these axons and their collaterals. (From Brown et al. 1978.)

Type I are those belonging to axons of Group Ib muscle afferent fibres. But the latter terminate in laminae V, VI and VII and do not follow a C- or L-shaped trajectory (see Chapter 12). Group Ib afferent fibre collaterals have been correctly identified from silver-stained sections by Réthelyi and Szentágothai (1973).

The interrupted sagittal column of arborizations from a single Type I axon runs for at least 7.5 mm; the upper limit is unknown. Neurones monosynaptically excited by a Type I axon will sample from its interrupted cylinder of terminals. The receptive fields of such neurones might be expected to reflect the longitudinal organization. There should be columns of neurones monosynaptically excited from Type I axons, the neurones within a column having overlapping receptive fields which all contain, as a minimum, the field of the Type I unit common to all the neurones. Unfortunately, detailed electrophysiological mapping of dorsal horn neurones excited by Type I units has not been performed. Such detailed mapping has only been carried out for neurones of the spinocervical tract which are excited by hair follicle afferent fibres (see Chapter 6). It is to be expected, however, that neurones receiving monosynaptic input from Type I axons will not disrupt the somatotopic organization of the dorsal horn.

It is surprising that more work has not been carried out on the central connexions of Type I axons. The Type I receptors have a distinctive morphology and characteristic response properties. They may be identified with certainty during an acute electrophysiological experiment. But only Tapper and his collaborators have attempted any analysis of the central projections of Type I axons at the spinal level.

P. B. Brown et al. (1973) recorded from dorsal horn neurones excited both monosynaptically and polysynaptically by Type I units. The receptive field areas of the neurones were fairly large, up to more than 60 cm^2 (Tapper et al. 1973). Brown et al. suggested that within these areas at least 10%–20% of the Type I receptors would contribute monosynaptic excitation to the neurone. This would represent as many as 20 Type I axons. It will be of interest to determine how such convergence is organized. For example, do a number (? 20) of collaterals from different axons converge and form a single 'flattened sphere' of arborizations, or is the distinctive flattened sphere arrangement of single collaterals smeared in either the longitudinal or transverse axes?

The morphological evidence presented in this chapter shows that Type I afferent fibres terminate in laminae III, IV and V near their point of entry into the spinal cord. Further rostrally they also terminate, presumably, in Clarke's column (Mann 1971). However, near their entrance the relay stations for Type I information are in laminae III–V. Only neurones with their somata or dendrites in these laminae are candidates for receiving monosynaptic excitation from Type I units. Tapper et al. (1973) recorded from positions in laminae III–VI, but it is not clear which of their sites yielded responses from Type I receptors. In a later report (P. B. Brown et al. 1975) they state that there were no significant differences between laminae for either the number of afferent systems converging onto individual neurones, or the distribution of classes of convergence. The axonal destinations of the neurones recorded by Tapper's group are not known.

The recognition that primary afferent depolarization evoked in cutaneous afferent fibre terminals by activity in cutaneous axons is organized in a quite specific way (Jänig et al. 1968b) leads to the prediction that some interneurones on the presynaptic inhibitory path should be excited by Type I, and also probably Type II, units. These neurones may have been included in those recorded by Tapper's group.

The post-synaptic pathway projecting through the dorsal columns is the only ascending somatosensory path known to carry information from Type I receptors. Angaut-Petit (1975b) recorded from axons of this pathway in the dorsal columns and showed that some of them responded to displacement of Type I receptors, an observation confirmed by the present author (unpublished work).

Spinal cord neurones that project to the dorsal column nuclei are, according to the retrograde horseradish peroxidase studies of Rustioni and Kaufman (1977), located in lamina IV and medial lamina V. These neurones may send their axons through either the dorsal columns or the dorso-lateral funiculus. It is not known whether those projecting through the dorso-lateral funiculus also include neurones responding to displacement of Type I receptors.

The neurones of the post-synaptic path to the dorsal column nuclei are well sited to receive monosynaptic excitation from Type I units. But it is not known whether such monosynaptic connexions exist: their existence may be expected, however. Input from Type I receptors in the glabrous foot and toe pad skin is distributed to the medial parts of laminae III–V. It is tempting to suggest that the neurones (of the post-synaptic path to the dorsal column nuclei) that are situated medially in lamina V should receive input from the Type I axons from glabrous skin. But the identified Type I projection to this system is from hairy skin; no reports of such a projection from glabrous skin have been made. However, we (Brown and Fyffe 1981) have shown that such a projection exists (see Chapter 8).

The spinothalamic tract in the cat takes its origin from cells in lamina I and the medial parts of lamina VII and dorsal lamina VIII. Lamina I neurones receive their input from the slowly conducting (Aδ) myelinated and the non-myelinated (C) primary afferent fibres (Christensen and Perl 1970). There is no evidence that they are excited by any faster-conducting afferent fibres. Although the spinothalamic tract has been the subject of much research activity in recent years there has been no detailed analysis of its primary afferent input and only the broad outlines are known (Willis et al. 1974, for the monkey). It is not clear whether Type I afferent fibres project to the system. It seems unlikely that neurones with somata in lamina VIII would receive monosynaptic excitation from Type I axons. The more superficial of lamina VII neurones may well send their dorsally directed dendrites into the region of termination of Type I afferent fibres, particularly the fibres from glabrous skin (see, for example, Fig. 1 in Scheibel and Scheibel 1968).

It must be very apparent to the reader by now that our knowledge of the central projections of Type I afferent fibres is very scanty indeed. In fact Type I units are enigmatic in a number of ways. (1) Their receptive field organization is puzzling. Individual receptors are excited by mechanical stimuli acting directly on them, and are, therefore, well suited to provide information about the location of a stimulus. But single axons usually innervate two or more Type I receptors, thereby reducing the discriminatory capability of the system. (2) They are the only cutaneous afferent units with axons conducting faster than the Aδ range that do not project through the dorsal columns directly (that is, with no synaptic interruption) from the cat's hind limb. (3) Their projection through the post-synaptic path to the dorsal column nuclei is to the rostral and ventral parts of these nuclei (Rustioni 1973). This suggests either that these afferents have a modulating role at the level of the dorsal column nuclei or that they project from the rostral dorsal column nuclei to parts of the brain other than the ventroposterior nucleus of the thalamus (Kuypers and Tuerk 1964; Busch 1961; Gordon and Jukes 1964). (4) Apart from the post-synaptic path to the dorsal column nuclei, the only other known ascending pathway from the cat's hind limb receiving Type I activity is the dorsal spinocerebellar tract. This suggests that at least one role for these afferents concerns the relationships between the body and space. Much needs to be done, however, to clarify the position with regard to the central projections of Type I units. It is a pressing problem.

5   Axons innervating slowly adapting Type II mechanoreceptors

As discussed at the beginning of Chapter 4, there are two distinct types of slowly adapting mechanoreceptors in mammalian skin innervated by large myelinated nerve fibres. They have been called Type I and Type II (Iggo 1966). The Type I receptors occur in both hairy and glabrous skin and contain Merkel cells (Iggo and Muir 1969; Smith 1970; Jänig 1971a, b). They are present in a wide range of vertebrate species and their electrophysiological response to a maintained displacement is characterized by an irregular discharge. For further details see Chapter 4.

Type II receptors (responses) were first clearly described by Witt and Hensel (1959), who were particularly concerned with their thermal sensitivity. Until the mid 1960s most reports either did not differentiate Type I and Type II responses (Maruhashi et al. 1952; Hunt and McIntyre 1960b) or confused them (Werner and Mountcastle 1965). Following the recognition that Type I and Type II receptors formed distinctly separate classes (Iggo 1966) Type II responses have been recorded from the hairy skin of cats (Burgess et al. 1968; Chambers et al. 1972), rabbits (Brown and Iggo 1967; Brown and Hayden 1971) and primates including man (Iggo 1963b; Perl 1968; Merzenich and Harrington 1969; Harrington and Merzenich 1970). They have also been recorded from the skin of reptiles (Kenton et al. 1971). In man Type II receptors are present in the glabrous skin (Knibestöl and Vallbo 1970; Knibestöl 1975; Johansson 1978); in cat, however, there are no convincing reports of their presence in the glabrous skin and the present writer has never seen any responses from the central pad or the toe pads of the hind foot that could be identified as coming from Type II receptors.

There appears to be a group of Type II receptors situated near the base of the claw. As early as 1964 Gordon and Jukes described neurones in the cat's gracile nucleus that responded with a main-

tained discharge to displacement of a claw (see also Brown et al. 1974). These neurones were undoubtedly responding to input from first-order afferent fibres innervating Type II receptors. Unpublished work by the present writer has shown that there is a group of receptors responding to claw movement that has all the characteristics of Type II receptors (see below); in fact when recording from dorsal roots the Type II claw units are relatively common, and certainly more frequent than Type II units from hairy skin. Recently Johansson (1978) has shown that Type II receptors in human glabrous skin may be subdivided into three classes on the basis of their selective sensibility to direction of skin stretch. One class (Johansson's C type) has a pronounced sensitivity to mechanical stimulation of the nail and often has an indentation-sensitive zone close to the proximal or lateral borders of the nail. Johansson's C type and the 'claw receptor' of Gordon and Jukes are analogous and form a subgroup of the slowly adapting Type II receptors.

A. Morphology of the Type II receptor

Unlike the Type I receptor, which has been the object of a number of recent light and electron microscope studies, the Type II receptor has only been studied by one group (Chambers et al. 1972). The Type II receptor is the Ruffini corpuscle (Ruffini 1894; Dogiel 1903). In cat hairy skin Ruffini endings are situated in the corium (dermis) and, as described in the classical light microscope studies, are spindle-shaped. Figure 5.1 is a reconstruction of a Type II ending from the cat's hairy skin. The ending varies in length from 0.5 to

2.0 mm, with a diameter up to 150 μm in the equatorial region and down to 30–40 μm near the poles. It is surrounded by a capsule, arising from the perineural sheath of the afferent nerve fibre, that consists of four or five layers of perineural cells. Inside the capsule the ending consists of an inner core and an outer envelope, the two being separated by a space apparently filled with 'fluid substances' (Chambers et al. 1972). The inner core consists of nerve terminals, connective tissue and cells. The cells give rise to membranes that divide the space surrounding the core into compartments. A single myelinated nerve fibre enters the organ, either at one of the poles or at the equatorial region; the myelin sheath is not lost until the inner core is reached. The nerve terminal is a club-like enlargement of the axoplasm that gives rise to numerous fine branches running to the poles of the ending. The terminal ramifications of axoplasm contact the collagenous fibrils of the inner core and also give rise to thorn-like processes of 0.2–1 μm diameter. The ending contains no specialized cells such as Merkel cells and presumably the nerve ending itself acts as the transducer.

According to Andres and Von Düring (1973) collagenous bundles coming from the subcutaneous and cutaneous layers enter the ending from both poles and therefore connect the receptor with the cutis or subcutis. Stretch of these collagenous fibrils will stretch the inner core; they are presumably the morphological basis of the Type II receptor's directional sensitivity to skin stretch.

As mentioned above, Type II receptors have not been found in cat glabrous skin but Type II responses have been recorded from monkey and human glabrous skin (Iggo 1963b; Perl 1968; Talbot et al. 1968; Knibestöl and Vallbo 1970; Knibestöl 1975; Johansson 1978). Type-II-like responses have been recorded upon movement of vibrissae and other sinus hairs of the cat's face (Gottschaldt et al. 1973) and the carpal tactile hairs (Nilsson and Skoglund 1965; Nilsson 1969b). Andres and Von Düring (1973) assume that the endings responsible are the straight lanceolate terminals that project many finger-like processes into the connective tissue of the hair shaft and the corium of the follicle, but this awaits confirmation. Ruffini-like endings also occur in joints (see Goglia and Sklenska 1969) and are presumably responsible for the slowly adapting responses of some joint

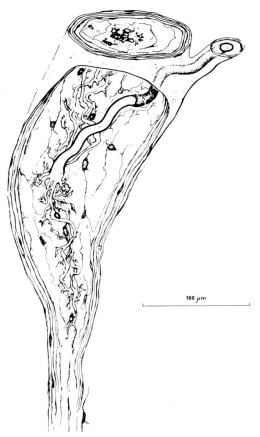

Fig. 5.1. Diagrammatic representation from serial semi-thin sections, of the structure of a slowly adapting Type II ending in cat's skin. (From Chambers et al. 1972.)

afferent units (Boyd and Roberts 1953; Skoglund 1956).

B. Physiology of Type II units

The response properties of the Type II receptors in hairy skin have been analysed in detail by Chambers et al. (1972) and Burgess et al. (1968). The following account draws largely upon those two reports.

In contrast to the Type I receptors, Type II units usually have a resting discharge, when first isolated, at a rate of between 5 and 20 impulses per second. This resting discharge is very regular and presumably arises from stretch of the ending at the 'resting' position of the limb. It may often be stopped by moving the limb so that the skin containing the receptor is released from stretch. Thus it is clear that the terms 'resting' or 'spontaneous' discharge are not really appropriate for the Type II units; the discharge is evoked by skin stretch and obviously depends on the position of the limb, etc. This may account for some of the variability in the two reports: Chambers et al. (1972) reported that 41 out of 45 units carried a discharge upon isolation, whereas Burgess et al. (1968) stated that slightly more than one-half of their sample of 89 units 'displayed appreciable resting activity'.

Examination of the receptive fields of Type II units reveals a characteristic, and for cutaneous receptors with myelinated axons a unique, class

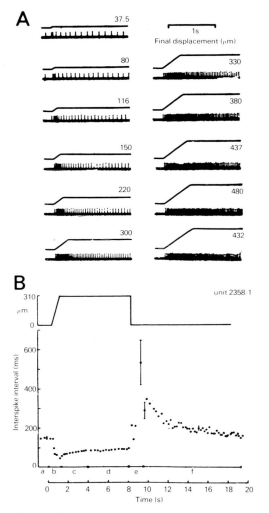

B

Fig. 5.2. Responses of a slowly adapting Type II unit to vertical displacement. **A** Single records of responses to the indicated displacements. **B** Graph of responses (each *point* the mean of six) to the vertical displacement shown in the *upper panel*. There are six phases: (*a*) resting discharge, (*b*) dynamic discharge, (*c*) adapting discharge, (*d*) adapted (static) discharge, (*e*) silent period during off-loading, (*f*) recovery of resting discharge. (From Chambers et al. 1972.)

feature: there is only a single spot-like skin area of mechanical sensitivity for each afferent fibre. Beneath this spot-like area lies a Ruffini ending. Although Type II units are easily excited by stretching the skin (and, therefore, may be excited from a distance) careful field examination has shown that, without a doubt, there is only a single receptor in each Type II afferent unit.

The conduction velocities of the axons of Type II units may range from 20 to 100 m s^{-1}, although most lie between 30 and 72 m s^{-1} with a mean value of about 54 m s^{-1} (Brown and Iggo 1967). Very similar values have been given by Burgess et al. (1968).

The characteristic response of a Type II unit to vertical displacement of the skin over the receptor is shown in Fig. 5.2. Chambers et al. (1972) identified five phases of the response superimposed upon the background activity. The first phase is a dynamic response during movement. The dynamic discharge frequency is determined by both the velocity and the amplitude of displacement, increasing as both variables are increased. Following this dynamic response, and during maintained steady displacement, there is first an adapting discharge during which the response rate slows down during about 8 s; this is followed by the static response, consisting of a very regular discharge whose frequency is linearly related to the amplitude of displacement over the range 100–350 μm. When the mechanical stimulus is removed suddenly, there is a cessation of firing and this silent period is followed by a recovery of the background activity.

Type II units are sensitive to stretching the skin and this sensitivity is directional. Units are excited by skin stretch along one axis and are silenced by stretching the skin along an axis at right angles to the axis producing the best response (see also Knibestöl and Vallbo 1970; Johansson 1978). This directional sensitivity led Chambers (1969) and Knibestöl and Vallbo (1970) to suggest a proprioceptive (kinaesthetic) function for them. This suggestion was not supported by Chambers et al. (1972) but has recently been championed by Johansson (1978). Certainly, the argument put forward by Chambers et al. against the suggestion, that is, that adjacent units do not always respond in the same way to a particular movement of the leg, does not seem a strong one: as long as the units respond consistently and their central connexions are appropriate then they could act as proprioceptors. There is the need for a well-controlled study to examine this problem.

Like most cutaneous mechanoreceptors Type II endings are affected by temperature (Witt and Hensel 1959; Chambers et al. 1972). They are excited by a rapid fall in skin temperature and their response is inhibited by a temperature rise. Type II units have static temperature sensitivity curves that are bell-shaped with peak sensitivities at about 26–36 °C. Iggo (1969) called the responses of both Type I and Type II units to temperature 'spurious'. Certainly the maximal rates of discharge that may be elicited by thermal stimulation are at least two orders of magnitude below the maximal rates that may be evoked by mechanical stimulation.

Type II claw units. Endings with Type II characteristics are found in the skin fold surrounding the claws in cats (Gordon and Jukes 1964) and in a similar position around the fingernails in human subjects (Johansson 1978). These receptors have been examined by the present writer. They may or may not show background activity, they have a single receptive spot for each afferent fibre and respond with a regular maintained discharge during maintained displacement of the skin containing the sensitive spot. They are very sensitive to movement of the claw. No histological work has been done on these receptors but it seems reasonable to assume that the endings will be the Ruffini corpuscle and to consider these units as a particular group of Type II units.

no excitatory convergence), and none of them had any inhibitory components in their receptive fields.

The projections of Type II units at spinal level are unknown. The spinocervical tract is the only ascending system that has been examined carefully enough to allow determination of the receptor population projection to it: there is no evidence that Type II units excite spinocervical tract cells (Brown and Franz 1969). Type II units probably project to the dorsal spinocerebellar tract (Mann 1971). It is not known whether they project to the ventral spinocerebellar tract, the spinothalamic tract or the post-synaptic dorsal column pathways.

Projections of Type II units onto spinal interneurones have not been described. P. B. Brown et al. (1973) in their study of convergence onto dorsal horn neurones did not consider the Type II units. In unpublished observations we (A. G. Brown, P. K. Rose and P. J. Snow) have observed neurones at lumbosacral level that appeared to be exclusively excited by Type II claw afferent fibres. These neurones could not be excited antidromically from the ipsilateral dorso-lateral funiculus; projections through other parts of the cord were not tested.

It can be seen that our knowledge of the central projections is very meagre. There is an urgent need for a series of studies that will provide the necessary information.

C. Central projections of Type II afferent fibres

The central projections of Type II units are not well known. According to Petit and Burgess (1968) all Type II units from the cat's hind limb project through the dorsal columns to the dorsal column nuclei. Brown et al. (1974) observed axons in the cat's medial lemniscus (presumed to have their somata in the dorsal column nuclei) that had properties characteristic of Type II units. They were interesting in that they all had only a single sensitive spot on the skin, indicating a one-to-one relation between the primary afferent unit and the post-synaptic neurone (that is, there was

D. Morphology of axons innervating Type II receptors

As with the slowly adapting Type I units from hairy and glabrous skin, it is pertinent to enquire whether the Type II units from hairy skin of the limbs and those with receptors in the skin around the base of a claw have axons that are morphologically similar after entering the cord. There are no a priori reasons for suspecting any differences, apart from axons from claw receptors having collaterals limited to the medial parts of the dorsal horn due to the somatotopic organization in the horn.

According to Brown and Iggo (1967) and Burgess et al. (1968) between 8% and 10% of the myelinated afferent fibres of the saphenous and sural nerves belong to Type II units. This represents about 15% of the larger cutaneous myelinated fibres conducting at velocities greater than the Aδ fibres. The addition of muscle and joint afferent fibres in the dorsal roots obviously reduces this percentage considerably. Type II fibres from the hairy skin of the thigh, leg and foot have been only rarely encountered when searching the dorsal root entrance zone with microelectrodes. But Type II fibres from claw receptors are much more common, indicating that they are relatively more numerous and perhaps more important. All of the Type II axons that have been injected with horseradish peroxidase (Brown et al. 1981) are of the claw variety. It is not known, therefore, whether the two types have a similar morphology, and only the Type II claw units will be covered in the following account.

I. Entry of axons into the spinal cord, branching and collateral distribution

The branching pattern of Type II axons is shown in Fig. 5.3. Type II axons follow the usual pattern and generally bifurcate soon after entering the spinal cord into an ascending and descending

branch, both of which move medially over the head of the dorsal horn as they ascend and descend respectively. A feature that seems to be more common in Type II axons than in others is that a collateral may be given off before the parent axon bifurcates. The ascending branch of Type II axons always ascended the dorsal columns (for at least 6 mm in our material) in a position no deeper than the level of the dorsal border of the dorsal horn, and usually 100–200 μm superficial to it.

Between 6 and 14 collaterals arose from the axon (mean 10) over distances of 5900 to 8300 μm. As with all primary afferent material these values represent lower limits. Intercollateral distances varied from 100 to 1800 μm (577 ± 345; mean ± s.d., $n = 89$). These intercollateral spacing values are similar to those for other primary afferent fibres that send their collaterals to the medial parts of the dorsal horn. Type II collaterals show no tendency to arise closer together near the dorsal root entrance of the parent axon than they do farther away from it; again this is unlike the hair follicle collaterals but similar to the Type I collaterals. Collaterals were spaced more closely on descending branches than on ascending ones, like those of Pacinian corpuscle and tendon organ afferents (see Chapters 3 and 13).

II. Morphology of collaterals and their arborizations

Like all primary afferent fibre collaterals, Type II collaterals have a distinctive morphology. They follow the general pattern and have a rostral trajectory as they descend from their point of origin towards their terminal arborizations; they usually enter the grey matter some 100 μm rostral to their point of origin and break up into their terminal branches a further 100–200 μm rostral yet again.

The typical morphology of Type II collaterals is shown in the photomontages of Fig. 5.4 and the reconstructions of Figs. 5.5, 5.6. A common feature is their tendency to divide either just before or shortly after entering the grey matter of the dorsal horn, which they do at its dorsal border or the junction of its dorsal and medial borders. The collaterals then pursue a more or less straight

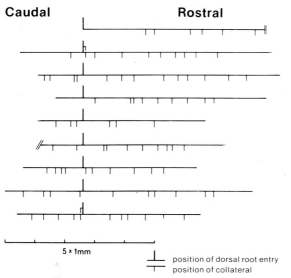

Caudal   **Rostral**

5 x 1mm

⊥ position of dorsal root entry
T position of collateral

Fig. 5.3. Diagrammatic representation of the branching pattern of axons of slowly adapting Type II units in the spinal cord. The total length of each axon stained is shown, together with the position of its entry into the cord through the dorsal root and the position of origin of each stained collateral. *Double vertical and sloping lines* indicate cut ends of stained axons. (From Brown et al. 1981.)

course through the dorsal three laminae, occasionally subdividing as they do so. In lamina IV the collaterals divide profusely: some turn and ascend back into lamina III (Fig. 5.6), others ramify more or less horizontally and the remainder carry on in the ventral direction. The result is a fairly dense arborization stretching from lamina III (often from its dorsal border) through lamina IV and into lamina V. The most ventral arborizations may reach the dorsal part of lamina VI. Type II collaterals, along with those from Pacinian corpuscle afferent fibres, form the most

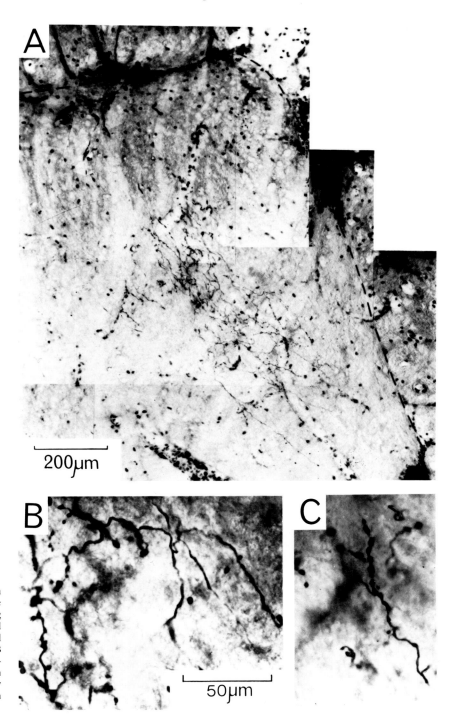

Fig. 5.4. A Photomontage, from 100-μm transverse sections, of the arborization of a slowly adapting Type II axon collateral. The dorsal and medial borders of the dorsal horn are shown as a dashed line. **B** and **C** Photomicrographs of terminal axons from a Type II unit in lamina III. There are many boutons *en passant*. (From Brown et al. 1981.)

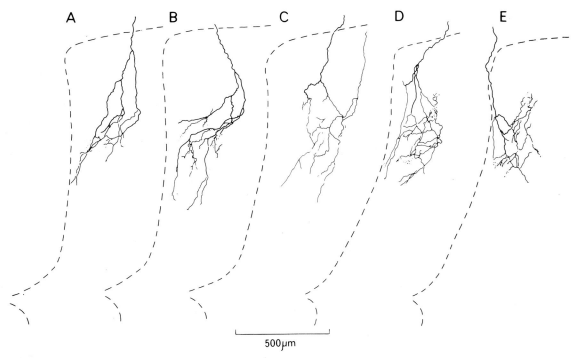

Fig. 5.5. Reconstructions, from transverse sections, of six adjacent collaterals from an axon innervating a slowly adapting Type II (claw) unit. **A** is the most caudal and **E** the most rostral. (From Brown et al. 1981.)

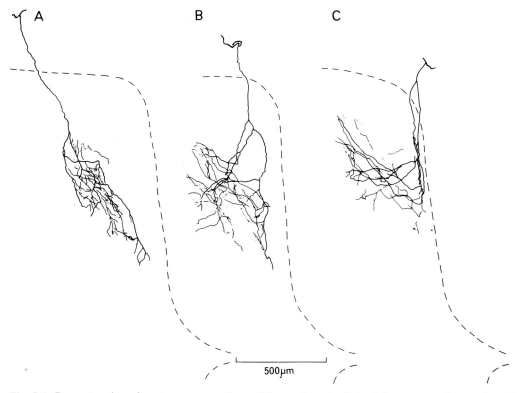

Fig. 5.6. Reconstructions, from transverse sections, of three adjacent collaterals from an axon innervating a slowly adapting Type II (claw) unit. **A** is the most caudal and **C** the most rostral. (From Brown et al. 1981.)

extensive terminal arborizations in the dorso-ventral direction of any cutaneous axon collaterals. Not all collaterals from Type II units have terminals extending so far. Thus some may have arborizations limited to laminae III and IV, while others, from the same axon, have arborizations in laminae IV, V and VI (see Fig. 5.5). In the transverse plane the terminal arborizations are some 500–600 μm in extent, occupying about one-third of the width of the horn.

In contrast to this extensive dorso-ventral and medio-lateral development of terminal arborizations, the rostro-caudal development is restricted. Type II collaterals form plates of terminals only some 100–300 μm thick in the longitudinal axis of the cord. The terminal arborizations of adjacent collaterals from the same axon are nearly always separated from one another by cord containing no terminals from that axon. Only where adjacent collaterals arise closer together than about 300 μm is there any chance of them forming a continuous slab of terminals in the sagittal plane: this is an uncommon occurrence. The collaterals from a single Type II axon, therefore, form a series of plates or sheets 100–300 μm thick across about a third of the dorsal horn in laminae III–V or III–VI; the sheets are in line in the longitudinal axis of the cord.

III. Synaptic boutons

Figure 5.7 shows photomicrographs of the terminal axons of Type II collaterals and the boutons they carry. Within the 100–300 μm thick sheets of collateral arborizations the terminal axons run in the plane of the sheets—in the transverse plane of the cord. They usually run dorso-ventrally at angles of up to 45° from the vertical from a more lateral position to a more medial one.

The distribution of terminal axons and synaptic boutons varies according to the lamina to which they project. There are more axons and more boutons in laminae III and IV than in laminae V and VI. The arrangement of boutons on the axons also varies according to their target laminae.

1. Lamina III and dorsal lamina IV

In these laminae (Fig. 5.7A, B, C) the boutons are usually arranged *en passant* with up to ten boutons on the last 50–60 μm of axon. Sometimes (Fig. 5.7A, B) groups of three to six

boutons *en passant* are intercalated along an axon, and occasionally boutons are offset from the main axon on short stalks. The bouton density in laminae III and IV is about 40–50 per 100 μm³.

2. Ventral lamina IV

Here there is an intermediate zone where the terminal axons and boutons are arranged in a fashion that is between that in the more superficial and that in the deeper layers. There are fewer boutons and *en passant* arrangements are rarer (Fig. 5.7D).

3. Lamina V and dorsal lamina VI

In these laminae there are fewer terminal axons than in more dorsal regions (Fig. 5.7E, F). Boutons are grouped together in twos and threes in *en passant* arrangements, often 100 μm or more away from the final bouton *terminal*, and occasional single boutons *en passant* are intercalated on the axon. The density of boutons is about 10–20 per 100 μm³, about half that in laminae III–IV.

IV. Organization of collaterals in the dorsal horn

The morphology of Type II axons and their collaterals is summarized in Fig. 5.8. The diagram represents the organization near the position at which the axon enters the spinal cord from the dorsal root and is comparable with similar diagrams for other afferents (see Chapters 2, 3, 4, 11, 12 and 13). If, as might be expected, Type II afferents send information to the dorsal spinocerebellar tract, then at more rostral levels collaterals to Clarke's column (dorsal nucleus) would be present.

Information from Type II receptors is distributed to the spinal cord in a characteristic way. Each collateral from a single axon distributes boutons to a wide and deep transversely oriented sheet of cord that includes laminae III–V and often the most dorsal part of VI. These sheets of tissue are some 100–300 μm thick in the sagittal plane and occupy about one-third of the transverse extent of the dorsal horn. Of the units with large cutaneous myelinated axons only the rapidly adapting units on the foot pads distribute information to the dorsal horn in this sheet-like fashion, although the sheets are 400–600 μm thick. Furthermore the collaterals from axons from rapidly adapting mechanoreceptors have terminal arborizations limited mainly to lamina III and also limited to up to about 400 μm in the transverse plane.

The sheets of terminals of Type II collaterals from a single axon are usually separated one from another by cord free from endings of that axon. These lengths of 'free' cord are usually a few hundred micrometres in length. All the collaterals

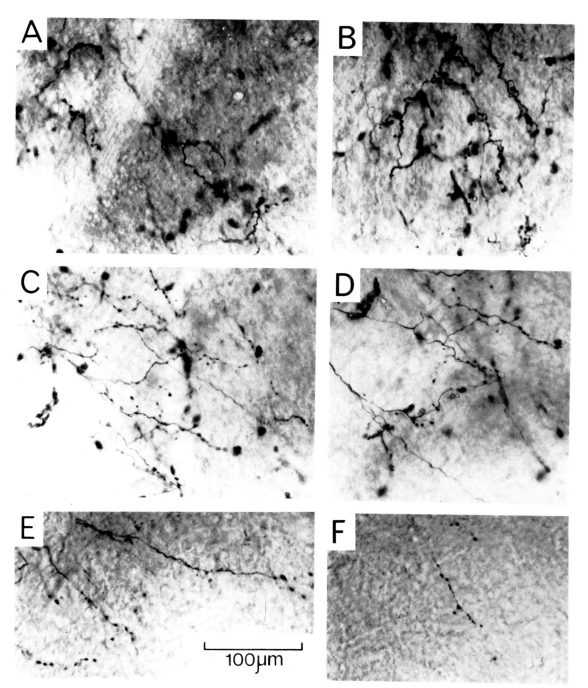

Fig. 5.7. Photomicrographs, from 100-μm transverse sections, of terminal branches of slowly adapting Type II collateral arborizations in lamina III (**A** and **B**) in lamina IV (**C** and **D**) and at the lamina V–VI border (**E** and **F**). For further description see the text. (From Brown et al. 1981.)

Rostral

Caudal

1mm

7mm

1mm

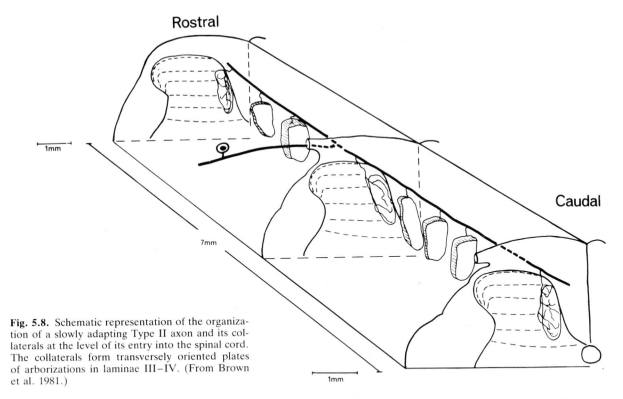

Fig. 5.8. Schematic representation of the organization of a slowly adapting Type II axon and its collaterals at the level of its entry into the spinal cord. The collaterals form transversely oriented plates of arborizations in laminae III–IV. (From Brown et al. 1981.)

from a single axon, however, produce terminal arborizations that are in line with one another in the sagittal plane and the general rule (that all collateral arborizations of single cutaneous axons are in line in the longitudinal axis of the cord) holds.

There are some interesting points concerning the somatotopic organization of the dorsal horn and the input from Type II units. Type II units consist of a single receptor and a single axon. Chambers et al. (1972) suggest that this limitation of a single receptive focus to a single axon may aid two-point discrimination. But Type II units are excited by skin stretch, which will depend on, among other things, the position of the limb. It therefore seems highly unlikely that Type II units are concerned very much with the localization of point stimuli applied to the skin. In fact, rather than being involved in this sort of 'static' situation much studied by electrophysiologists it is most likely that Type II units are concerned with 'dynamic' situations involving active touch in which kinaesthetic information is paramount. The apparent restricted receptor focus for Type II units is illusory, and this is reflected in the central organization of the collaterals. Input from Type II units cuts across the precise transverse organiza-

tion of the hair follicle afferent collaterals in lamina III (and also the somewhat more coarsely organized collaterals of Type I units) and smears somatotopic arrangement. Type II input also is distributed to more dorsal laminae than most other cutaneous information. Thus, any system of spatial localization built on the principles of a fine-grain topographical organization of the dorsal horn (particularly in the transverse plane), which appears to be how hair follicle afferent input and the spinocervical tract are organized (see Chapters 2, 6 and 7), is largely ignored by the Type II input. Only in the most general way does Type II input fit into the scheme of organization laid down by the inputs from hair follicle receptors and rapidly adapting mechanoreceptors in lamina III: single Type II claw units project to about one-third of the transverse extent of the dorsal horn. It is of interest that the other type of cutaneous afferent unit from skin that is easily excited at a distance from the location of the receptor, the Pacinian corpuscle unit, also has a central collateral organization that cuts across the fine-grained arrangement of the collaterals from hair follicle receptors and rapidly adapting mechanoreceptors.

The transverse sheets of Type II collaterals cut

across the longitudinally oriented dendrites in laminae III and IV (Scheibel and Scheibel 1968; Chapters 6 and 9). Many contacts made between Type II units and dendrites in laminae III and IV, like those made by axons from rapidly adapting mechanoreceptors with dendrites in the same laminae and between Ia afferents and moto-neuronal dendrites (see Chapters 3 and 14), will presumably be of the 'crossing-over' variety, although dorsally projecting dendrites do exist (Chapter 8). In laminae V and VI there should be more opportunity for 'climbing'-type contacts as the dendrites in these laminae take on a more dorso-ventral and medio-lateral organization.

When the input to a neurone is carried on axon terminals that run at right angles to the dendrites of the neurone there is an interesting functional result: all contacts made between the pre-synaptic and post-synaptic elements will be at about the same electrotonic distance from the soma of the post-synaptic cell. This will be so irrespective of whether the contacts are made on one or many dendrites, and if the contacts are excitatory the post-synaptic potential produced by their activation will have a simple time course reflecting the position of the synapses. This point is more fully discussed in Chapter 14. In laminae III and IV single dendrites may be 1–2 mm in length. It is possible, therefore, that a single neurone might have dendrites cutting across, and making contact with, three or four collateral arborizations from a single Type II afferent fibre.

Monosynaptic connexions between Type II afferents and spinal cord neurones will be possible for neurones with their cell bodies or dendrites in laminae III to VI. In other words, an enormous number of neurones, and many different types, are candidates for receiving such monosynaptic excitation. Even motoneurones may extend their dendrites into lamina V (see Fig. 1 in Cullheim and Kellerth 1976; and Fig. 14.1 in the present work). But at the time of writing no set of neurones receiving monosynaptic excitation from Type II afferent fibres has been identified. In some early experiments using Procion Yellow injection we (A. G. Brown, P. K. Rose and P. J. Snow, unpublished observations) stained two neurones that appeared to receive only Type II excitation, but whether it was monosynaptic was not clear. The dendritic trees spread widely across the dorsal horn and were restricted to a sheet in the transverse plane that closely followed the arrangement of Type II claw afferent collaterals.

The dearth of evidence on central connexions of Type II units, together with the extent of their terminal arborizations in the spinal cord, makes any speculation about their possible connexions meaningless. All that can be done is to point out the sad state of affairs and hope it acts as a spur to future research. The necessary electrophysiological experiments should not prove too difficult: Type II responses are quite characteristic and easily recognized.

6 Spinocervical tract neurones

The recognition of a third major somatosensory pathway carrying information from the trunk, limbs and tail is recent (Morin 1955). In addition to the dorsal column-lemniscothalamic pathway and the spinothalamic tract there is a path that projects through the lateral cervical nucleus and, via the medial lemniscus, to the thalamus. Its spinal part has been identified as the spinocervical tract (Lundberg and Oscarsson 1961; Lundberg and Norrsell, cited in Lundberg 1964a). The spinocervico-lemniscothalamic pathway is present in a large number of mammalian species, including primates, and is particularly well developed in the cat.

The literature on the spinocervical tract has been reviewed in detail (Brown 1973) and more recent review articles have also appeared (Boivie and Perl 1975; Brown and Gordon 1977). For the purposes of the present chapter I shall not repeat the detailed material that may be found in those articles, except where it is of particular relevance to spinal cord organization. I shall, however, take the opportunity to include some of the more recent results that are only to be found in original papers.

A. Physiology of the spinocervical tract

I. Types of unit in the tract

The spinocervical tract is under the control of a number of neuronal pathways descending from the brain (Taub 1964; Fetz 1968; Brown and Franz 1969; Brown and Martin 1973; Brown et al. 1973, 1977a). The actions of these pathways include the depression (inhibition) of transmission from particular cutaneous afferent fibres to the

tract. Operationally this action leads to differences in the response properties of spinocervical tract neurones when recorded under different conditions, such as in spinal versus decerebrate preparations (Wall 1967; Brown 1973). By careful examination of the receptive field properties of spinocervical tract neurones in different preparations (Brown and Franz 1969) and the use of reversible cold block of the cord (Brown 1973) it has been possible to determine the characteristics of the different types of unit present in the tract.

There are four categories of spinocervical tract neurones in the lumbosacral cord (Brown 1973):

Type I neurones are excited by hair movement. Under no conditions are they caused to fire by maintained mechanical stimulation of the skin. They are excited exclusively by myelinated cutaneous afferent fibres: non-myelinated afferent fibres do not excite them (Brown et al. 1975), although they may be excited by noxious heat (Brown and Franz 1969). This latter response is presumably due to input in small myelinated axons (Martin and Manning 1972). Type I neurones receive monosynaptic excitation from Type T hair follicle afferents (Brown and Franz 1969; Brown 1971, 1973).

Types II and III neurones are similar in that they both respond to hair movement and also to pressure on and pinch of the receptive field, the responses to maintained pressure and pinch being slowly adapting. They are excited by non-myelinated afferent fibres in addition to myelinated ones (Brown et al. 1975). Type II units have axons with low conduction velocities (Brown and Franz 1969; Brown 1971) and receive monosynaptic input from Type G hair follicle afferents. Type III units, on the other hand, have a wide range of axonal conduction velocities and receive monosynaptic excitation from Type G and T hair follicle afferents and possibly Type D too (Brown 1973).

Type IV spinocervical tract neurones are not excited by hair movement under any conditions. They are excited by noxious stimuli when descending control systems are inoperative or acting only weakly (Brown and Franz 1969; Brown 1971).

Type I spinocervical tract neurones form about 30% of the total; Types II and III make up most of the remaining 70%. Type IV units always form a small minority of any sample of spinocervical tract units, usually less than 5% (Brown 1971; Bryan et al. 1973; Cervero et al. 1977). The higher proportions found by Brown and Franz (1969) (8% in decerebrate or anaesthetized cats and as many as 28% in spinal cats) probably reflect sampling bias. Thus the great majority of spinocervical tract cells are excited by hair movement and receive monosynaptic inputs from some hair follicle afferent fibres.

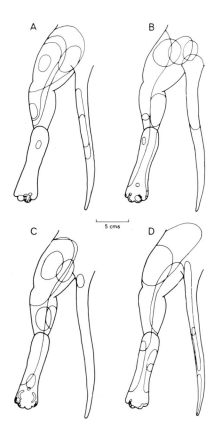

Fig. 6.1. Excitatory receptive fields of spinocervical tract neurones. **A** Type II units; **B** Type I units; **C** and **D**, Type III units. Receptive fields on the toes are small and fields generally become larger on the more proximal parts of the limb. Some fields, which include parts of the foot, are very large indeed. For the significance of the different types see the text. (From Brown and Franz 1969.)

Figure 6.1 shows the receptive fields (hair movement fields) of different types of spinocervical tract neurones. Comparison of these fields with those of hair follicle afferent units (see Fig. 2.2) demonstrates that there must be considerable convergence from many hair follicle units onto single spinocervical tract neurones. Convergence will be most marked for spinocervical tract neurones with large fields including parts of the leg, thigh and hip, but even when the fields are on toes they are usually at least twice the size of the primary afferents' fields.

II. Actions of descending control systems

The descending neuronal systems that affect transmission through the spinocervical tract all appear to act in the same way. Their actions differ from those of systems acting on the dorsal column nuclei (see Brown and Gordon 1977). The operational effects of the descending control make the tract neurones more specific in their responses to cutaneous input. When the descending systems are active, Type I neurones only respond to movement of tylotrichs, Type II neurones respond only to movement of guard hairs, and the responses of Types II, III and IV units to noxious stimuli are severely or completely inhibited (Brown 1971). Figure 6.2 shows the effects of descending activity on the spontaneous and pressure-evoked discharges of spinocervical tract neurones. The actions of segmental inhibitory systems appear to be similar to those of the descending systems (Brown et al. 1973).

When the descending systems are stimulated electrically, inhibitory effects on transmission through the spinocervical tract are produced (Brown et al. 1973; Brown and Martin 1973; Brown and Short 1974). This inhibition has a time course of up to 200 ms or more with maximal action at 20–40 ms (Fig. 6.3), that is, the time course is similar to that of pre-synaptic inhibition in the mammalian spinal cord. Polysynaptic excitatory inputs from myelinated afferent fibres and the excitatory actions of non-myelinated fibres are strongly inhibited by the descending systems (Fig. 6.4). The monosynaptic excitatory inputs to spinocervical tract neurones are much less affected, and possibly unaffected, by the descending systems (Brown et al. 1973; Brown and Martin 1973).

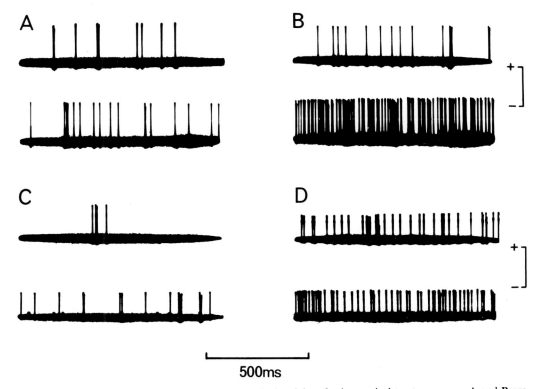

Fig. 6.2. Effects of descending control systems on the resting and evoked activity of spinocervical tract neurones. **A** and **B** are from a single unit, and **C** and **D** from a different unit; both are Type III units. In each pair of records the upper trace shows the response in the decerebrate cat, where there is tonic activity in some descending systems, and the lower trace shows the responses after cooling of the spinal cord (in the lower thoracic/upper lumbar region), which blocks the descending activity. **A** and **C** are records of resting activity and **B** and **D** are responses evoked by squeezing the skin of the receptive fields with a small toothed clip. Both units had higher rates of discharge in the spinal state under both conditions. The amplitude calibration is 4 mV for both units. The recordings were taken from spinocervical tract axons as they ascended the dorso-lateral funiculus in the lumbar cord. (From Brown 1971.)

There are a number of descending pathways that control transmission through the spinocervical tract. Brown et al. (1973) showed that they descended the cord bilaterally in both dorsal and both ventral funiculi (see Fig. 6.3). The origins of the paths are largely unknown. Fetz (1968) showed that electrical stimulation of the medullary pyramids may inhibit some dorsal horn neurones. Stimulation of the first and second somatic sensory areas of the cerebral cortex inhibits transmission through the spinocervical tract (Brown and Short 1974). By using intracortical microstimulation Brown et al. (1977a) showed that the inhibition can be evoked from localized cortical areas, especially from cytoarchitectonic areas 4γ, 4δ and 3a. Taub (1964) demonstrated that electrical stimulation of cerebellar nuclei, the mesencephalic tegmentum and a central ponto-bulbar area could all inhibit transmission through

the tract. More recently, Brown and Martin (1973) showed that activity *ascending* the dorsal columns and relaying through the dorsal column nuclei could lead to descending effects on the tract. Part of the central pathway for the latter effect includes the brain stem and cerebellum. It is obvious, therefore, that many neuronal systems control the spinocervical tract.

III. Transmission of information through the tract

The spinocervical tract is concerned, above all, with hair movement. Nearly all of its neurones are excited by movement of hairs and none of them receive excitatory input from sensitive mechanoreceptors in the glabrous skin of foot and toe pads. As shown in Chapter 2, hair follicle

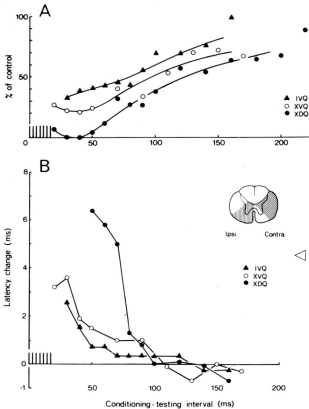

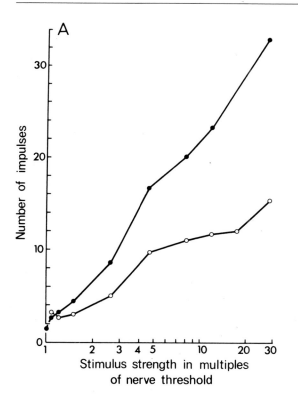

Fig. 6.3. Time course of descending inhibitory action on spinocervical tract cell discharges (polysynaptic input). The graphs show the responses of a neurone evoked by electrical stimulation of a cutaneous nerve when conditioned with a short tetanus (indicated by the *vertical bars* at the beginning of each abscissa) to the ipsilateral ventral cervical cord (IVQ), contralateral ventral cervical cord (XVQ) and contralateral dorso-lateral cervical cord (XDQ). In **A** the number of impulses and the percentage of control values are plotted against the conditioning-testing intervals. In **B** the change in latency of the first impulse evoked by the testing shock is plotted against the conditioning-testing interval. There are marked increases in latency. Each *point* represents the mean of at least five observations. (From Brown et al. 1973.)

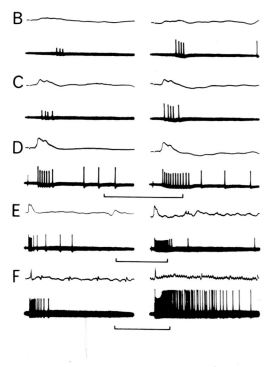

Fig. 6.4.

receptors code the rate of hair movement very precisely. Spinocervical tract neurones have responses to hair movement that are very similar to those of primary hair follicle afferent units (Fig. 6.5). Stimulus–response relationships of spinocervical tract neurones to constant-velocity hair movement are shown in Fig. 6.6. The main difference between the responses of hair follicle units and spinocervical tract neurones is a higher exponent of the power function for the central neurones, indicating an increase in sensitivity. Some of this increase may be a peripheral effect due to innervation of single hair follicles by more

than one primary afferent fibre and to overlapping receptive fields that converge onto a spinocervical tract neurone. Some may be due to properties of the synapses between hair follicle afferents and the tract neurones or to properties of the neurones themselves.

Transmission between hair follicle afferent fibres and spinocervical tract neurones is very secure. Hongo and Koike (1975) have shown that a single impulse in a hair follicle afferent fibre is capable of evoking a large excitatory postsynaptic potential in a spinocervical tract neurone. Furthermore, we (A. G. Brown, P. K. Rose

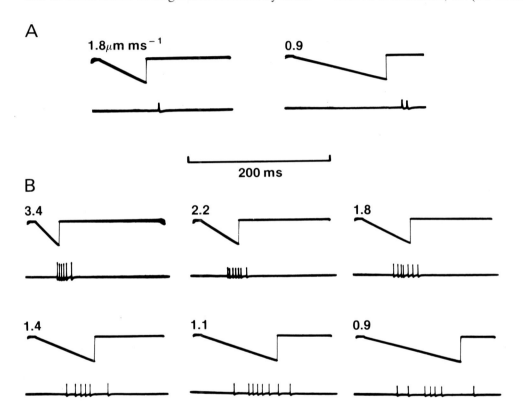

Fig. 6.5. (*Above*) Responses of spinocervical tract neurones to hair movement. **A** impulses evoked by rapid movement at the 'off' of the stimulus (insensitive unit); **B** trains of impulses produced by different constant rates of hair movement. (From Brown and Franz 1969.)

◁ **Fig. 6.4.** (*Opposite*) Effects of descending impulses on the responses of a spinocervical tract neurone (Type III) to electrical stimulation of a cutaneous nerve. In A the number of impulses evoked by electrical stimulation of the medial plantar nerve is plotted against the strength of stimulation in multiples of threshold (T) for the whole nerve. The filled circles are the responses in the spinal state (descending systems reversibly blocked by cooling the cord) and the open circles are the

responses in the decerebrate state (descending systems tonically active). Each *point* is the mean of three to six responses. At all strengths of stimulation above 1.2T more impulses are evoked in the spinal state, the difference becoming more marked with stronger stimuli. **B–F** are original records of individual responses; the *left-hand column* shows responses in the decerebrate state and the *right-hand column* responses in the spinal state. The upper record in each pair is the afferent volley recorded at the dorsal root entrance zone, the lower record the response of the unit. Strengths of stimulation were: **B** 1.07T; **C** 1.5T; **D** 4.7T; **E** 12.0T. **F** shows the responses evoked by a stimulus supramaximal for the C fibres. This last response, which is not plotted in **A**, illustrates the marked inhibition of the responses to C fibre stimulation when the descending systems are active. Time scales: **B–D** 50 ms; **E** 100 ms; **F** 500 ms. (From Brown 1971.)

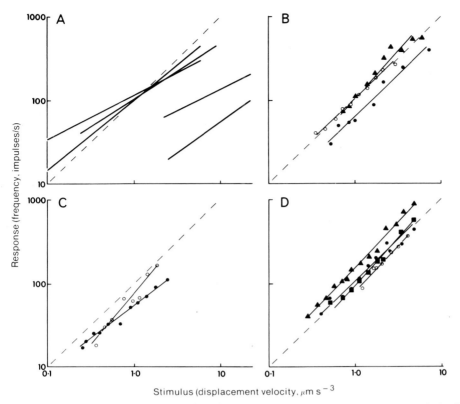

Fig. 6.6. Stimulus–response relationships of spinocervical tract neurones to constant-velocity hair movement. **A** Responses of hair follicle afferent units (from Brown and Iggo 1967), for comparison. **B** Spinocervical tract units free from descending control (spinal preparation). **C** Spinocervical tract neurones of the Type I category. **D** Type III units. The dashed line has a slope of unity. Symbols represent different neurones. (From Brown and Franz 1969.)

and P. J. Snow, unpublished observations) have shown that this tight coupling extends to poly-synaptic connexions. In experiments in which an intracellular microelectrode was used to stimulate single dorsal root ganglion cells (hair follicle afferents) and a second, extracellular microelectrode was used to record the responses of a spinocervical tract neurone, one-to-one following of the neurone's response was observed at 300–400 Hz with central latencies of between 6 and 11 ms — far too long to be monosynaptic.

Spinocervical tract neurones of Types II, III and IV respond to noxious mechanical stimulation of the skin, especially when the descending control systems are inoperative. Also, all types of spinocervical tract neurones may respond to noxious heat (Brown and Franz 1969, 1970; Brown 1971). Recently Cervero et al. (1977) have confirmed these earlier reports and extended the observations to show that some spinocervical tract neurones may be inhibited by noxious heat and others may show excitation followed by inhibition upon repetition of the stimulus. Cervero

et al. (1977) suggest that the spinocervical tract is indirectly involved in nociception, perhaps providing signals that help in the recognition, discrimination and peripheral localization of potentially damaging stimuli. It is certainly difficult with the current state of knowledge to make any more clearly defined suggestions about the possible role of the spinocervical tract in nociception. It is, perhaps, worth noting that Kennard (1954) showed that section of the dorsal quadrant of the spinal cord led to some modification in the response of cats to harmful stimulation. She suggested that fibres essential for the recognition of painful stimuli ascend this part of the cord. But such lesions interrupt many pathways in addition to the spinocervical tract, including descending ones.

In summary, the pre-eminent role of hair follicle afferent fibres in exciting spinocervical tract neurones should be stressed. The close anatomical relation between the terminal arborizations of hair follicle afferent fibres and the dendritic trees of spinocervical tract neurones will be described in this chapter and Chapter 7. The role of the spinocervico-lemniscothalamic system in nociception is uncertain but may be important under certain, as yet unknown, conditions. Some cutaneous receptors do not excite the spinocervical tract. These include the sensitive mechanoreceptors in glabrous skin (Pacinian corpuscles, rapidly adapting mechanoreceptors, slowly adapting Type I receptors), the Type I and II slowly adapting receptors in hairy skin and the Type II receptors at the claw bases. It has been shown in earlier chapters that these afferent units distribute much of their information to parts of the cord other than lamina III where most of the dendrites of spinocervical tract neurones are situated.

B. Anatomy of the spinocervical tract

I. Location of neurones

The first problem in locating spinocervical tract neurones is to identify them. Electrophysiological methods are undoubtedly the best. Spinocervical tract neurones send their axons to the lateral cervical nucleus; they may be identified by antidromic firing from just below the nucleus (stimulation of the ipsilateral dorso-lateral funiculus at C-3) associated with lack of antidromic excitation from positions rostral to the lateral cervical nucleus (rostral C-1 or higher). This method of identification was introduced by Lundberg and Norrsell (cited in Lundberg 1964a) and Taub and Bishop (1965) and is the method used in the present writer's laboratory.

The most important criteria for demonstrating antidromic firing are: (1) 'collision' between an antidromic and an orthodromic impulse (Darian-Smith et al. 1963; Gordon and Miller 1969), which can be used with both extracellular and intracellular recording; and (2) for intracellular recording only, the rise of an antidromic action potential from a flat baseline with no preceding excitatory post-synaptic potential. When demonstrating antidromic excitation of spinocervical tract neurones it is also necessary to section the dorsal columns caudal to the C3 stimulating electrodes in order to prevent orthodromic firing of the cells evoked by stimulating ascending primary afferent fibres in the dorsal columns.

The criterion of antidromic firing from below the lateral cervical nucleus and absence of such firing from above the nucleus is very strict. It depends upon the assumption that all spinocervical axons terminate in the lateral cervical nucleus—an assumption that is not necessarily correct. However, many neurones with cell bodies in the dorsal horn and axons ascending the ipsilateral dorso-lateral funiculus satisfy the criterion: they may be allocated to the spinocervical tract without doubt. But in most experiments, especially when a high spinal section has been performed to render the preparation free from descending influences, it is not possible to place stimulating electrodes at the most rostral levels in C-1. Under these circumstances, with stimulation at mid or even caudal levels of C-1, spinocervical tract axons may be excited antidromically, albeit with high strengths of stimulating current.

When spinocervical tract axons are stimulated at C-1 their conduction velocities measured between the C-1 and the C-3 stimulating electrodes are much lower than their velocities between C-3 and the recording site in the lumbosacral cord. Brown and Franz (1969) accepted an axon as belonging to the tract if either the C-1 stimulus was ineffective, or the conduction velocity between C-1 and C-3 was 50% or less than that from C-3 to the recording site. In more recent experiments this criterion has been relaxed somewhat so that a reduction in conduction velocity of 33% is now accepted. It is necessary to stress, however, that the vast majority of spinocervical tract neurones are not fired antidromically from C-1.

The relaxation of the antidromic firing criterion to include neurones with axons fired from C-1 allows the inclusion in the tract of neurones with axons ascending the dorso-lateral funiculus that give off collaterals to the lateral cervical nucleus but then carry on to the brain with a reduced conduction velocity. Such axons are thought to exist, possibly projecting to the dorsal column nuclei (Dart and Gordon 1973; Craig 1978). Neurones with axons giving collaterals to the lateral cervical nucleus and then projecting to the brain with little or no reduction in conduction velocity will not be included as belonging to the spinocervical tract, even with the relaxed criteria. It is not known how many neurones that properly belong to the tract are overlooked because of these practical difficulties. In any electrophysiological experiment in which neurones are recorded from the lumbosacral cord up to 10% may have response properties similar to identified spinocervical tract neurones, but be excited antidromically from C-1 with no conduction velocity reduction between C-1 and C-3. It is not possible to know whether these axons give collaterals to the lateral cervical nucleus.

It is important to understand the necessity for proper identification of spinocervical tract neurones. Several reports, purporting to show the location of spinocervical tract neurones, have appeared in which the neurones are not rigorously identified. Thus in the first systematic intracellular study of spinocervical tract cells, Hongo et al. (1968) identified them as follows: (1) antidromic invasion upon stimulation of the ipsilateral spinal half (except dorsal columns) or dissected dorsal part of the lateral funiculus at the level of the lower thoracic region; (2) monosynaptic excitation from cutaneous afferent fibres; (3) location of the microelectrode tip at depths of 1.1–1.8 mm from the cord dorsum. The first and second criteria do not exclude the 10% or so of neurones with axons projecting beyond the lateral cervical nucleus and possibly include propriospinal neurones. The third criterion cannot be used if the location of spinocervical tract neurones is being studied. However, most of the cells recorded by Hongo et al. (1968) probably were spinocervical tract neurones—but some doubt remains.

Bryan et al. (1973) have presented evidence on the location of 105 neurones that they identified as belonging to the spinocervical tract. All but 12 of these were recorded with extracellular microelectrodes. These authors suggested that spinocervical tract neurones are located in Rexed's laminae II to VI or even deeper, with the majority in laminae IV and V. Only 31 neurones, however, were tested for antidromic activation from C-1 and the rest of the sample could have been contaminated with neurones projecting beyond the lateral cervical nucleus. Thus Bryan et al. (1973) have a rather higher proportion of their sample of neurones situated in lamina VI or deeper than do other workers (Brown et al. 1976, 1980b; Cervero et al. 1977). These deep neurones probably do not belong to the spinocervical tract (see also Craig 1978).

A completely different approach to the location of spinocervical tract neurones has been used by Craig (1976, 1978): the retrograde transport of horseradish peroxidase after injection into the lateral cervical nucleus in both cats and dogs. Labelled neurones were located predominantly in lamina IV; they were certainly not as widely distributed as indicated by Bryan et al. (1973). Retrograde horseradish peroxidase studies require cautious interpretation, but one of the main problems—take-up of the enzyme by axons injured during the injection—was unlikely to have complicated Craig's results because the location of stained neurones was more limited, not less, than that indicated by the electrophysiological results of Bryan et al. (1973). It is possible that axons giving collaterals to the lateral cervical nucleus and then projecting to the brain did not pick up enough of the enzyme to label their somata. This possibility was recognized by Craig (1976), but when the lateral cervical nucleus is flooded with horseradish peroxidase (Craig used injections of small volumes, 0.1–0.4 μl total) similar results are obtained, as will be described below.

In our own studies on the location of spinocervical tract neurones we have used three methods: intracellular staining, extracellular recording and retrograde transport of horseradish peroxidase. The most direct method is intracellular staining with either Procion Yellow (Brown et al. 1976) or horseradish peroxidase (Brown et al. 1977b) after electrophysiological identification of the neurones. It is the most accurate method available but it is limited to the neurones with large cell bodies. Spinocervical tract neurones with axons conducting at less than 30 m s^{-1} have rarely been injected, due to our inability to maintain stable impalements in such neurones for long enough. Such cells presumably have smaller somata than those with axons conducting faster than 30 m s^{-1}. The intracellularly stained sample, therefore, does not include these cells, which make up about 30% of the total recordable population of spinocervical tract neurones (Bryan et al. 1973; Brown et al. 1976).

Figure 6.7 shows the locations of 44 stained spinocervical tract neurones on the outline of a standard L-7 dorsal horn. There are certain difficulties in producing a composite diagram of this type. The size and shape of the dorsal horn and the relative sizes and arrangements of the various laminae all vary from segment to segment and within segments in the same cord. Variation between cords is even more marked. In Fig. 6.7 cells are placed on the standard horn in terms of their relative positions between (1) the medial and lateral borders and (2) the dorsal border and the most ventral extent of the dorsal columns, in their own horn (see Brown et al. 1976 for details). All stained neurones are in laminae III, IV and V. Most (30; 68%) are in lamina IV, fewer (13; 30%) are in lamina III, and only a single neurone (2.3%) is in lamina V. None is deeper than lamina V; this may reflect the fact that during an experiment one rarely takes the microelectrode below the position where an extracellularly recorded potential starts to become smaller, but withdraws it and tracks down again in an attempt to impale the cell. In other words the more superficial parts of the cord are more thoroughly searched than the deeper ones.

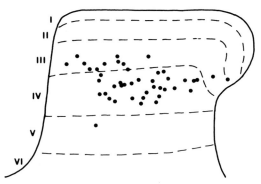

Fig. 6.7. Locations of intracellularly stained spinocervical tract neurones in the dorsal horn. The positions of 44 neurones are shown. Neurones have been placed on a standardized dorsal horn according to their positions in their own horn (for details see the text).

Because of the limitations of intracellular staining (restriction of the sample to the larger neurones and a tendency to concentrate on the more superficial parts of the dorsal horn) an indirect approach has been made (Brown et al. 1976, 1980b). In this method extracellular recording is used and attempts made to record all spinocervical tract neurones within particular parts of the cord. This is a valid approach because spinocervical tract neurones are scattered in the dorsal horn (Hongo et al. 1968; and our own experience) and the extracellular potentials of even the smallest cells may be picked up at distances of at least 150 μm from the point of intracellular penetration with a microelectrode. By making grids of electrode tracks through the dorsal horn, with tracks 250 μm apart in rows 250 μm apart, all or all but a very few, spinocervical tract neurones should be recorded. Histological reconstruction is aided by leaving microelectrode tips in situ at the end of each row, thereby allowing the locations of the extracellularly recorded neurones to be estimated with a fair degree of accuracy.

Figure 6.8 shows the estimated positions of 60 spinocervical tract neurones within segments L-7–S-1, the positions being the locations of the largest potentials recorded from the cells. There is a slightly wider distribution than in the stained sample (Fig. 6.7), with a larger proportion (10%) in lamina V and one cell in lamina VI. But nearly 90% are in laminae III and IV, most being in IV. This experiment was typical of all similar types of experiments (see, for example, Text-figure 1 in

Brown et al. 1976), and the results are in good agreement with those of Cervero et al. (1977) for a pooled sample of 57 neurones from 13 cats. The distribution is more localized than suggested by Bryan et al. (1973). Bryan et al. (1973) suggested that there may be a component of the tract with cell bodies deeper in the horn and with axons having low conduction velocities. We have not been able to confirm this in our experiments and analysis of the extracellular material has shown that neurones with low conduction velocities are randomly dispersed through laminae III to V.

Even with the most accurate electrode marking techniques, however, extracellular recording is not a precise way of locating neurones. The data gathered in the author's laboratory over the years indicate that for spinocervical tract cells the error in the dorso-ventral axis may be as much as ±150 μm, and it is similar in the two horizontal axes. Any dimpling of the cord surface by the microelectrode will produce a dorsal shift in the apparent position of the electrode tip: we were always careful to avoid this. But even without dimpling, the vertical error is enough to move an estimated placement from one lamina to an adjacent one.

Because of these deficiencies of the extracellular recording method, and also as an independent check that we were able to record all spinocervical tract cells extracellularly, we used the retrograde horseradish peroxidase in a novel way (Brown et al. 1980b). The lateral cervical nucleus of one side was flooded with the enzyme, after cutting the dorsal columns at C-4 to

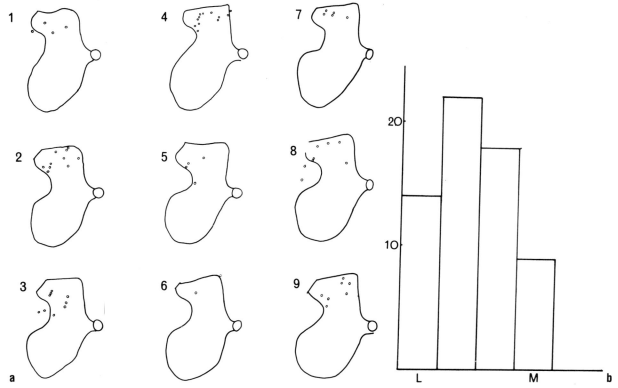

Fig. 6.8. Locations of spinocervical tract neurones estimated from extracellular recording. **A** Estimated positions of 60 neurones located in a grid of microelectrode tracks in the L-7–S-1 segments. The grid consisted of nine rows of tracks, with a spacing of 250 μm between rows and 250 μm between tracks within the rows. Each cross section of the dorsal horn represents a row of tracks: 1 is the most rostral row, 9 the most caudal. **B** Numbers of cells in the different quarters of the horn from lateral (L) to medial (M). This figure should be compared with Fig. 6.9, which shows the locations of spinocervical tract neurones on the opposite side of the spinal cord determined by the retrograde horseradish peroxidase method. (From Brown et al. 1980b.)

prevent retrograde transport down axons belonging to the post-synaptic dorsal column pathway. The aim was to label all spinocervical tract cell bodies. In the same animals extracellular grids of microelectrode tracks were made in the contralateral lumbosacral cord to record spinocervical tract neurones. Figures 6.8 and 6.9 are from such an experiment, Fig. 6.8 being the locations of tract neurones determined electrophysiologically and Fig. 6.9 the locations determined by retrograde horseradish peroxidase. The electrophysiological method recorded 60 neurones in a 2-mm length of L-7 cord; the enzyme transport method also revealed 60 neurones on the opposite side of the same length of cord. All but four of the retrogradely labelled cells were in laminae III and IV; three of these four were dorsal to lamina III and one was in lamina V. The similarity between the two sets of results is striking and has also been found in other experiments of the same type.

We had feared that the retrograde horseradish peroxidase experiments would label large numbers of neurones that did not belong to the spinocervical tract, because of the large volumes of enzyme injected to ensure all tract axon terminals had the chance to pick it up. Obviously, any non-spinocervical tract neurones that were stained formed a very small minority. It is possible, however, that some of the neurones revealed were not 'true' spinocervical tract cells. In 1968, Fedina et al. reported that transmission through the lateral cervical nucleus could be inhibited from widespread inputs in forelimb and hind limb nerves. For the hind limbs the pathway to the lateral cervical nucleus ascended the cord in the ventro-lateral funiculi (mainly contralaterally). In other words, there are bilateral ascending pathways to the lateral cervical nucleus other than the spinocervical tract. Full details of the inhibitory paths are not known. But there is the real possi-

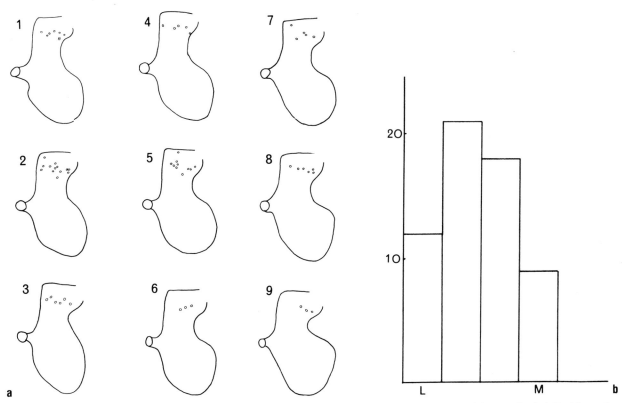

Fig. 6.9. Locations of spinocervical tract neurones determined by the retrograde horseradish peroxidase method. **A** Positions of the cells on transverse sections of the dorsal horn; cells within 250-μm slices of the spinal cord have been pooled for each drawing to correspond with the electrophysiological recording grid made on the opposite side of the cord and shown in Fig. 6.8. **B** Numbers of cells in the different quarters of the horn from lateral (L) and medial (M). Sixty neurones were located by this method and the numbers and locations agree remarkably with the results of electrophysiological recording shown in Fig. 6.8. (From Brown et al. 1980b.)

bility that injections of horseradish peroxidase into the lateral cervical nucleus may lead to labelling of neurones giving axons to these pathways if they are not interrupted by synapses.

It is, therefore, of some interest that in our retrograde material marginal cells in lamina I have been labelled on both sides of the cord. Ipsilaterally the labelled marginal cells represent between 12 and 18% of the total in different experiments (the three dorsal cells in Fig. 6.9 include one marginal cell). On the side contralateral to the injection a similar number of marginal cells together with cells in deeper laminae (VII and VIII) were stained, as were a few neurones in laminae III–V. Obviously some of these cells could have been stained because of spread of enzyme beyond the lateral cervical nucleus (Molenaar and Kuypers 1978). The contralateral cells may be cells of origin of the inhibitory pathway to the lateral cervical nucleus. On the ipsi-

lateral side some of the stained neurones may also belong to this pathway. Marginal cells could be in this category, or be genuine spinocervical tract cells, in which case they would be Type IV neurones since marginal cells are excited exclusively by nociceptive inputs (Christensen and Perl 1970; Cervero et al. 1979a). According to Kumazawa et al. (1975) some marginal cells send their axons towards the brain in the contralateral ventro-lateral cord, and they contribute to the spinothalamic tract (Trevino and Carstens 1975). But some marginal cells were apparently stained by Craig (1976) after horseradish peroxidase injection into the lateral cervical nucleus (see his Fig. 2, cervical cord) and they are also stained after injections into the medulla (Rustioni and Kaufman 1977; Molenaar and Kuypers 1978).

The conclusions that may be drawn from these three types of experiments are: spinocervical tract cells are concentrated in lamina IV and to a lesser extent in lamina III; about 10% may be in lamina V; very few cells lie outside laminae III–V; marginal cells of lamina I are candidates as cells of origin of either the spinocervical tract or the inhibitory pathway to the lateral cervical nucleus, and may project to both pathways.

II. Density and distribution of neurones

The location of spinocervical tract neurones in laminae III, IV and to a lesser extent V, with very few cells outside these layers, leads to the formation of a sheet of neuronal somata across the dorsal horn. Within this sheet the cells are scattered such that individual cells are easily isolated and recorded with microelectrodes. As shown in the preceding section both systematic microelectrode recording and retrograde horseradish peroxidase methods will reveal all spinocervical tract

neurones and may therefore be used to determine their density and distribution.

Figure 6.10, from the same experiment as Figs. 6.8 and 6.9, shows the horizontal distribution of spinocervical tracts cells in a 2-mm length of L-7–S-1 cord as determined, on one side, by electrophysiological methods and on the other by retrograde horseradish peroxidase transport. Figure 6.10A corresponds with Fig. 6.8 and Fig. 6.10B presents the same data as Fig. 6.9. On each side of the cord there are 60 neurones, a remarkable coincidence. In other experiments the numbers of spinocervical tract neurones revealed by the two methods have agreed to within 10%. In segments L-7–S-1 there are between 20 and 40 neurones in each millimetre length of cord.

Earlier experiments using only electrophysiological methods (see Brown 1976) had suggested that there are more spinocervical tract neurones in the lateral part of the horn than in the medial

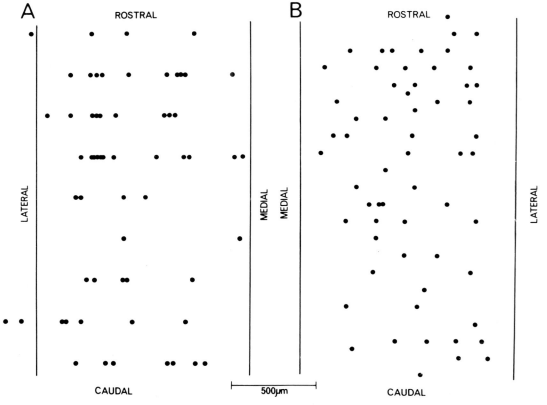

Fig. 6.10. The distribution of spinocervical tract neurones. **A** Plan view of the spinal cord showing the estimated positions of spinocervical tract neurones recorded in a grid of microelectrode tracks with spacings of 250 μm in the grid. The locations of these neurones in transverse sections of the cord are shown in Fig. 6.8. **B** Plan view of the opposite side of the same spinal cord to show the positions of spinocervical tract neurones determined by the retrograde horseradish peroxidase method. The positions of these cells in transverse sections of the dorsal horn are shown in Fig. 6.9. On each side of the cord 60 neurones were located. (From Brown et al. 1979.)

part. The evidence from our much more extensive series of experiments performed subsequently, shows that this is not so. Figures 6.8 and 6.9 are typical in showing rather more neurones in the middle two quarters of the dorsal horn.

It has been possible to determine the total number of spinocervical tract neurones in the lumbosacral enlargement of the cord. In cats with horseradish peroxidase injection sites covering all the lateral cervical nucleus and cord sections, to minimize transport down non-spinocervical axons, counts have been made of labelled cells. In segments L-4–S-2 between 650 and 900 neurones have been counted and 90–135 of these were marginal cells. Figure 6.11 shows photomicrographs from one such experiment and illustrates clearly how the neurones of the tract form a sheet of cells in the dorsal horn. Figure 6.12 shows histograms from four similar experiments that illustrate the distribution of spinocervical tract neurones through segments L-4–S-2. These experiments provided typical numbers of cells in those parts of the cord (L-7–S-1) that had been the subject of previous intensive electrophysiological study. Most cells are in segments L-7–S-1 and the numbers drop off both rostral and caudal to these segments. There are even fewer cells in thoracic segments. This observation is reassuring in that it shows that the number of cells labelled is not a function of the distance travelled by the enzyme, as it would be if insufficient time had elapsed between the injection and the termination of the experiment. In these experiments the animals survived 37–48 h after the injection.

The numbers of spinocervical tract cells determined by retrograde horseradish peroxidase transport (total numbers labelled minus marginal cells) agree well with previous estimates made from fibre counts. Van Beusekom (1955) concluded that the tract contains between 2000 and 3000 axons on each side. Heath (1978) recorded from axons of the tract at upper cervical levels in order to determine the relative numbers of units representing different parts of the body. In a sample of 247 axons 50.2% had forelimb receptive fields, 33.6% hind limb fields and the remaining 16.2% had fields on the trunk and tail. With about 750 neurones to represent the hind limb, there will be about 1100 for the forelimb and some 350 for the trunk and tail, giving a total of about 2200 neurones on each side. Obviously 2000–3000 is about the right order of magnitude.

At first sight the above numbers are surprising. Anyone used to working on the dorsal columns and their nuclei, the ventrobasal thalamus or the somatic sensory areas of the cerebral cortex would expect a relatively much greater forelimb representation than a hind limb one. Thus in the medial lemniscus (mainly axons from the dorsal column nuclei) Brown et al. (1974) found 70% had receptive fields on the forelimb and only 9% on the hind limb. But the spinocervical tract is not organized in this way. It has a much more even representation over the whole body; the forelimb predominance is not so well marked.

These differences between the spinocervical and dorsal column-lemniscal systems in the relative numbers of neurones given over to different parts of the body should provide clues to their functions. Traditionally the dorsal column system has been thought to play an important role in the discriminatory aspects of somaesthesis, although contrary opinions have been expressed recently (Wall 1970; see Brown and Gordon 1977 for a discussion). No satisfactory hypotheses for the functional role of the spinocervico-lemniscothalamic system have yet been made. In view of its lack of input from sensitive receptors in glabrous skin, a role in fine discriminatory analysis seems highly unlikely. The spinocervical tract represents, above all, the hairy skin. The system is highly developed in carnivores which have sophisticated motor skills. Brown et al. (1973) suggested that timing the occurrence of stimuli was an important function for the system and Heath (1978) has taken this suggestion further and developed the idea that the spinocervical tract might be involved in the regulation of movement, particularly running.

III. Somatotopic organization

Within the lumbosacral enlargement of the spinal cord a map of the hind limb is laid out across the dorsal horn. There have been a number of studies of the topographical organization of the dorsal horn (Wall 1960; Bryan et al. 1973; Brown and Fuchs 1975) and the gross picture has been established. Bryan et al. were the only authors to attempt identification of their dorsal horn neurones (they identified them as spinocervical tract cells, but see above) and they concluded that the map is laid out so that rostrally located cells

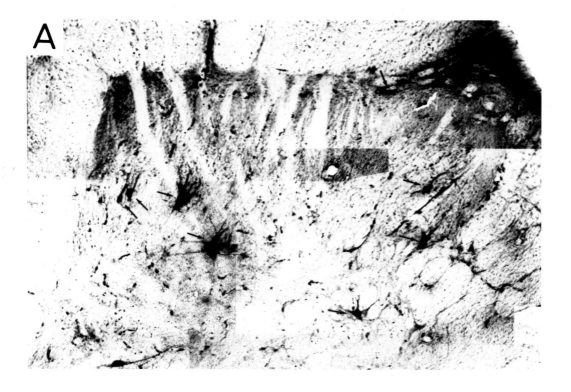

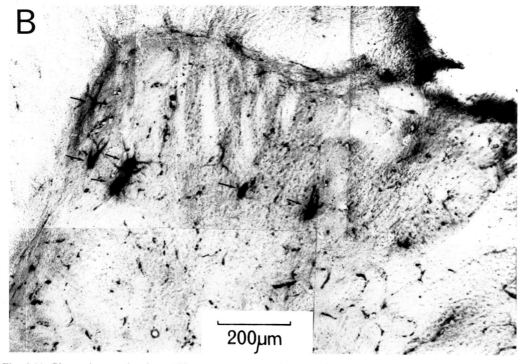

Fig. 6.11. Photomicrographs, from 100-μm transverse sections, to show spinocervical tract neurones (arrows) labelled by the retrograde horseradish peroxidase method. The organization of spinocervical tract neurones to form a sheet of cells in the dorsal horn is clearly seen. (From Brown et al. 1980b.)

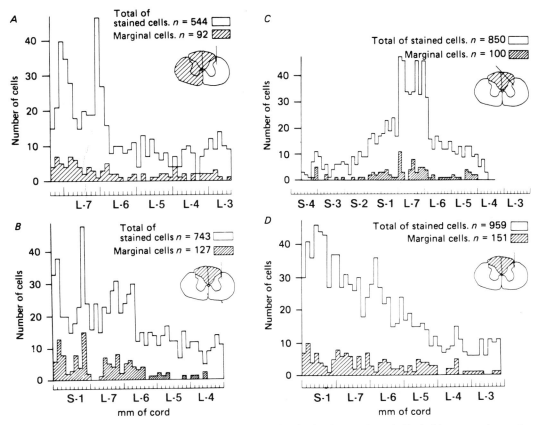

Fig. 6.12. The density and distribution of spinocervical tract neurones in the lumbosacral cord. Each histogram shows the distribution of spinocervical tract neurones from a single cat. A lateral cervical nucleus of each cat had been flooded with horseradish peroxidase in order to allow all spinocervical tract axon terminals to pick up the enzyme. Most neurones are found in segments L-7–S-1. Marginal cells (which may not belong to the spinocervical tract: see text) are shown cross-hatched. (From Brown et al 1980b.)

have receptive fields on the embryological anterior part of the limb and caudally located neurones have fields on the embryological posterior part of the limb. In this respect they agree with Wall (1960), but there is disagreement about the representation in the transverse plane of the cord. Wall suggests that medial cells have distal fields and lateral cells proximal ones. Bryan et al. conclude that medial cells receive input from the ventral surface of the limb and lateral cells from the dorsal surface.

The discrepancies undoubtedly arise in part from the pooling of rather scanty data from separate animals. The results of Brown and Fuchs (1975), although also pooled data, go some way to resolving the discrepancies. As shown in their Figure 1 and summarized in their Fig. 2, the medio-lateral representation depends on the segmental level. In segments L-6 to rostral S-1, medial neurones have distal and ventral fields,

the only exceptions being some representation of dorsal toes in medial L-6, while lateral cells have proximal and dorsal fields. In L-5 and caudal S-1, medial cells may receive information from more proximal parts of the limb, usually from its ventral surface; lateral neurones still receive input from proximal and dorsal skin. These results of Brown and Fuchs (1975) for the map in the dorsal horn are similar to those of Werner and Whitsel (1967, 1968) for the somatotopic representation in the dorsal columns and the first somatic sensory area of the cerebral cortex.

The spinocervical tract is ideal for topographical studies. All tract neurones within a given part of the cord may be recorded and large numbers of neurones may be recorded in an individual cat. Very detailed maps may be generated, the only restriction being the stamina of the investigators! Figures 6.13 and 6.14 show the receptive field organization in the sheet of spinocervical tract

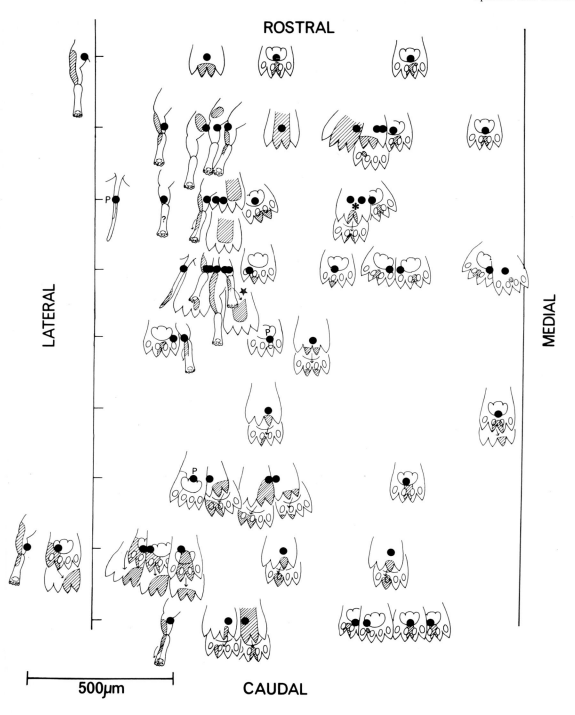

Fig. 6.13. Somatotopic organization in the spinocervical tract. Receptive fields are shown for the 60 neurones recorded in a grid of microelectrode tracks at 250-μm spacings (same experiment as shown in Figs. 6.8 and 6.10A). The organization into longitudinal columns of cells with overlapping receptive fields may be clearly seen. In this part of the L-7–S-1 cord ventral surfaces of the toes are represented medially, dorsal surfaces of the toes in the middle of the horn and more proximal and dorsal parts of the hind limb laterally. The *asterisk* indicates two cells with identical receptive fields. Their positions are shown by separate *filled circles*. The *star* represents a receptive field common to two cells, one of which (with *arrow* leading from it) also extended to the postero-lateral foot. The two cells with fields on the tail appear to be misplaced in the map. (From Brown et al. 1980b.)

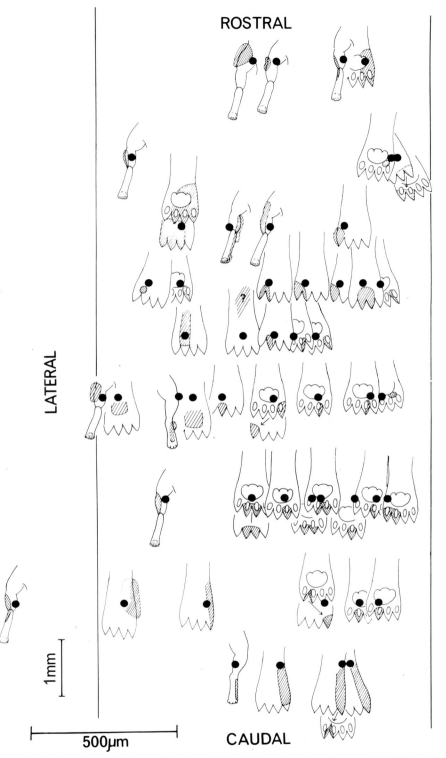

Fig. 6.14. Somatotopic organization in the spinocervical tract. Plan view of the spinal cord to show the receptive field positions of neurones recorded from rows of microelectrode tracts with spacings of 250-μm within the rows and spacings of about 1 mm between rows. The representation of ventral toe skin medially, with dorsal and proximal leg and thigh laterally is apparent. The representation of toe 5 is caudal to that for toe 2. The organization into columns of cells having overlapping fields may also be observed. (From Brown et al. 1980b.)

neurones in L-7 and L-6–S-1 respectively. Within these segments lateral cells have proximal and dorsal fields, and medial cells have distal and ventral fields. The maps agree with the results of Brown and Fuchs (1975).

The most striking feature of the receptive field maps is their arrangement into longitudinal columns with overlapping fields. Within a column there is only a gradual shift of the fields. In the transverse plane the gradient in the somatotopic map is very steep; in L-7, for example, medial cells have fields on the toes and lateral cells have fields on the proximal thigh and hip, the leg and foot being represented in between. Only a minority of neurones adjacent to one another in the transverse plane has overlapping receptive fields.

Hair follicle afferent fibres have monosynaptic excitatory connexions to spinocervical tract neurones. The terminal arborizations of hair follicle afferent fibres are arranged in longitudinally running sheets through lamina III (see Chapter 2). The arrangement of spinocervical tract neurones into columns of cells with overlapping receptive fields is a reflexion of the organization of the hair follicle afferent terminals that supply their major input.

The thickness of the longitudinal columns of spinocervical tract neurones may be assessed from receptive field maps such as those of Fig. 6.13 or others in which even finer grids of microelectrode tracks have been made (Brown et al. 1980b). When neurones are adjacent in the transverse plane up to about one-third of them have overlapping receptive fields; when adjacent in the sagittal plane about 90% of them have overlapping fields. Therefore, most receptive field columns are only a single cell wide, although a number of columns (theoretically as many as one-half) may be two cells in width. Further analysis is probably unwise because extracellular recording fails to localize neurones accurately enough. The problem will be returned to below when experiments will be described in which adjacent pairs of neurones were stained so that their dendritic tree relationships could be examined in detail.

IV. Morphology of neurones

1. Somata and dendritic trees

Intracellular staining of spinocervical tract neurones with either Procion dyes or horseradish peroxidase is, as mentioned previously, limited to the larger cells. Even within this group, however, spinocervical tract neurones have a very varied morphology (Jankowska and Lindström 1973; Brown et al. 1976, 1977a; Jankowska et al. 1976). They certainly do not constitute a homogeneous group, although they do share some common characteristics.

Spinocervical tract neurones have somata with volumes of 20×10^3 to 120×10^3 μm^3. These measurements from intracellularly stained cells represent the upper end of the range (cells with axonal conduction velocities of 24–79 m s^{-1}). Cells with axonal conduction velocities of less than 30 m s^{-1} make up about 30% of the population of tract neurones but have not been stained with intracellular techniques to any extent as they do not withstand the prolonged intracellular penetration for the requisite length of time. Such cells presumably have small somata.

The somata vary in shape. They are usually elongated in the dorso-ventral direction and also in the sagittal plane. Cells situated very far laterally in the dorsal horn are usually flattened dorso-ventrally (see Fig. 6.18).

The dendritic trees also vary greatly in shape, branching pattern, density of branches etc. Originally we (Brown et al. 1976) tried to classify the dendritic trees on the basis of their outlines as seen in reconstructions from transverse sections, but this proved to be a not very useful exercise.

The complexity of branching of dendritic trees varies from neurone to neurone. Some spinocervical tract neurones have dendritic trees with few (four or five) primary dendrites, each branching only a few times. Two neurones of this type are shown in Fig. 6.25. Other neurones may have as many as ten or more primary dendrites that branch profusely (Fig. 6.15A). Characteristically all spinocervical tract neurones have well-developed dorsally directed dendrites. Many neurones have their dendritic trees limited almost exclusively to dendrites that ascend in the dorsal direction (Figs. 6.15B, 6.24, 6.25, 6.26, 6.27). This latter type of neurone corresponds with the type described by Scheibel and Scheibel (1968) as characteristic of lamina IV and presumably also corresponds with the 'large antenna type neurons' in lamina IV described by Réthelyi and Szentágothai (1973).

The dorsally directed dendrites of spinocervical

tract neurones, except those with cell bodies deep in the dorsal horn, ascend through lamina III. They have ample opportunity to come into contact with synaptic boutons of hair follicle afferent fibres. Upon reaching the border between lam-

inae III and II the dendrites turn and run along the border in the sagittal plane. This is especially well seen in sagittal sections (Fig. 6.16A) or in reconstructions from such sections (Figs. 6.15B, 6.24). The dendrites seldom enter lamina II.

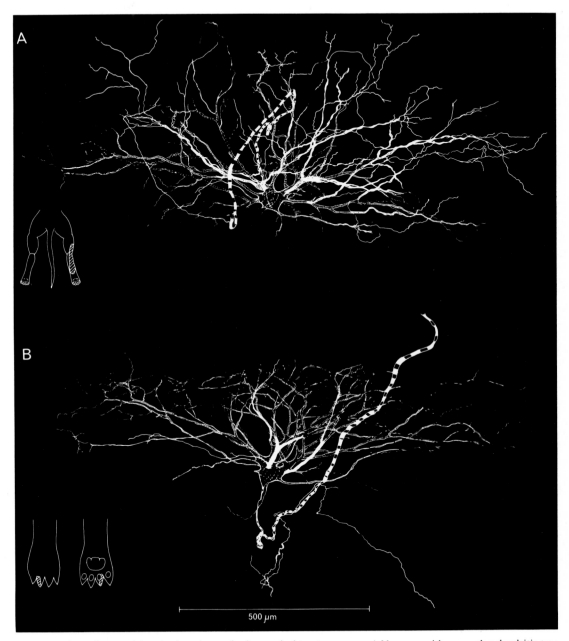

500 µm

Fig. 6.15. Reconstructions, from serial sagittal sections, of spinocervical tract neurones. **A** Neurone with a complex dendritic tree containing about ten primary dendrites, each giving arise to branches of up to the seventh or eighth order. The receptive field is shown in the inset figurine. **B** Neurone with a dendritic tree limited to dorsally projecting dendrites that turn and run in the sagittal plane at the border between laminae II and III. The receptive field is shown in the inset figurine. In this and all similar figures the solid (white) dendrites are the nearest to the observer, dendrites with the lightest shading are furthest away, etc. Axons are indicated by *dashes* between *continuous lines* and axon collaterals by either *continuous lines* (as in this figure) or *dashed lines* (as in Fig. 6.17.)

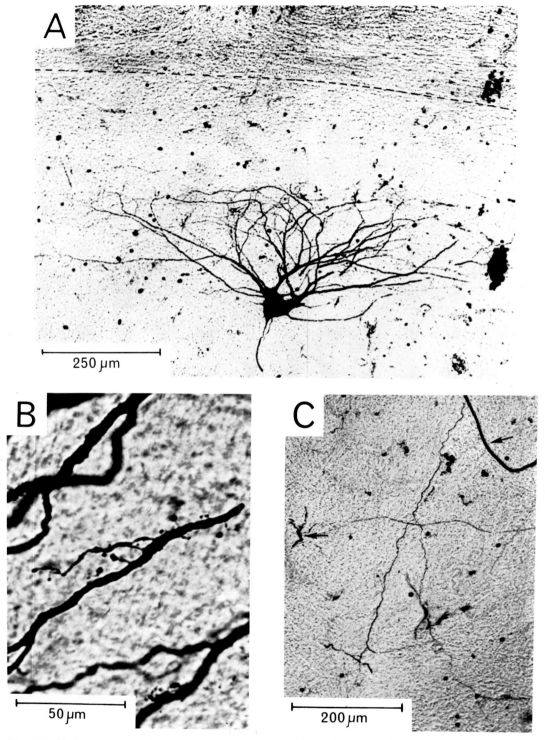

Fig. 6.16. Photomicrographs of spinocervical tract neurones stained with horseradish peroxidase. **A** Sagittal section through the soma of a neurone. Note how the dendrites ascend towards the dorsal border of the dorsal horn (indicated by the *dashed line*) but at about 200-μm deep, turn and run parallel to it. **B** Dendrites of a spinocervical tract neurone showing dendritic spines. **C** Axon collaterals from spinocervical tract neurones. Two axons are shown (*arrows*), each giving off collaterals. The collateral running from top to bottom of the micrograph can be seen to divide a number of times. All sections are 50-μm thick. (From Brown et al. 1977b.)

Therefore spinocervical tract neurones probably do not receive direct excitatory input from non-myelinated axons to any great extent. The responses of these neurones to noxious stimuli are presumably mediated via interneurones.

In addition to their dorsally directed dendrites, many spinocervical tract neurones have dendrites ramifying at the level of the cell body and also penetrating ventral to the cell body (Fig. 6.17). Where these dendrites are in laminae IV and V they would have plenty of chances to come into contact with many different types of cutaneous afferent fibres. But spinocervical tract neurones only receive monosynaptic inputs from hair follicle afferent fibres, as far as is known. They are not excited by Pacinian corpuscles, rapidly adapting receptors in the foot pads, or by either type of slowly adapting sensitive mechano-receptor. Hair follicle afferent fibres have their terminal arborizations limited almost exclusively to lamina III, so dendrites of spinocervical tract cells in laminae IV and V (or deeper) must be receiving inputs from other sources, that is, from various interneurones, either excitatory or inhibitory.

The dendritic trees vary in their medio-lateral and rostro-caudal spreads according to the position of the neurones in the dorsal horn. All cells have dendritic trees that are more extensive in the sagittal plane than in the transverse plane of the cord. Cells in the medial third of the horn have the most restricted dendritic trees: in the transverse plane the trees measure about 200–450 μm across, in the sagittal plane 550–1000 μm. Cells in

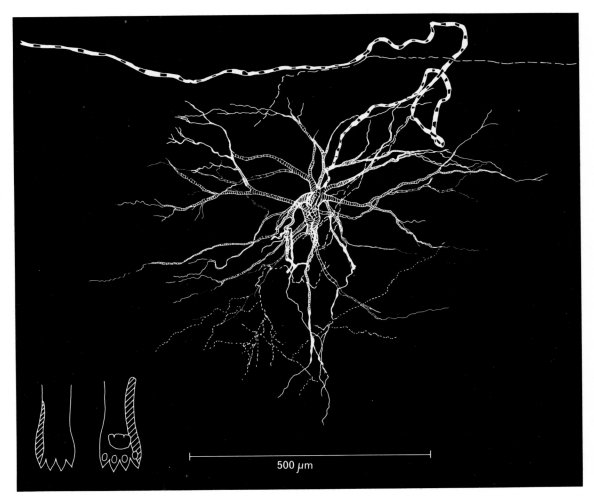

Fig. 6.17. Spinocervical tract neurone with well-developed ventrally directed dendrites. This neurone, reconstructed from serial sagittal sections, had a long (1300 μm) caudally directed collateral, part of which is shown. The receptive field is shown on the inset.

the middle third of the horn have dendritic trees with transverse spreads of 200–650 μm and sagittal spreads of 800–1400 μm. Neurones in the lateral third of the horn have dendritic trees that are very restricted in the transverse plane, 200–450 μm, but greatly elongated in the longitudinal direction, 1400–2200 μm (Fig. 6.18). The ratios between the rostro-cadual and the medio-lateral spreads of the dendritic trees of spinocervical tract cells range from 2.0 for medially situated neurones to 7.5 for laterally situated ones. These measurements are significant when considering relationships between the neurones and the terminal arborizations of hair follicle afferent fibres, and the somatotopic organization within the sheet of spinocervical tract neurones (see below).

2. Dendritic spines

An important result provided by intracellular injection of horseradish peroxidase has been the demonstration of dendritic spines on spinocervical tract neurones in the adult cat (Jankowska et al. 1976; Brown et al. 1977b). It has been known, at least since Ramon y Cajal (1909), that dorsal horn neurones in kittens have spines on their dendrites. Scheibel and Scheibel (1968) noted, in kittens, that neurones with cell bodies in lamina IV have well-developed spines on their dorsally directed dendrites but that laterally running dendrites have fewer, smaller spines. The well-developed spines on the dorsal dendrites can be as long as 12 μm and complexly curved or

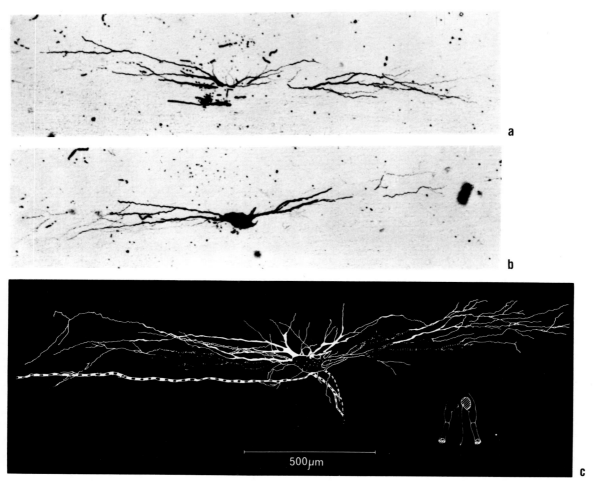

500μm

Fig. 6.18. Spinocervical tract neurone situated in the lateral part of the dorsal horn. **A** and **B** Photomicrographs of adjacent serial 50-μm sagittal sections. **C** Reconstruction of the complete dendritic tree. The dendritic tree is enormously elongated in the sagittal plane (2200 μm). The receptive field is shown in the *inset* in **C**.

branched with multiple terminal enlargements.

Spinocervical tract neurones must now be numbered amongst the dorsal horn neurones with this type of spine arrangement. Figure 6.19 shows camera lucida drawings of spines seen on spinocervical tract cell dendrites and Fig. 6.16B is a photomicrograph of the spines. The observations of Scheibel and Scheibel (1968) on kittens have been confirmed for adult cats: dorsally directed dendrites of spinocervical tract neurones have long spines, often with stalks 5–12 μm long, which often branch, terminating in swellings 2–3 μm in diameter (Fig. 6.19A–C). Laterally and ventrally directed dendrites have fewer spines which are usually shorter than those on dorsal dendrites (Fig. 6.19D).

The implication of this result, in agreement with Scheibel and Scheibel (1968), is presumably that differences in the development of spines on different dendrite systems of the same cell indicate differences in input. The dorsally directed dendrites with well-developed spine systems are ideally situated to receive the input from hair follicle afferent fibres. As mentioned above, the input to the lateral and ventral dendrites is likely to be from various interneurones. The Scheibels

(1968) suggest that the corticospinal tract might provide input to the laterally directed dendrites. This is unlikely since stimulation of the sensorimotor cortex produces effects more consistent with pre-synaptic inhibition than with the post-synaptic type (Brown and Short 1974; Brown et al. 1977a). Evidence for differential location of synapses on spinocervical tract cells is lacking at the moment. It could be provided by horseradish peroxidase injections into pairs of neuronal elements.

3. Axons and axon collaterals

Axons of spinocervical tract neurones nearly always arise from the cell body. Occasionally an axon arises from the base of a first-order dendrite. The initial few hundred micrometres of the axon is usually thin and pursues a tortuous path close to the cell body (Fig. 6.20). This initial part of the axon is generally confined to within ±250 μm of the parent cell body in the sagittal plane. In other words, although it traverses an irregular path, often of some considerable length, in the grey matter near the cell soma, it is confined within a thin transverse sheet of tissue (Fig. 6.20A, B).

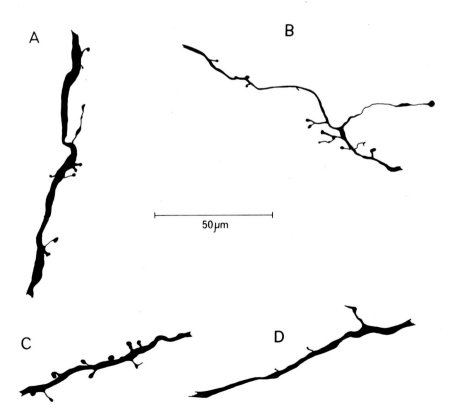

Fig. 6.19. Camera lucida drawings of dendritic spines of spinocervical tract neurones. **A–C** Spines on dorsally directed dendrites. Note the long necks to many spines, some of which are branched. **D** Spines on a ventrolaterally directed dendrite. Note the relatively sparser distribution and the simpler nature of the spines, with most having short necks.

50 μm

The irregular initial course of the axons from neurones in lamina IV was noted by Scheibel and Scheibel (1968). While following this tortuous path the axon becomes thicker before entering the ipsilateral dorso-lateral funiculus, where it turns rostrally (often at almost a right angle: see Figs. 6.17, 6.20B) to ascend the cord.

The great majority of spinocervical tract axons give off collaterals from their first 2–3 mm. The minority (about 14%) show no sign of axon collaterals. All of this latter group responded to hair movement but not to pressure on the skin, and may constitute a special subset of neurones (see below).

Axon collaterals arise as the axon runs in the grey matter close to the parent cell body and also as it ascends in the dorso-lateral funiculus (Fig. 6.20). Up to six collaterals may arise in the grey matter (usually two or three) and up to four have been observed arising in the dorso-lateral funiculus. The most rostral level at which a collateral has been observed is 5.5 mm from the soma (Fig. 6.20A). When *axons* of the spinocervical tract were injected with horseradish peroxidase at upper lumbar levels no collaterals were demonstrable (Brown et al. 1977b). Presumably there is a limit to how far from the cell an axon collateral will arise. Collaterals arise at approximately right angles from the parent axon (Fig. 6.22A).

Most collaterals branch within 500 μm of their origin, though a few may run for more than 1 mm in either the rostral or caudal direction and in either grey or white matter before doing so (Fig. 6.17). After further branching the axon collaterals break up into their terminal arborizations.

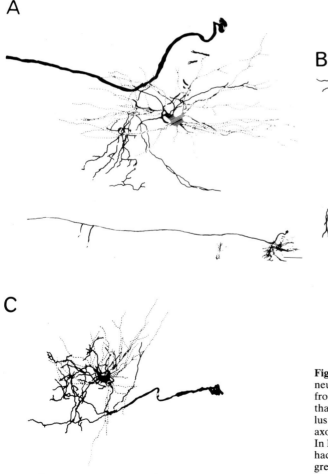

A

C

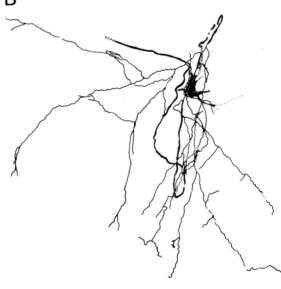

B

Fig. 6.20. Axons and axon collaterals of spinocervical tract neurones. A and B are reconstructed from sagittal sections, C from transverse sections. The neurone in A has four collaterals that arise from the axon as it ascends the dorso-lateral funiculus. Because of the marked tortuosity of its course, the main axon could not be reconstructed as it ran close to the cell body. In B the dendrites have been omitted for clarity. This neurone had six collaterals arising from the main axon as it ran in the grey matter close to the parent cell. In C, lateral is to the right. In this figure axons and collaterals are shown as *continuous lines*, dendrites as *dashed lines*. (Modified from Brown 1976.)

500μm

Collaterals that arise from the initial part of the axon in the grey matter usually distribute their terminal arborizations within about 600 μm of the cell body in the sagittal and transverse planes. Usually the arborizations are situated between the level of the cell body and up to 500 μm deep to it (Fig. 6.21). Axon collateral terminations are infrequent within the dendritic tree of the parent cell. Thus most of the terminal arborization of a spinocervical tract cell's axon collaterals are situated directly under the dendritic tree of the parent neurone, almost like a mirror image of it, in laminae IV, V and sometimes VI.

Collaterals that arise from the axon as it ascends the dorso-lateral funiculus enter the dorsal horn and break up to arborize in a position

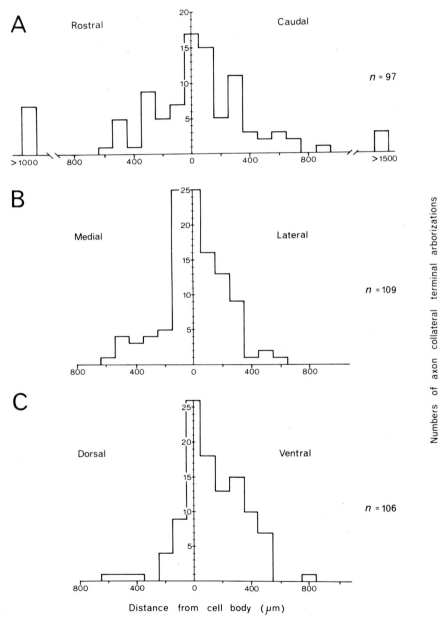

Fig. 6.21. The distribution of spinocervical tract axon collateral terminal arborizations. Each histogram shows the distribution of arborizations with reference to the position of the cell body (*zero* on the *abscissae*). **A** Rostro-caudal distribution; **B** the medio-lateral distribution; **C** the dorso-ventral distribution. Note the preponderance of terminals ventral to the cell body. (From Brown et al. 1977b.)

corresponding, in the sagittal plane, with the positions of the initial collateral arborizations. The somatotopic organization of the dorsal horn into longitudinal columns of neurones having overlapping receptive fields is thereby maintained.

Wall (1967) has suggested that cells in lamina IV excite cells in lamina V, since he observed that the deeper neurones responded to cutaneous afferent fibres some 0.9–2.0 ms later than the more superficial cells. P.B. Brown et al. (1975), however, could find no systematic differences in latency between cells they located in laminae IV and V. But spinocervical tract neurones (laminae III and IV) do send collaterals to terminate in laminae IV and V and their terminal boutons may lie in close association with neuronal somata (see below, and Jankowska et al. 1976). The anatomical substrate for a 'cascade' such as described by Wall (1967) is present.

The demonstration that spinocervical tract neurones have axon collaterals at the local, segmental, level leads to a fundamental change in emphasis when considering the possible functions of the system. Several possibilities now have to be admitted; not only is the spinocervical tract an ascending somatosensory pathway but it also has local actions. A copy of the message that is forwarded to the lateral cervical nucleus is also passed to cells in the dorsal horn. There is no evidence for recurrent effects back onto the spinocervical tract via this local pathway. The question immediately arises as to whether the ascending information should be thought of as a copy of the segmental message rather than vice versa. One is reminded both of Lundberg's (1971) ideas on the possible role of the ventral spinocerebellar tract in comparing and feeding to the brain information about inputs to motoneurones, and of the ideas that various ascending pathways to the cerebellum carry information about the activities of pools of interneurones in the cord (see, for example, Oscarsson 1973).

The need to identify the neurones that receive input from the spinocervical tract is important in the context of the functional role of the axon collaterals. The synaptic actions of the collaterals should be excitatory, assuming that all terminals of a mammalian spinal neurone have similar actions (not necessarily a correct assumption). It is likely that the neurones receiving input from the spinocervical tract are on spinal reflex pathways. Alternatively the neurones could belong to other

ascending pathways, and Jankowska et al. (1979) suggest that neurones with axons ascending the dorsal columns may receive input via the spinocervical tract (see Chapter 8).

4. Synaptic boutons

In well-stained axon collaterals synaptic boutons may be seen on the fine terminal branches. The boutons are of two kinds: disc-like expansions 2.5–4.0 μm in diameter at the ends of collaterals (boutons *terminaux*) (Fig. 6.22B); and a number (six to ten) of elliptical swellings along the last 30–50 μm of collaterals (boutons *en passant*) (Fig. 6.22C).

Jankowska et al. (1976) and J. Rastad (personal communication) have seen, in electron micrographs, boutons of the *en passant* type along the terminal parts of spinocervical tract axon collaterals, where they were in contact with neuronal somata and proximal dendrites. In Fig. 6.22B two boutons *terminaux* are in close apposition to a nerve cell body in lamina V. We have previously published an illustration of two boutons of a spinocervical tract cell apparently on the soma and a dendrite of a Procion-Yellow-stained dorsal horn neurone (see Fig. 1E, F in Snow et al. 1976). Whether such synapses could provide a powerful synaptic drive to the post-synaptic cell seems unlikely—the boutons are not very large and there are few of them.

C. Relationships between the anatomy and the physiology of spinocervical tract neurones

I. Receptive field position and dendritic trees

Relationships between receptive field location and dendritic tree morphology of spinocervical tract neurones might be expected, since the neurones are laid out in a somatotopic map and the spread of a neurone's dendritic tree depends upon its position in the horn. But there are few clear correlations (Brown et al. 1976). The most obvious relationship is for neurones in the lateral third of the dorsal horn. They have dendritic trees restricted in the transverse plane and enormously

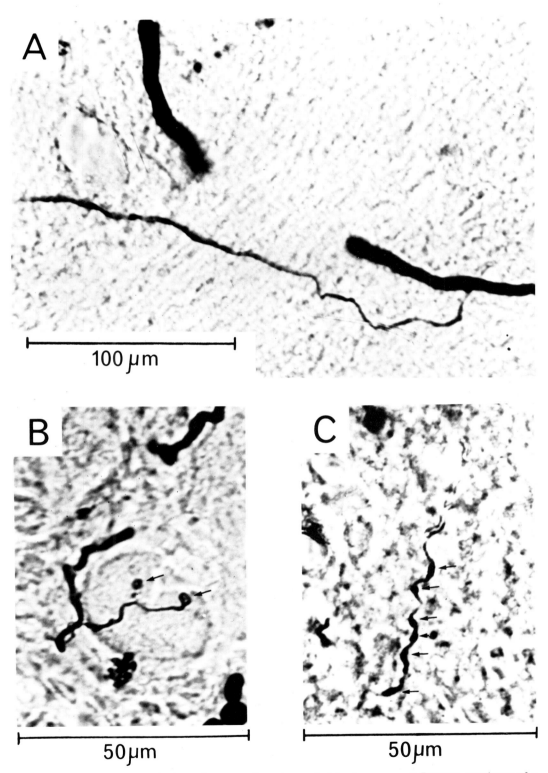

Fig. 6.22. A Collateral arising at a right angle from the axon of a spinocervical tract neurone. **B** Boutons *terminaux* of a spinocervical tract axon collateral (*arrows*). The boutons are close to or on a cell body, which may be seen in this unstained 30-μm thick section. **C** *en passant* type of bouton formation. The very fine axon gives rise periodically to elliptical swellings (*arrows*). (From Brown et al. 1977b.)

elongated in the sagittal plane, and all have receptive fields that include part of the hip, thigh or leg (in segments L-6–S-1).

II. Receptor input and morphology

1. Dendritic trees

There is little, if any, correlation between the dendritic tree morphology of a spinocervical tract neurone and the nature of its input from primary afferent fibres. The dendritic tree morphology depends more on the position of the cell in the dorsal horn than on anything else (see above).

The great majority of spinocervical tract neurones is excited by hair movement and receives monosynaptic excitation from hair follicle afferent fibres. These monosynaptic connexions have to be made in lamina III, which is where the boutons of the afferent fibres are located. The dorsally directed dendrites of spinocervical tract cells run through lamina III and one of their main functions will be to receive this input.

A small minority of spinocervical tract neurones does not receive an input from hair follicle afferent fibres but is excited exclusively from nociceptors (Brown and Franz 1969; Brown 1971; Cervero et al. 1977). These neurones might be expected to have a different dendritic tree morphology. They certainly have well-developed ventrally directed dendrites (Fig. 6.23) and they tend to be situated in the deeper parts of lamina IV (not as deep in the horn as suggested by Bryan et al. 1973). But other neurones that do receive hair follicle inputs may have a similar morphology. Furthermore, it is of interest that the dorsally directed dendrites of the cells receiving only nociceptive input do not penetrate into lamina II where the non-myelinated afferent fibres terminate.

2. Axon collaterals

Although most spinocervical tract neurones have axons that give off collaterals, a minority does not. Those with no axon collaterals were all similar in responding to hair movement but not to pressure and pinch of the skin. Such neurones with no slowly adapting responses to maintained mechanical stimulation are known to receive cutaneous A fibre input but no C fibre input (Brown et al. 1975).

It seems reasonable to conclude that those spinocervical tract neurones with no axon collaterals form a particular subgroup. The position is not absolutely clear, however, as some neurones with axon collaterals also responded only to hair movement and not to pressure or pinch. This result was possibly due to depression of a C fibre input by anaesthetic agents. The appropriate control experiments using unanaesthetized spinal cats have not been performed.

What is clear, however, is that some part of the spinocervical tract is purely for transmitting information towards the brain and has no segmental function. This division of the tract into two component parts, one with and one without segmental functions, is intriguing. If that part with a segmental function is made up of the tract neurones with a C fibre input (as suggested above) then an

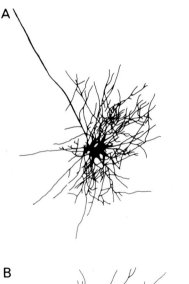

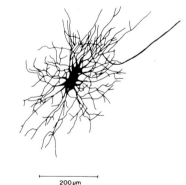

Fig. 6.23. Dendritic trees of spinocervical tract neurones excited exclusively by noxious input (Type IV neurones). Reconstructions are from transverse sections and the neurones had been injected with Procion Yellow. Note the well-developed ventrally directed dendrites on both neurones.

important role for descending control systems becomes apparent. Descending systems are particularly efficacious in switching off the actions of the nociceptive input to spinocervical tract neurones. The descending systems could, therefore, effectively isolate the segmental apparatus from the slowly adapting nociceptive components of spinocervical cell discharges. The responses to hair movement would largely remain but may be much less effective segmentally than they are at the level of the lateral cervical nucleus.

3. Relationships between dendritic trees and receptive fields of adjacent neurones

Spinocervical tract neurones are organized in a sheet across the dorsal horn. In the sheet a map of the hind limb is laid out. Cells are arranged in longitudinal columns with individual neurones in the columns having overlapping receptive fields. In the transverse plane the gradient of the map is very steep. Finally the dendritic trees of spinocervical tract neurones are elongated in the sagittal plane, that is, in the axes of the longitudinal columns of neurones. All of these points have been discussed in detail in the preceding sections.

The present section describes the results of experiments in which adjacent spinocervical tract cells were injected with horseradish peroxidase. Consideration of the points in the previous paragraph led to the following expectations: neurones adjacent in the sagittal plane would have overlapping receptive fields and interdigitating dendritic trees; neurones adjacent in the transverse plane would have either (1) non-overlapping receptive fields and dendritic trees that did not interdigitate but which were contained within their own private volume of cord, or (2) overlapping receptive fields and interdigitating dendritic trees. In these experiments (Brown et al. 1980c) cells were defined as adjacent if their cell bodies were contained within a single 50-μm thick section or were in two adjacent serial sections of 50 μm thickness: that is, the cells were within ±50 μm of each other in either the sagittal or transverse planes.

The results from these experiments were particularly clear-cut. Fourteen pairs of neurones were stained: five sagittal pairs and nine transverse pairs. All five sagittal pairs had receptive fields that either overlapped (two pairs) or were contained one within the other (three pairs), and all five pairs of neurones had interdigitating dendritic trees. Two sagittal pairs of neurones are shown in Figs. 6.24 and 6.25, where the intertwining nature of the dendritic trees is apparent. Even when the cell bodies of a pair of neurones were as far apart as 660 μm there was dendritic interdigitation and receptive field containment (Fig. 6.25). For the nine pairs of neurones adjacent in the transverse plane the situation was more complicated, but equally clear. Three pairs had non-overlapping receptive fields and their dendritic trees did not interdigitate. With the somata of the pair as close together as 135 μm the dendritic trees could still be contained within their own private volume of dorsal horn with no interdigitation, and no receptive field overlap (Fig. 6.26). Six transverse pairs of spinocervical tract neurones had interdigitating dendritic trees. In four of these pairs the receptive fields were accessible for complete examination; they either overlapped (two pairs) or one field of the pair was contained within the other (two pairs), as shown in Fig. 6.27.

These experiments show that when the dendritic trees of adjacent spinocervical tract neurones interdigitate then their receptive fields overlap completely or in part. Conversely, when the fields occupy areas of skin that do not overlap then the cells' dendritic trees will occupy quite separate volumes of dorsal horn.

With the information now available on the average spreads of the dendritic trees of spinocervical tract neurones in different parts of the dorsal horn, together with that on the density of the neurones in the lumbosacral cord, some predictions may be made. On average the dendritic trees of spinocervical tract neurones will interdigitate with one another if (1) the cell bodies are separated in the sagittal plane by up to 750 μm in

---

Overleaf (Page 102)
Fig. 6.24. Dendritic trees and receptive fields of adjacent ▷ spinocervical tract neurones. Reconstructions of a pair of neurones adjacent in the sagittal plane are shown. The dendritic trees interdigitate and the receptive field of the neurone to the left of the figure is contained within that of the neurone on the right. (From Brown et al. 1980c.)

(Page 103)
Fig. 6.25. Dendritic trees and receptive fields of adjacent ▷ spinocervical tract neurones. These two neurones were 660 μm apart in the sagittal plane but their dendritic trees interdigitated and the field of the neurone on the right was contained within that of the neurone on the left. (From Brown et al. 1980c.)

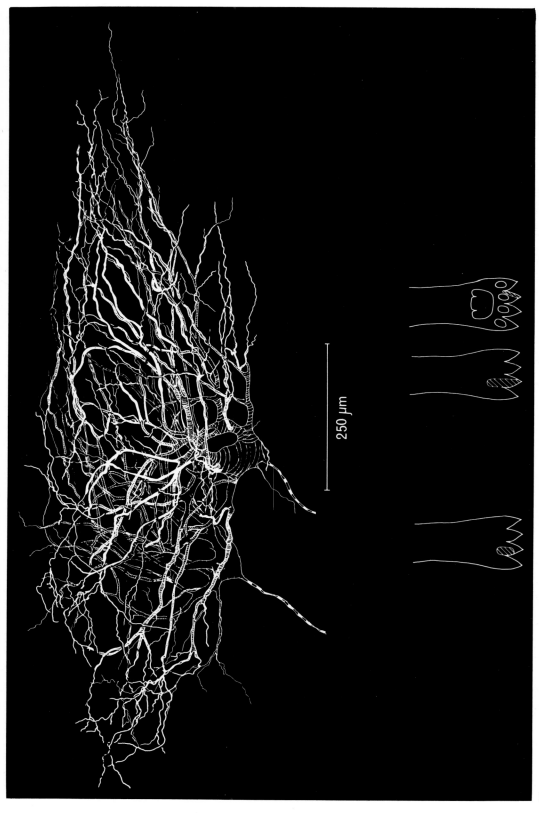

250 µm

Fig. 6.24.

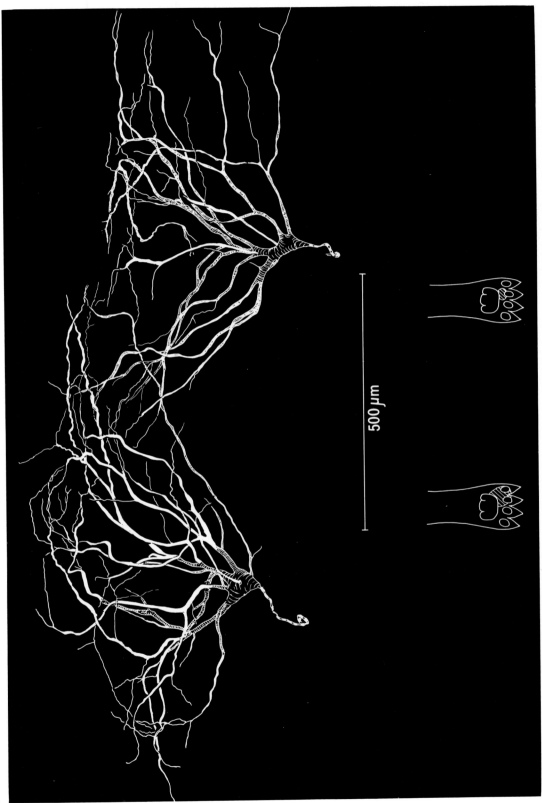

Fig. 6.25.

the medial third of the horn, by 11 000 μm in the middle third and by 18 000 μm in the lateral third; (2) the somata are separated in the transverse plane by up to 325 μm, 425 μm and 325 μm for the medial, middle and lateral thirds of the lumbosacral cord respectively. The situation is complicated in the transverse plane, however, by further possible restrictions on the spread of dendritic trees. Thus hair follicle afferent terminal arborizations, which supply input to the neurones, form sagittally running sheets of about the same width as the dendritic trees. Where two sheets run side by side it is possible that tract neurones sample from only one of the sheets. Certainly, spinocervical tract neurones very close together in the transverse plane (135 μm, see above) may have dendritic trees that do not interdigitate. The limits given above should, on average, hold; cells farther apart than these limits should have non-interdigitating dendritic trees.

It is possible to estimate the maximum number of spinocervical tract neurones that will have dendritic trees interdigitating with a given spinocervical tract neurone. From the medial to lateral thirds of the horn in L-6–S-1 the maximum numbers are about 25, 80 and 85 respectively. The differences between the thirds reflect the spreads of the dendritic trees not the cell densities. The numbers will fall off quite sharply in more rostral and caudal parts of the lumbosacral enlargement due to the reduction in cell density that takes place. The greater part of dendritic interdigitation takes place in the longitudinal axis of the cord due to the elongation of the trees in the sagittal plane. It is obvious how the longitudinal columns of spinocervical tract neurones with overlapping receptive fields are built up.

4. Relationships between dendritic trees and hair follicle afferent fibre collaterals

One unexpected correlation between the dendritic trees of spinocervical tract neurones and hair follicle afferent fibre collaterals is that both the longitudinal spread of the trees and the intercollateral spacing depend on their position in the dorsal horn. Furthermore, they are both of the same order of magnitude. Thus in the medial horn dendritic trees spread about 770 μm in the sagittal plane and the intercollateral spacing of hair follicle afferents is about 720 μm on the average. In the lateral horn the values are about 1800 μm and 1200 μm respectively.

This result has an important implication. If there is no systematic gradient across the width of the dorsal horn in the numbers of neurones relative to the numbers of hair follicle afferent fibres, then the convergence factor between hair follicle afferents and spinocervical tract neurones will be constant. The interest of this lies in a suggestion made by Vierck (1973) that the ability to distinguish the size of a passively applied disc could be performed either by edge detection or by counting the number of primary afferent fibres activated. Vierck suggested that the first strategy might be used by the dorsal column pathway, where surround (lateral) inhibition is highly developed, and the second strategy might be used by pathways ascending the dorso-lateral funiculus (spinocervical tract). A system of neurones receiving excitatory input from a set of primary afferent fibres with the same convergence factor for all the neurones would reflect, by the number of neurones active, the number of primary afferent fibres active. That is, it could count the number of receptive fields stimulated.

The total sagittal extent of a sheet of terminals from a single hair follicle afferent fibre is unknown. In Chapter 2 a suggestion of at least 1.5–2.0 cm was made (but see Wall and Werman 1976; Imai and Kusama 1969). Values of up to 3–4 cm may be more realistic. In L-7–S-1 a 1-cm sheet of hair follicle arborizations will contain or be dorsal to the somata of 50–75 spinocervical tract neurones; a 3–4-cm sheet will be similarly related to 100–150 cells (Brown et al. 1980c). Therefore, the divergence factor from a single hair follicle afferent to the neurones of the spinocervical tract may be as large as 1 to 100–150. This factor might be larger if neurones 'off beam' of the sheet of terminal arborizations send their dendrites into it.

Divergence factors of 1 to 100–150 mean that a single hair follicle afferent might contact as many as a fifth to an eighth of the total population of spinocervical tract neurones in the lumbosacral enlargement of one side. This seems a very high

Fig. 6.26. Dendritic trees and receptive fields of adjacent ▷ spinocervical tract neurones. Reconstructions of the trees of a pair of neurones adjacent in the transverse plane are shown. The cell bodies were only 135 μm apart and yet the dendritic trees did not interdigitate and there was no receptive field overlap. The receptive fields are shown at the bottom of the figure in positions relative to their neurone. (From Brown et al. 1980c.)

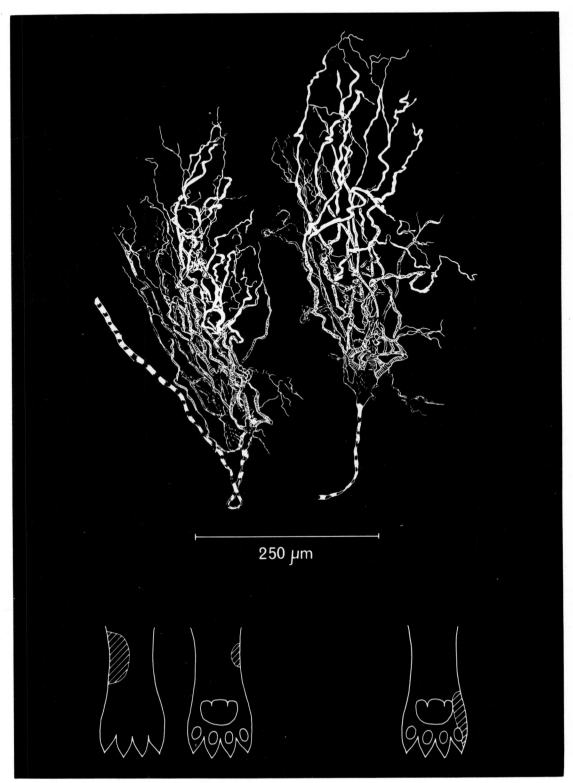

250 μm

Fig. 6.26.

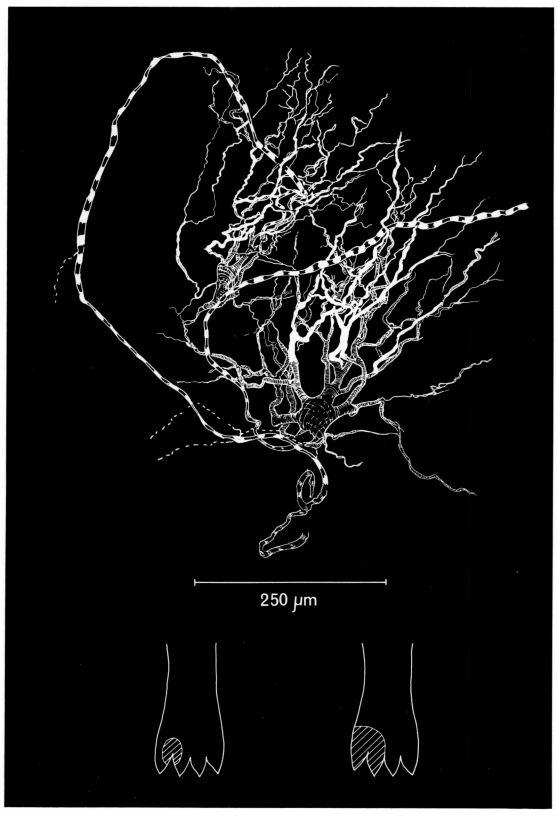

250 μm

Fig. 6.27.

proportion. But other indirect evidence from receptive field maps of spinocervical tract cells (such as Figs. 6.13, 6.14) supports this estimation.

The important point that emerges from the above analysis is that movement of hairs on, say, one or two toes, or the dorsum of the foot, may potentially cause the firing of a large proportion of the total spinocervical tract cell population, certainly an eighth to a fifth of them. The spinocervical tract is thus superbly equipped to monitor the occurrence of hair movement, and also, but to a much lesser extent, to localize it. This conclusion, taken with other evidence of (1) extremely secure synaptic coupling from hair follicle afferent fibres, (2) the more even distribution of receptive field representation in the spinocervical tract compared with the dorsal column-lemniscothalamic system, supports our earlier suggestion (Brown et al. 1973) that the spinocervico-lemniscothalamic system may be concerned with timing the occurrence of hair movement.

◁ **Fig. 6.27.** Dendritic trees and receptive fields of adjacent spinocervical tract neurones. This pair of neurones, adjacent in the transverse plane, had interdigitating dendritic trees and, as shown below, overlapping cutaneous receptive fields. (From Brown et al. 1980c.)

7 Relationships between hair follicle afferent fibres and spinocervical tract neurones

In the previous chapter some aspects of the relationships between hair follicle afferent fibres and spinocervical tract neurones were discussed on the basis of indirect evidence. It was concluded that, in the cat's lumbosacral spinal cord, between 50 and 150 spinocervical tract neurones might have their somata and/or their dendrites within the sagittal column of terminal arborizations from a single hair follicle afferent fibre, and that a single hair follicle afferent fibre might, therefore, contact as many as 12 to 20% of the total population of spinocervical tract cells. Also, it was shown that the somatotopic map formed by the set of spinocervical tract neurones is, essentially, a reflexion of the organization of the collateral arborizations of hair follicle afferent fibres.

To provide a fuller understanding of how spinocervical tract neurones sample from a population of hair follicle afferent fibres more direct evidence is needed. For example, it is generally thought that these neurones do not have a subliminal fringe to their excitatory receptive field (Wall 1960; Brown 1971; but see Lundberg and Oscarsson 1961). If this is indeed the case, then it is pertinent to ask how connexions made between hair follicle afferent fibres from the periphery of the receptive field compare with those from the centre, in both position and number. The absence of a subliminal fringe might be due to an even distribution of synapses (over the receptive surface of the neurone) from hair follicle afferent fibres innervating all parts of the receptive field. Hongo and Koike (1975), however, have demonstrated differences in transmission characteristics between hair follicle afferent fibres and spinocervical tract neurones according to the position of the primary afferent's field within that of the neurone. They suggested that afferent fibres with centrally located fields should have synapses on the soma and more proximal dendrites and that there may be more of them (or they may

have more powerful actions), whereas afferent fibres from the peripheral part of the neurone's receptive field should have more distally located synapses and fewer of them (and possibly with weaker actions). A related question concerns the arrangement of contacts upon the dendritic trees: if a single hair follicle afferent fibre makes contact with only a single major dendrite and its branches, then strategically placed inhibitory synapses (at the base of the major dendrite) could selectively inhibit input from that afferent fibre. There is no electrophysiological evidence for such an arrangement on spinocervical tract neurones: monosynaptic connexions between hair follicle afferent fibres and the neurones seem particularly free from interference (Brown 1971; Brown et al. 1973, 1975; Brown and Martin 1973).

In an attempt to address problems such as these we (Brown and Noble 1979, 1981) have performed more direct experiments. Single hair follicle afferent fibres were injected with horseradish peroxidase and the lumbosacral cord was then searched for spinocervical tract neurones whose receptive fields contained or were just separate from the field of the afferent fibre. The neurones were impaled and injected with the enzyme. The results from these experiments are described below. The results were very clear and only one factor made interpretation difficult in some instances: this was the lack of contrast between the reaction product in the hair follicle arborization and the neuronal soma and dendrites, especially proximal, thick dendrites. This led to a probable under-estimation of the numbers of possible contacts between the two stained elements.

A. Anatomy of the relationships between hair follicle afferent arborizations and spinocervical tract neurones

I. Relationships where the afferent fibre and the neurone had receptive fields on different areas of skin: the negative results

When the receptive fields of the two elements (afferent fibre and central neurone) were located on separate areas of skin no contacts were observed between them, even when the fields were closely adjacent. Usually in this situation the terminal arborizations of the collaterals of the hair follicle afferent fibre were contained in a quite separate volume of cord to that of the spinocervical tract neurone's dendritic tree; sometimes there was overlap between the two, but no contacts were observed.

In recent years there has been considerable interest in the idea of 'non-functioning' or 'silent' synapses (see Mark 1970, 1974a, b). Experiments on the dorsal horn of the spinal cord (Merrill and Wall 1972; Basbaum and Wall 1976; Wall 1977; Devor et al. 1977; Devor and Wall 1978; Mendell et al. 1978) have provided evidence that such synapses might occur here and that they may be revealed under certain circumstances, e.g. after the removal of more powerful synaptic inputs by section of appropriate dorsal roots. The evidence, however, is equivocal with regard to whether previously 'silent' synapses are revealed or whether new connexions are made following denervation. Most of the apparently new connexions upon activation have latencies indicative of polysynaptic pathways, although Mendell et al. (1978) did demonstrate some short-latency effects that could have been within the monosynaptic range. It seems likely that some of the connexions revealed following partial denervation of a neurone are exposed because of the increased sensitivity of such neurones, so that inputs that normally produce only a relatively small component of excitation become sufficiently effective to cause firing. There are, however, sufficient pieces of evidence to allow the conclusion that some dorsal horn neurones receive inputs that, in the usual physiological preparations, do not cause the cell to fire,

and these inputs may be revealed by both acute and chronic denervation (and also by pharmacological methods that increase cell excitability: Wall 1977).

It has become of importance that the spinal cord neurones exhibiting such connexions be identified. The phenomenon has similarities with effects that can often be seen with intracellular recording from dorsal horn neurones when the membrane potential has deteriorated somewhat. In these circumstances areas of receptive field that previously only produced excitatory postsynaptic potentials upon stimulation now lead to action potential discharges (A. G. Brown and R. E. W. Fyffe, unpublished observations). These effects are commonly seen in dorsal horn neurones that send their axons into the dorsal columns (see Chapter 8); such cells have well-marked subliminal fringes to their receptive fields. But subliminal fringes have not been described for spinocervical tract neurones.

The absence of synaptic contacts between hair follicle afferent fibres and spinocervical tract neurones when their receptive fields are on quite separate areas of skin is, therefore, not surprising. Such contacts might be present between hair follicle afferent fibres and dorsal horn neurones with pronounced subliminal fringes, such as the neurones with axons projecting to the dorsal columns. The 'silent' synapses revealed by Wall and his co-workers on dorsal horn neurones are from afferent fibres with receptive fields some distance away from the natural receptive field of the neurone, not from surrounding skin. They may be demonstrated by electrical stimulation of distant skin (Mendell et al. 1979) in 14% to 79% of neurones with 'lamina IV and V' characteristics. Unfortunately Mendell et al. made no attempts to determine the identities of their neurones in terms of axonal projections or the individual types of afferent unit exciting them. The vast majority of 'silent' or 'long-ranging' afferent connexions demonstrated by Wall's group have had the properties of polysynaptic linkages. Double-staining experiments such as those described in the present chapter would not provide any information about these connexions. More direct evidence is urgently required on the interesting phenomena described by Wall's group.

II. Relationships where the receptive field of the neurone contained the field of the afferent fibre: the positive results

When the receptive field of the hair follicle afferent fibre was contained within that of the spinocervical tract neurone (and the two elements were satisfactorily stained) then terminal arborizations from the axon were always, in part at least, within the dendritic tree of the cell. Contacts were always observed between the two.

1. Positions of terminal arborizations of afferent fibres and dendritic trees of neurones

As described in Chapter 2, hair follicle afferent collaterals form 'flame-shaped arbors' in the spinal cord. These are the end-on views, seen in transverse sections, of long columns or sheets of a continuous arborization produced by the collaterals from a single axon. The arborizations, although present throughout lamina III and most or all of lamina IV, carry synaptic boutons only in lamina III and the most dorsal parts of IV (and occasionally the deepest part of II). It is only in these laminae that contacts between hair follicle axons and spinocervical tract cells can take place. For the vast majority (95%) of the neurones these contacts will be made on dorsally directed dendrites. When the soma is in lamina III (25%) or the most dorsal part of lamina IV then contacts will be possible on the soma and the more proximal parts of ventrally directed dendrites (see Figs. 7.2, 7.4).

The widths of hair follicle afferent arborizations and spinocervical tract neuronal dendritic trees are similar in extent, if anything the collateral arborizations being rather thinner (150–400 µm compared with 200–550 µm: see Chapters 2 and 6). It is of interest to ask whether the two are always in register in the transverse plane or whether they may be out of register. In fact none of our sample of ten pairs showed complete coincidence of the two elements: there was always overlap between the two but part of the dendritic tree always occupied a region of the dorsal horn that contained no endings from the afferent fibre (see Fig. 7.6). It will be remembered (Chapter 6) that between one-third and one-half of spinocervical tract neurones adjacent in the transverse plane of the cord have interdigitating dendrites and overlapping receptive fields. It may

be concluded that where a spinocervical tract neurone sends its dendrites into only part of the transverse extent of a hair follicle collateral arborization and makes contacts with it, then any adjacent spinocervical tract cell that also sends its dendrites into that arborization to make contacts will also have dendrites that interdigitate with the dendrites of the other neurone. Adjacent spinocervical tract cells with non-interdigitating dendritic trees have receptive fields on separate areas of skin: they would not both make contacts with the same hair follicle afferent fibre. This conclusion is illustrated in Fig. 7.1.

2. Number of afferent collaterals distributed to each cell

There is a striking correlation between the intercollateral spacings on hair follicle afferent fibres and the longitudinal spread of dendritic trees of spinocervical tract cells. The two sets of values vary according to the transverse locations of the terminal arborizations and the dendritic trees. Thus in the medial part of the dorsal horn collaterals arise from hair follicle afferents about every 720 µm on the average and spinocervical tract cell dendritic trees are about 770 µm in rostro-caudal extent; in the lateral horn both values are about 1200 µm. It is tempting to speculate that when connexions are made between a hair follicle afferent and a spinocervical tract cell they are all made by a single collateral from the axon.

Examination of our material (ten stained pairs with contacts) revealed that this suggestion is likely to be correct. There was no evidence for a single neurone receiving contacts from more than one collateral of a hair follicle afferent. Even where collaterals were closer together than the average and more than one ran through the dendritic tree of a neurone, only one of the collaterals had terminals on the spinocervical tract neurone. It will be shown that a similar result holds for connexions between Ia afferent fibres and motoneurones (Chapter 14). This sort of arrangement may well turn out to be a general principle of nervous organization in the vertebrate and is reminiscent of the usual arrangement between a motor axon and an extrafusal muscle fibre in the adult, although in this instance a single postsynaptic cell (muscle fibre) only receives innervation from a single pre-synaptic neurone (motoneurone).

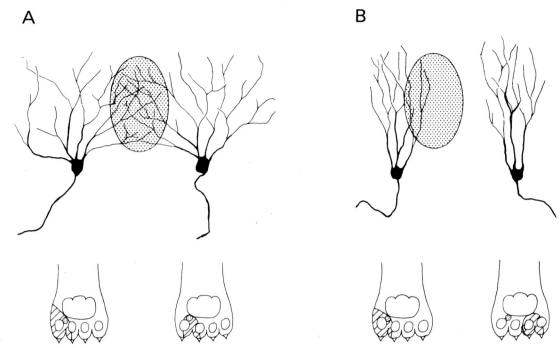

Fig. 7.1. Diagrammatic representation of the relations between dendritic trees of adjacent spinocervical tract neurones and the terminal arborizations of hair follicle afferent fibres. In **A** the dendritic trees interdigitate and the track cells' receptive fields overlap; the hair follicle afferent contacts both dendritic trees. In **B** there is no dendritic interdigitation and no receptive field overlap for the track cells; the hair follicle afferent fibre contacts only the cell on the left.

3. Contacts between afferent fibres and neurones

In our material all presumed contacts between hair follicle afferent fibres and spinocervical tract neurones have been identified by light microscopy. Obviously this limits the strength of the conclusions that may be drawn. Only electron microscopical examination would provide unequivocal results as to whether a particular structure has all the necessary features for identification as a synapse—and then no information about its function would be forthcoming. There is no doubt, however, that useful results may be obtained with the light microscope, especially with regard to the general plan of organization of the contacts, their numbers and position. In examining our histological material we took particular care not to identify an apparent contact as a synapse unless (1) the axonal element showed a discrete bouton-like swelling, and (2) there appeared to be contact between the swelling and the neurone's soma or dendrites. It is highly likely that by adopting these criteria the number of contacts was under-estimated. Any such under-estimation should not affect the general conclusions.

a) *Numbers and positions of synapses and their relationships to receptive field positions.* The clearest correlations were observed between the numbers and sites of hair follicle synaptic boutons upon spinocervical tract neurones and the relative positions of their receptive fields. When the primary afferent fibre had a receptive field near the centre of the tract cell's field there were many contacts (at least 40 and 60 respectively in the pairs shown in Figs. 7.2–7.5) and these contacts were on more proximal parts of the dendritic tree. On the other hand, when the primary afferent fibre had its receptive field located near the periphery of the tract cell's field then there were fewer contacts (between 2 and 13: Figs. 7.6, 7.7) and they were situated on more distal parts of the dendritic tree.

For the pair shown in Figs. 7.2 and 7.3 the receptive field of the spinocervical tract cell was on the plantar surface of toes 2 and 3; the hair follicle afferent fibre had its receptive field at the centre of the neurone's field. The spinocervical tract neurone, rather unusually, had very well-developed ventrally directed dendrites and it was onto two of these and their branches that the

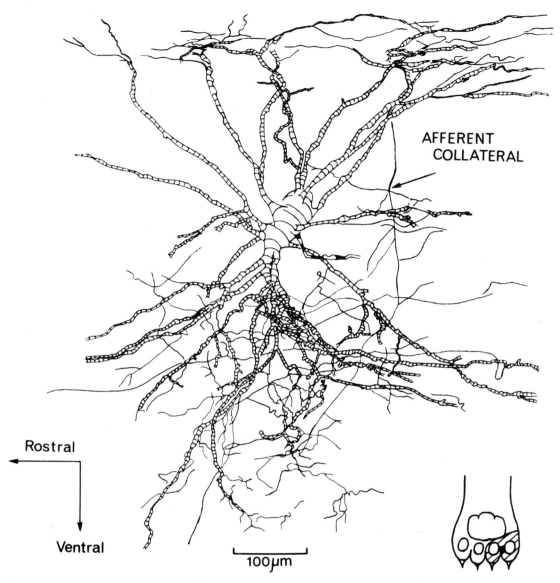

Fig. 7.2. Reconstructions, from sagittal sections, of a spinocervical tract neurone and part of a hair follicle afferent collateral that makes contact with it. As shown by the inset figurine the receptive field of the hair follicle axon was centrally placed in the field of the tract neurone. Synaptic contacts (see Fig. 7.3) were located on the proximal parts of the ventrally directed dendrites. The neurone was situated in lamina III and the contacts were made close to the III–IV border. (From Brown and Noble 1981.)

Opposite page (top)
Fig. 7.3. Photomicrographs and reconstructions of contacts made between a hair follicle afferent fibre and a spinocervical tract ▷ neurone. The afferent–neurone pair is that shown in Fig. 7.2. In the photomicrographs the *arrows* indicate sites of synaptic contacts: a, fine axonal branches, s, dendritic spines. Note the 'climbing' type of contacts on the dendrites and, in **B**, contacts on dendritic spines. (From Brown and Noble 1981.)

Opposite page (bottom)
Fig. 7.4. Reconstructions, from sagittal sections, of a spinocervical tract neurone and part of a hair follicle afferent collateral ▷ arborization. The afferent's receptive field was centrally placed in that of the neurone and about 60 contacts were identified between the two. The small *arrows* and *numbers* indicate sites of contacts, some of which are shown in more detail on Fig. 7.5. In this afferent–neurone pair the synaptic contacts were rather widely spread on the dendritic tree. (From Brown and Noble 1981.)

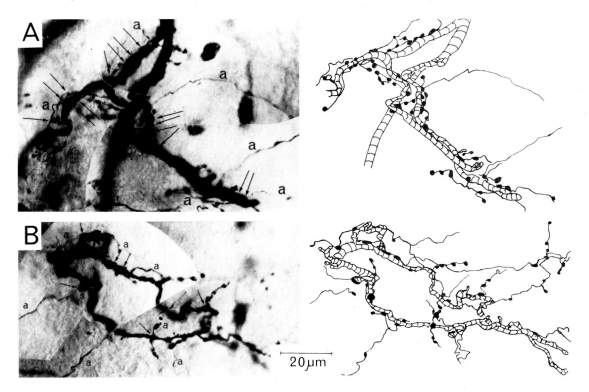

Fig. 7.3.

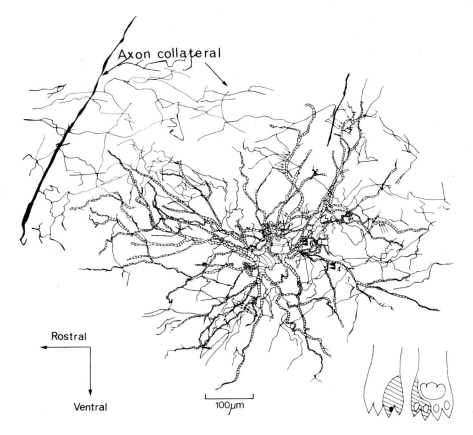

Fig. 7.4.

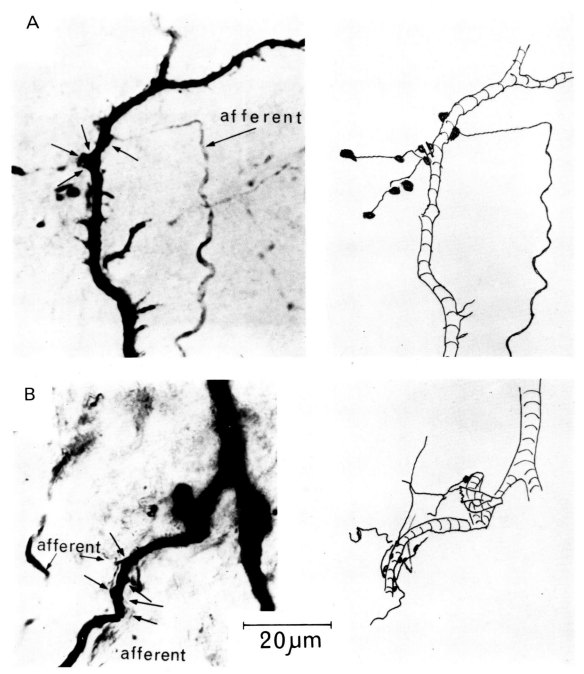

Fig. 7.5. Details of some of the contacts between the afferent–neurone pair shown in Fig. 7.4. In the photomicrographs the *arrows* indicate sites of contacts. (From Brown and Noble 1981.)

contacts were made. The contacts were from within about 20–30 μm of the soma out to about 200 μm on dendrites up to the fourth order. At least 40 contacts were observed.

Another afferent–neurone pair with the pri-

mary afferent's field centrally located is shown in Figs. 7.4 and 7.5. The tract cell had a field on both dorsal and ventral surfaces of the lateral two toes and adjoining parts of the foot; the hair follicle afferent fibre had its field near the geometrical centre of the neurone's field. About 60 contacts were counted between these elements and they were spread rather widely on five main dendrites and their branches: four of the dendrites were directed dorsally and caudally, and one was directed ventrally (again there was a rather well-developed ventral dendritic system). Contacts were located on dendrites of the first to the sixth order at distances from about 30 μm to about 500 μm from the soma.

The afferent–neurone pairs shown in Figs. 7.6 and 7.7, in contrast, had primary afferent fields situated near the periphery of the neurones' fields. In all of these pairs (and in those not illustrated) there were fewer contacts between the two (between 2 and 13) and they were situated at least 200 μm from the cell body and could be as far as 800 μm from it.

b) *Types and arrangements of synaptic contacts.* In addition to the correlations between numbers and locations of hair follicle synapses on spinocervical tract cells on the one hand and the positions of the receptive fields on the other, there were also correlations between the types and arrangements of the synapses and the positions of the fields. The main type of synaptic arrangement in all pairs was the 'climbing-type' of association where a series of boutons *en passant* made contacts along the length of a segment of dendrite. The 'crossing-over type' of arrangement, where the terminal axon runs essentially at right angles to a series of dendrites, giving boutons to each, was seen but was much less common.

The 'climbing' type of synaptic organization was extremely common where the hair follicle axon's field was centrally located in the tract neurone's field (Figs. 7.3, 7.5). As many as seven boutons from an individual fine branch of the terminal arborization could be arranged along a segment of dendrite some 25 μm in length, and other fine axonal branches often gave other 'climbing-type' boutons to the same branch in close proximity (Fig. 7.3). Another feature of these pairs of elements was also common: this was a 'climbing type' of arrangement of synapses running along a dendrite, but with the individual boutons being borne on short branches, or stalks, given off a fine axonal branch rather in the manner of the rungs of a ladder (Fig. 7.8).

For neuronal pairs where the axon's field was peripherally located in the tract cell's field, synaptic contacts were sometimes single and isolated from other contacts between members of the pair (Fig. 7.6). More usually there were small groups of two to four boutons spaced closely together on a dendrite (Fig. 7.7B,D). Boutons *terminaux* were more common for these pairs.

Spinocervical tract neurones are well endowed with dendritic spines and an obvious question to ask is whether hair follicle afferent fibres make contact upon the spines. Contacts upon spines were, indeed, commonly observed, the boutons apparently forming a cap on the head of the spine in some instances (Fig. 7.3A) or just contacting part of the head in others (Fig. 7.3B). The proportion of contacts upon spines was, however, very small in comparison with the numbers contacting the dendrites at other places. Contacts upon dendritic spines were, in our small sample, only seen in those pairs of elements with a centrally located hair follicle receptive field and several tens of synaptic contacts between the two. It may be tentatively concluded that the spine synapses might be particularly efficacious in producing excitatory responses.

4. Conclusions

Figure 7.9 summarizes the general organization of the hair follicle afferent–spinocervical tract cell relationship. In addition to illustrating the correlations described above between numbers and positions of contacts and the positions of the two receptive fields, the diagrams also show how the contacts are distributed to different primary dendrites and their branches. In general, only a small fraction of the primary dendrites had branches receiving contacts from a single hair follicle afferent, even when the number of contacts was relatively large. For the most widely spread set of contacts (that shown in Fig. 7.4) five of the 11 primary dendrites had branches upon which contacts were made. Usually only two or three dendrites were involved in synaptic contact with a single hair follicle afferent fibre.

Obviously there is some grouping of the contacts made by a single hair follicle afferent fibre upon the dendritic tree of a single spinocervical tract neurone. Strategically placed inhibitory synapses, at the bases of the appropriate dendrites, would be extremely effective in reducing the effects of input from such single fibres. But, as mentioned at the beginning of this chapter, there is no electrophysiological evidence that such mechanisms occur: monosynaptic exci-

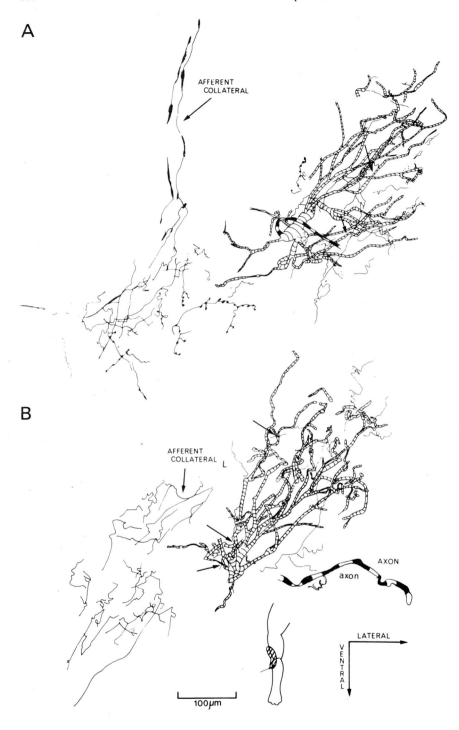

Fig. 7.6. Reconstructions, from serial transverse sections, of a spinocervical tract neurone and collateral arborizations from a hair follicle afferent fibre. The receptive field of the afferent was peripherally located in the field of the neurone as shown in the figurine drawing. Each part of the figure (**A, B**) shows a half of the cell's dendritic tree. Only five contacts were observed and their sites are indicated by *arrows*. (From Brown and Noble 1981.)

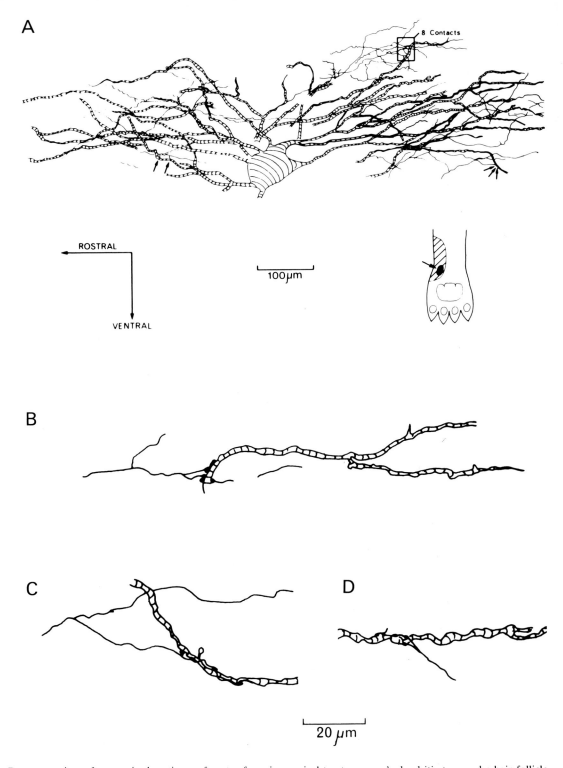

Fig. 7.7. A Reconstructions, from sagittal sections, of parts of a spinocervical tract neurone's dendritic tree and a hair follicle afferent collateral arborization. In this pair the hair follicle axon had a receptive field located peripherally in the neurone's field (see the figurine) and the contacts were few and located peripherally on the dendrites (indicated by *box* and *arrows*).

B–D Details of some of the contacts made between this pair of neuronal elements. The contacts are clustered together at discrete parts of the dendrites. (From Brown and Noble 1981.)

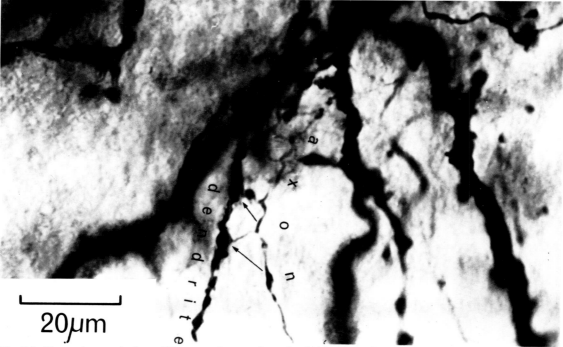

Fig. 7.8. Photomicrograph, from 100-μm section, to show the 'ladder-like' effect between a terminal axon of a hair follicle afferent fibre and the synaptic boutons distributed to a spinocervical tract cell's dendrite. The boutons appear to be at the ends of the 'rungs' of the ladder (*arrows*). (From Brown and Noble 1981.)

tation of the cells is very resistant to interference and no subliminal fringe can be demonstrated.

The results described in this section have provided anatomical support for the electrophysiological observations and suggestions made by Hongo and Koike (1975). These authors stimulated single hair follicle afferent fibres and recorded intracellularly from spinocervical tract neurones. They noted that when the primary afferent fibre had its field centrally located in the neurone's field the excitatory post-synaptic potentials were larger and had a faster rise time than when the field was peripherally located. They suggested that the former result was due to a larger number of synapses more proximally located in comparison with the latter. This is indeed the case.

The results raise a number of problems for an understanding both of the function of the system in the adult animal and of the mechanisms involved in the formation of the contacts. As described above, the absence of any obvious subliminal fringe implies that movement of hairs in the periphery of the tract cell's receptive field is as effective, or nearly so, as movement of hairs near the centre of the field. And yet hair follicle

afferents from the peripheral sites make fewer and more distal contacts upon the cell. Hongo and Koike (1975) showed that single fibre excitatory post-synaptic potentials evoked from peripheral locations were of smaller amplitude and slower rise time than those evoked from the centre. This apparent paradox might be resolved if it is realized that stimulation of a single hair follicle afferent fibre is an almost impossible natural event: movement of even a single hair will excite several hair follicle afferent fibres since single follicles are innervated by several axons and the resulting temporal and spatial summation will probably be sufficient to fire the neurone. Even so, careful receptive field stimulation might reveal differences in efficacy between central and peripheral locations. There may also be greater convergence onto spinocervical tract neurones from the periphery of their fields.

The number of hair follicle afferents converging upon a single spinocervical tract cell is unknown. Since a single hair follicle afferent may contact a large minority of the total population of spinocervical tract neurones in the lumbosacral enlargement (see Chapter 6) it must be assumed that the convergence factor is large, perhaps

A

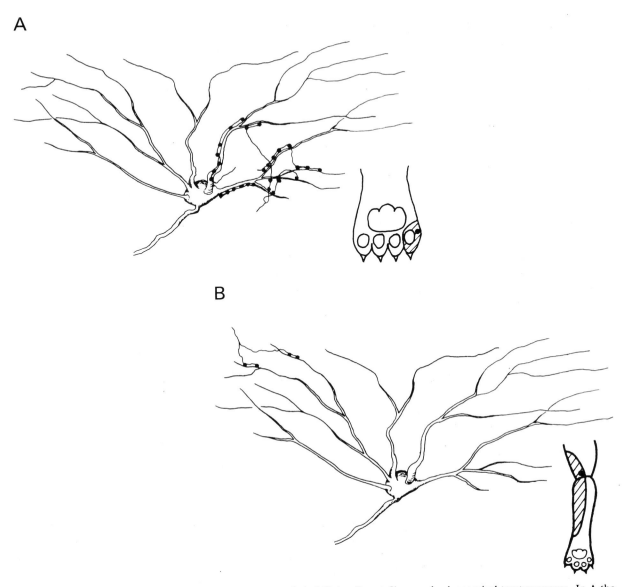

B

Fig. 7.9. Summary diagrams of the relationships between hair follicle afferent fibres and spinocervical tract neurones. In **A** the primary afferent has a receptive field centrally located in the neurone's field and contacts are made on the proximal dendrites (and soma). There are many contacts, usually limited to one or two primary dendrites and their branches. In the drawing 28 contacts are shown but there may be many more. In **B** the afferent fibre has a receptive field peripherally located in the neurone's field and there are few contacts, located on distal dendrites.

several hundred to one. And yet the present results imply a highly ordered organization of the contacts, with grouping of synapses on particular dendrites, and localization and number of synapses dependent on receptive field location.

The hair follicle afferent–spinocervical tract cell system should provide a useful model with which to study the little-known factors that determine how synaptic contacts are formed and maintained.

8 Neurones with axons ascending the dorsal columns

The dorsal columns (posterior columns, posterior funiculi, fasciculus gracilis and fasciculus cuneaatus) are commonly considered simply from the point of view that they contain ascending axons of primary afferent fibres whose cell bodies are located in the dorsal root ganglia. This view is manifestly incorrect. Indeed it has been known since the last century (Edinger 1889) that some dorsal column fibres arise from neurones in the grey matter of the spinal cord. Although some of the non-primary axons in the dorsal columns have short axons, ascending and descending for only a segment or two, some have been recognized for many years as ascending as far as the dorsal column nuclei (Rothmann 1899; Münzer and Wiener 1910). Other long axons connect the spinal enlargements with each other (Barilari and Kuypers 1969) and in rodents a part of the corticospinal tract descends through the dorsal columns (King 1910; Ranson 1913b, 1914b; Simpson 1914, 1915a, b; Reveley 1915; Douglas and Baar 1950). Finally, it has recently been shown that some neurones in the dorsal column nuclei send their axons down the dorsal columns (Dart 1971; Dart and Gordon 1973; Burton and Loewy 1977; Armstrong et al. 1979).

Recent interest in non-primary ascending fibres in the dorsal columns stems from the reports of Uddenberg (1968a,b), who recorded from single fibres in the cuneate fascicle excited from cutaneous and deep nerves of the forelimb. This was soon followed by a similar demonstration of an ascending pathway from the hind limb running in the gracile fascicle (Petit et al. 1969; Petit 1971; Angaut-Petit 1975a, b). At about the same time the non-primary axonal projection through the dorsal columns was re-investigated by anatomical degeneration techniques (Rustioni 1973, 1974) and the cells of origin were soon demonstrated by retrograde transport of horseradish peroxidase (Rustioni and Kaufman 1977).

Non-primary axons ascending the dorsal columns do not all project to the dorsal column nuclei. It is likely that there are projections to the nucleus intercalatus, nucleus Z, vestibular nuclei, the external cuneate nucleus, the solitary nucleus, area postrema and the tegmental region (Pompeiano and Brodal 1957; Brodal and Angaut 1967; Morest 1967; Rustioni 1973, 1974; Rustioni and Molenaar 1975; Rustioni and Kaufman 1977). It is therefore important to bear in mind that the neurones to be discussed in the present chapter probably do not belong to a single system. Because of the close anatomical association of the various target nuclei in the medulla it is difficult to identify the projection of any individual neurone in both anatomical and physiological studies. Detailed identification of this degree has not yet been achieved.

Ascending input to the dorsal column nuclei via non-primary axons is not limited to those axons running up the dorsal columns. Some axons ascending the dorso-lateral funiculus project to the dorsal column nuclei (Gordon and Grant 1972; Dart and Gordon 1973; Rustioni 1973; Rustioni and Molenaar 1975). This group of neurones presents difficulties for experimental study, for the reasons mentioned in the preceding paragraph and also because of the close association of their axons with those of the spinocervical tract in the dorso-lateral funiculus. Indeed it is possible that some neurones project to both the lateral cervical nucleus and to the dorsal column nuclei.

It will be realized, therefore, that the dorsal columns, far from being a simple tract of ascending first-order afferent fibres, are very complex indeed. They contain axons of a number of different systems, only some of which project to the dorsal column nuclei. The rest of this chapter will be concerned with neurones whose cell bodies are in the spinal grey matter and whose axons ascend the dorsal columns.

A. Physiology of neurones with axons ascending the dorsal columns

I. Response properties

There have been few electrophysiological studies of neurones whose axons ascend the dorsal columns, and in none of them have the cutaneous receptive fields been examined with the detail necessary to provide more than an indication of the cutaneous receptors involved. In the two largest series of studies (Uddenberg 1968a, b; Petit 1971; Angaut-Petit 1975a, b) recordings were made from axons in the dorsal columns and the point has been made (Burton and Loewy 1977) that these axons might have been *descending* the cord. This, although a possibility in all experiments where axons are recorded from, is extremely unlikely in view of the short latencies of most responses to peripheral nerve stimulation and (in Angaut-Petit's experiments) the fact that similar responses were recorded caudal to a spinal transection.

In Uddenberg's sample of units with receptive fields on the forelimb there seems to be homogeneity of response properties (at least as far as one can tell from the rather cursory description given in the 1968b paper). All units responded to hair movement with a rapidly adapting discharge and, in addition, had slowly adapting discharges to maintained pressure on the skin. Pinching the skin evoked a further increase in the discharge. Units could also be weakly excited by moving the joints: Uddenberg could elicit no response by moving the claws or by applying a vibratory stimulus, and this suggests that there is no excitatory input from the slowly adapting Type II receptors at the claw bases or from Pacinian corpuscles. On the other hand sensitive spots on the skin could be found and slowly adapting responses could be elicited from glabrous skin by light pressure. Both of these latter observations indicate a contribution from slowly adapting Type I receptors to the cells' excitatory input—a conclusion confirmed for hind limb units by Angaut-Petit (1975b) and ourselves (Brown and Fyffe 1981b).

The neurones with hind limb receptive fields do not form a homogeneous group with regard to response properties. Angaut-Petit (1975b) was able to divide her sample of 92 units into several categories: about 16% were activated solely by light mechanical stimuli such as hair movement, a 10-mg von Frey hair or by tapping; most units (77%) responded to a wide range of stimuli, from hair movement to noxious mechanical and heat stimuli; a few units were excited only by noxious stimuli. Some neurones, at least, were shown to respond to electrical stimulation of non-myelinated cutaneous nerve fibres. In unanaesthetized spinal preparations both the background activity and responses to noxious stimulation were greater than in anaesthetized preparations.

At first sight the response properties of these post-synaptic dorsal column units described by Angaut-Petit appear the same as those of spinocervical tract neurones. Only in one respect does there appear to be difference. Angaut-Petit (1975b), in agreement with Uddenberg (1968b), describes responses in some units to displacement of slowly adapting Type I receptors in hairy skin. These receptors have not been observed to excite spinocervical tract neurones.

We (Brown and Fyffe 1981b) have confirmed the results of Angaut-Petit with regard to the response properties of these cells and in addition have observed some further differences between them and neurones of the spinocervical tract. When receptive fields are on the foot and toes they often include glabrous skin. These neurones respond to light mechanical stimulation of the glabrous skin, for example with a camel-hair brush, with a rapidly adapting discharge and in addition often respond quite well to a vibratory stimulus or to tapping on the frame supporting the animal. These observations suggest that rapidly adapting mechanoreceptors and/or Pacinian corpuscles in the foot and toe pads project onto the neurones and excite them. As will be shown below some of the neurones are ideally situated to receive such inputs.

The sizes of receptive fields of post-synaptic dorsal column neurones appear similar to those of spinocervical tract neurones, at least when the cells are recorded extracellularly (Angaut-Petit 1975b; Brown and Fyffe 1981b). A striking feature revealed by intracellular recording, however, is the presence of a marked subliminal fringe, from which excitatory post-synaptic potentials can be evoked, surrounding the field from which action potentials may be elicited. If the neurone's membrane potential fell after microelectrode impalement, then impulses could be evoked from this surrounding area, and the cutaneous area from which the cell could be fired increased enormously (see Fig. 8.9). Spinocervical tract neurones do not have such a subliminal fringe and their receptive fields are very resistant to size changes, not being affected by anaesthetic depth or descending neuronal systems (Wall 1960, 1967; Brown 1971).

In addition to cutaneous input other primary afferent fibres excite these neurones. As mentioned above, Uddenberg (1968b) demonstrated excitation upon bending of the joints and also upon electrical stimulation of high-threshold fibres of muscle nerves. However, he failed to find any effects from stimulation of low-threshold (Group I) muscle afferent fibres. Recently Jankowska et al. (1979) have made an intracellular study of lumbosacral neurones with axons in the dorsal columns. They have shown that about half of the cells receive excitation from Group I muscle afferent fibres as well as confirming excitation from high-threshold muscle and joint axons.

II. Input from non-primary sources

Jankowska et al. (1979) have investigated the possibility that neurones of the post-synaptic dorsal column system might receive inputs from a number of non-primary sources. Evidence was found suggesting excitation from corticospinal tract fibres, axon collaterals of spinocervical tract cells and a system of axons originating (or terminating, it was not possible to decide which) between segments Th-9 and C-3–C-4. It is an interesting suggestion that spinocervical tract neurones might excite post-synaptic dorsal column cells. All cutaneous afferent fibres that excite spinocervical tract neurones appear also to activate neurones with axons ascending the dorsal columns. If such a connexion is confirmed then the interactions between dorso-lateral tract and dorsal systems are made at the earliest opportunity. The two sets of systems may be linked at both the spinal segmental level and the level of the dorsal column nuclei (see Chapter 6, Sect. B.II.).

III. Axonal conduction velocity

Dorsal column axons have conduction velocities in the range 10–85 m s^{-1} (Brown 1968; Petit and

Burgess 1968). The non-primary fibres have conduction velocities throughout this range (16–71 m s^{-1} in the gracile fascicle: Angaut-Petit 1975a; 40–70 m s^{-1} in the cuneate fascicle: Uddenberg 1968b). Axons from neurones with hind limb fields usually conduct at less than 50 m s^{-1} (Angaut-Petit 1975a; Brown and Fyffe 1981b). The non-primary dorsal column pathway does not, on the average, conduct as quickly as the spinocervical tract, where many axons conduct at more than 50 m s^{-1} and between 80 and 100 m s^{-1} is not uncommon (Brown and Franz 1969; Bryan et al. 1973). Any information common to the two pathways will, in general, reach high cervical levels earlier through the spinocervical than through the dorsal column tract.

B. Anatomy of neurones with axons ascending the dorsal columns

I. Location

The cells of origin of the post-synaptic dorsal column pathway have been demonstrated by the retrograde transport of horseradish peroxidase after injections of the enzyme into the dorsal column nuclei, in both cat and monkey (Rustioni and Kaufman 1977; Rustioni 1977). As indicated in Chapter 1, the neurones are located mainly in lamina IV and adjoining laminae, with a particular concentration of cell bodies in the medial part of lamina V (Fig. 8.1). When the enzyme injections were confined to one side of the medulla and within the boundaries of the dorsal column nuclei the labelled cells were all ipsilateral. Unfortunately Rustioni's experiments did not differentiate between those cells that send their axons to the dorsal column nuclei via the dorsal columns and those (Gordon and Grant 1972; Dart and Gordon 1973; Rustioni 1973; Rustioni and Molenaar 1975) that project via the dorso-lateral funiculus.

Intracellular injection of horseradish peroxidase into neurones shown both electrophysiologically and by direct examination of the stained axon to project through the dorsal columns has revealed the locations of this group (Brown and Fyffe 1981b). Figure 8.2 shows that, in agreement

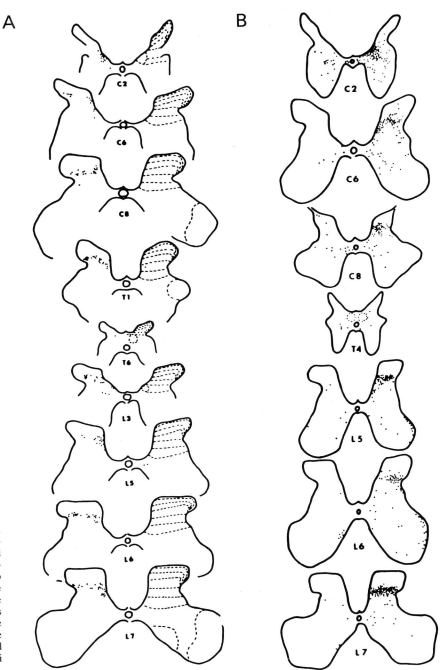

Fig. 8.1. The location of the cells of origin of the post-synaptic dorsal column pathway as determined by retrograde transport of horseradish peroxidase in cat (**A**) and monkey (**B**). Injections of horseradish peroxidase were made into the dorsal column nuclei, on the left side in **A** and on the right side in **B**. The projection in the cat is strictly ipsilateral, but there are contralateral cells marked in the monkey. (**A** from Rustioni and Kaufman 1977; **B** from Rustioni 1977.)

with the findings of Rustioni and Kaufman (1977), most cells are in lamina IV. There is a considerable number (about 30%) in or at the ventral border of lamina III and a concentration of cells in the medial part of lamina V. Like spinocervical tract neurones these cells form a sheet across the dorsal horn (see Chapter 6, Sec. B.I). The proportions of cells in the different laminae are about the same in the two systems, the main difference being the aggregation of somata in medial lamina V in the post-synaptic dorsal column system. This deeper, medially located set of neurones receives input from glabrous skin of the foot and toe pads (see Sect. B.III.2 below) and this input is absent in the spinocervical tract.

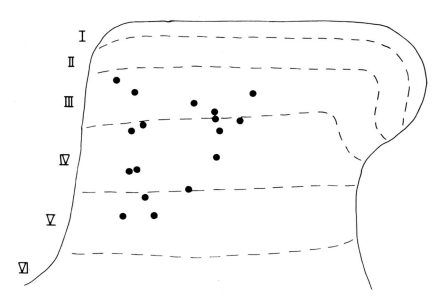

Fig. 8.2. The location of intra-cellularly stained neurones with axons projecting through the dorsal columns. The positions of the cells have been placed on a standard dorsal horn outline according to their relative positions from the medial, lateral and dorsal border and the central canal. (From Brown and Fyffe 1981b.)

II. Density

There is no detailed information on the density of post-synaptic dorsal column neurones comparable with that for spinocervical tract cells. When recording from axons in the dorsal columns about 10%–15% may be identified as non-primary (Angaut-Petit 1975a); a similar figure has been observed by the present writer in unpublished work. When the cells are being recorded in the dorsal horn (Brown and Fyffe 1981b) they require considerably more looking for than do spino-cervical tract neurones. This is due, however, to their lack of extensive extracellular field potentials rather than to their scarcity. It would seem reasonable to assume that the non-primary dorsal column pathway is made up of about the same number of neurones as the spinocervical tract, perhaps some 2000–3000 on each side with 550–800 of these in the lumbosacral enlargement.

III. Cellular anatomy

1. Size of cell bodies

It is considerably more difficult to obtain good intracellular microelectrode penetrations of most post-synaptic dorsal column cells than of spino-cervical tract neurones and most other cells in laminae III–V of the dorsal horn. This suggests that they might have relatively small somata, and horseradish peroxidase staining has confirmed

this. Cell bodies range from 20–30 μm up to about 50–60 μm. Some cells are elongated so that although only about 20 μm across in one direction they may be up to 60 μm at right angles to it (Fig. 8.3).

2. Dendritic trees

The dendritic trees of non-primary dorsal column neurones are clearly related to the position of the cell body in the dorsal horn. Three types of neurones can be distinguished on the basis of their dendritic tree organization.

Neurones with their cell bodies in lamina III and at the III–IV border have dendritic trees that are developed mainly, but not exclusively, in the dorsal direction (Figs. 8.3–8.5). The dorsally directed dendrites are contained within a narrow cylindrical or cone-shaped volume with the dendritic tree restricted in lateral, medial, rostral and caudal directions to total extents of only 100–300 μm. This restriction was not dependent on the position of the cell in the transverse plane—cells in the middle of the horn (Figs. 8.4, 8.5) as well as those near the edge (Fig. 8.3) showed this restriction. All of these more superficial cells had dendrites that reached into lamina II (substantia gelatinosa), often extending throughout its thickness and into lamina I (Fig. 8.3).

At the opposite extreme from lamina III neurones are those in the medial parts of lamina V and deep IV. These neurones have very extensive dendritic trees developed in the transverse

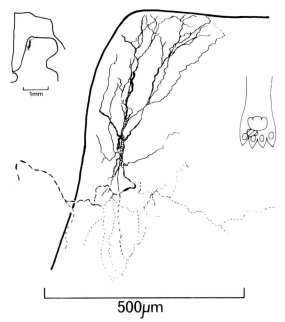

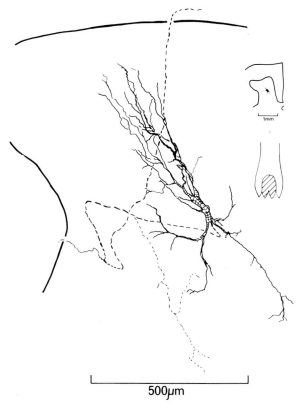

Fig. 8.3. Reconstruction, from transverse sections, of a post-synaptic dorsal column neurone with its soma in lamina III. The dendrites extend dorsally into lamina I. The axon and its collaterals, which arborize in lamina IV, are shown as *dashed lines*. The position of the cell in the dorsal horn and the location of the receptive field are shown in the *inset figures*. (Modified from Brown and Fyffe 1981b.)

Fig. 8.4 Reconstruction, from transverse sections, of a dorsally located (lamina IV) post-synaptic dorsal column neurone. Most of the dendritic tree is directed dorsally and reaches into lamina II. The axon, after giving off collaterals, ascends through the dorsal laminae and comes to lie dorsal to the horn (*dashed line*). The position of the cell in the dorsal horn and the location of the receptive field are shown in the *inset figures*. (Modified from Brown and Fyffe 1981b.)

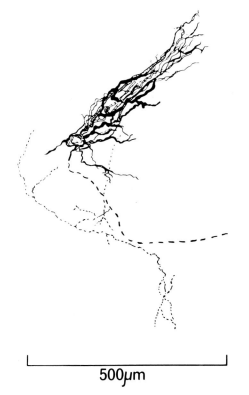

⊲ **Fig. 8.5.** Another example of a neurone with its axon projecting through the dorsal columns and situated dorsally in the spinal grey matter (at the lamina III–IV border). The dendritic tree occupies a narrow cone-shaped volume of tissue in laminae II and III (see Fig. 8.10 for overall position and details of the axon and its collaterals). The location of the receptive field is shown in the figure on the right.

plane of the cord and radiating out from the cell body (Figs. 8.6, 8.7). The trees extend for up to 1 mm, from the medial edge of the dorsal horn to about the junction of the lateral and middle thirds and from the upper border of lamina III to the level of the central canal (ventral border of lamina VI or even into lamina VII). Most of these cells have a well-developed set of dendrites that run along and parallel with the medial border of the dorsal horn towards the central canal (Figs. 8.6, 8.7). Although very extensive in the transverse plane of the cord, these neurones are restricted in the parasagittal plane and are only about 200–300 μm in rostro-caudal spread.

Both of these sets of neurones, those in lamina III and medial lamina V etc., are clearly different in their dendritic tree organization from spino-cervical tract neurones. The latter all have trees well-developed in the parasagittal plane whereas the post-synaptic dorsal column cells considered so far are restricted in this direction.

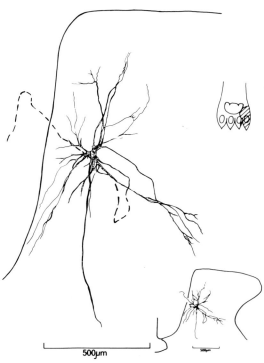

Fig. 8.7. Similar reconstruction to that shown in Fig. 8.6. (Modified from Brown and Fyffe 1981b.)

In addition these post-synaptic dorsal column cells have only six or seven primary dendrites whereas spinocervical tract cells often have more than this.

A third type of post-synaptic dorsal column neurone is situated in lamina IV. The dendrites are mainly directed dorsally; the dendritic trees are about 500 μm in transverse extent and in the longitudinal direction are either limited to about 200–300 μm. (Fig 8.8) or are more extensive but still only about 500 μm long (Fig. 8.9). The dendrites of these neurones reach into lamina II and may extend throughout its thickness (Fig. 8.8). The neurones have ten or more primary dendrites.

A feature that clearly distinguishes the dendritic trees of non-primary dorsal column neurones from those of the spinocervical tract is that when the soma is in lamina III or IV the dorsally directed dendrites penetrate into lamina II, often throughout its complete thickness. Only a minority of spinocervical tract neurones have dendrites that extend into the substantia gelatinosa and then only its inner portion (lamina II$_i$). These post-synaptic dorsal column neurones pre-

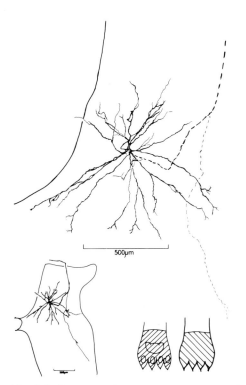

Fig. 8.6. Reconstructions, from transverse sections, of post-synaptic dorsal column cells with somata in the medial parts of laminae V and (deep) IV. The dendritic trees radiate out from the somata and are restricted to the transverse plane. Their positions in the dorsal horn and receptive fields are shown in the *inset figures*. (Modified from Brown and Fyffe 1981b.)

sumably receive some inputs from within the substantia gelatinosa and this input is not given directly to spinocervical tract cells. An obvious, but not necessarily correct, conclusion would be that the non-primary dorsal column neurones with dendrites in lamina II receive excitation from peripheral C fibres, which are believed to terminate there (see Chapter 10).

3. Axonal projections

A necessary criterion for inclusion of a neurone in the post-synaptic dorsal column category is that it should send its axon into the dorsal columns. In our experiments (Brown and Fyffe 1981b) we initially identified these neurones by electrophysiological methods before injecting horseradish peroxidase into them. The main electrophysiological criterion was antidromic excitation (collision test) from the upper cervical cord in preparations with bilateral section of the dorso-lateral funiculi caudal to the site of stimulation. We were, therefore, surprised and initially rather dismayed to find some neurones identified electrophysiologically as belonging to the system which upon microscopic examination were seen to have axons projecting into the ipsilateral dorsolateral funiculus. Were our electrophysiological methods not rigorous enough? Two of these neurones, however, were observed to have axons that initially entered the dorso-lateral funiculus but then re-entered the grey matter of the dorsal horn and crossed it to enter the dorsal columns (Fig. 8.10).

This observation shows that the initial projection of an axon is not a satisfactory guide to the path it finally takes and makes interpretation of anatomical data, per se, open to serious doubt. Even when the intracellular horseradish peroxidase technique is used (and this is the best method available at present) only about 1 cm of axon is revealed: this may not be sufficient to allow the projection to be determined. In our experiments we have seen a number of cells that behaved, electrophysiologically, as though they should have had an axon in the dorsal columns and yet the histological material showed the axons projecting into the dorso-lateral funiculus for up to 1 cm. Possibly they passed across into the dorsal columns at a higher level, but there is no anatomical evidence to support this.

Further intriguing questions are posed by this observation. For example, under what conditions

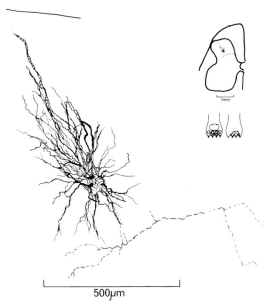

Fig. 8.8. Reconstruction, from transverse sections, of a post-synaptic dorsal column neurone with soma in lamina IV. The dendritic tree reaches dorsally into lamina II and ventrally into lamina V. Most of the dendrites are directed dorsally. (Modified from Brown and Fyffe 1981b.)

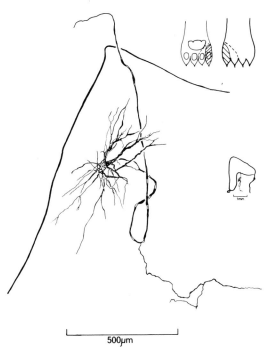

Fig. 8.9. Similar reconstruction to that shown in Fig. 8.8.

do axons enter one tract and then change to another, perhaps crossing a considerable thickness of grey matter in order to do so? What are

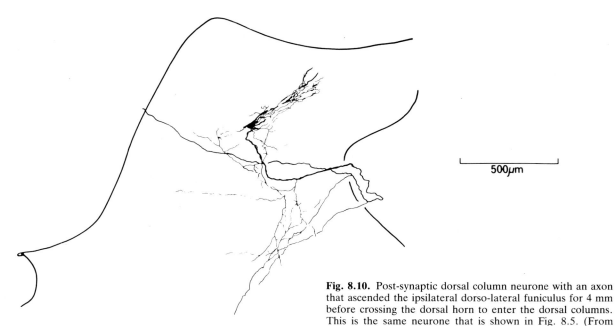

Fig. 8.10. Post-synaptic dorsal column neurone with an axon that ascended the ipsilateral dorso-lateral funiculus for 4 mm before crossing the dorsal horn to enter the dorsal columns. This is the same neurone that is shown in Fig. 8.5. (From Brown and Fyffe 1981b.)

the guiding mechanisms that can bring such change about? Are there any functional implications for the phenomenon? Mere contact guidance would seem an inappropriate mechanism to allow an axon to change from one tract to another, and to suggest that the axon 'made the wrong choice' initially seems trivial. The neurones that projected into the dorso-lateral tract were not situated laterally in the dorsal horn (both were in the middle third of the horn), so position of the cell body does not seem to be a determining factor. Both of the axons that made this particular journey gave off collaterals as they ascended the dorso-lateral funiculus and, so far, we have seen very few collaterals arising from non-primary axons deep in the dorsal columns. It is possible, but seems unlikely, that a reason for initial projection to the dorso-lateral cord might be to allow collaterals to be given off rostral to the cell body.

Those axons entering the dorsal columns more or less directly did so through either the medial border of the dorsal horn, where they tended to take up a deep position in the columns (Figs. 8.3, 8.5, 8.8, 8.9), or through the dorsal border of the horn, when they came to lie in that part of the columns dorsal to the grey matter (Figs. 8.6, 8.7). The trajectory of the axon did not depend on the position of the cell body: ventrally located neurones might send their axons through the dor-

sal border of the horn and dorsally located neurones might send theirs either through the medial border or the dorsal border.

4. Axon collaterals

Most post-synaptic dorsal column neurones have axons that give off collaterals during their initial course in the grey matter near the cell body. Between one and three collaterals are given off and usually they arborize ventral to the parent cell (Figs. 8.3–8.5), where they spread over a wider extent than is covered by the cell's dendritic tree. Some cells have collaterals which enter the dorso-lateral funiculus where they descend for a few millimetres: their final destinations are unknown. Unfortunately, for technical reasons there is little evidence about the extent and termination of these collaterals from the non-primary dorsal column axons.

Like the majority of spinocervical tract neurones post-synaptic dorsal column cells have locally arborizing collaterals in addition to a main axon that ascends the spinal cord. They can, therefore, influence neurones in the locality of their cell bodies and up to a few millimetres away. The identity of any target cells is unknown. It is obvious, however, that spinocervical tract cells will not receive input from any cells excited by slowly adapting Type I receptors, rapidly adapting mechanoreceptors in glabrous skin or Pacinian corpuscles.

C. Organization of the post-synaptic dorsal column pathway

I. Correlations between form and function of the neurones

In contrast with spinocervical tract neurones, where there are almost no correlations between structure and function, some correlations may be made for the non-primary dorsal column pathway. The wider spectrum of cutaneous input to post-synaptic dorsal column cells is reflected in their distribution in the dorsal horn: when a cell responds to light mechanical stimulation of the glabrous skin, indicative of input from rapidly adapting mechanoreceptors or Pacinian corpuscles, the dendritic tree is located in the medial parts of the dorsal horn in laminae III–VI, where such input is distributed (see Chapter 3).

Neurones with transversely oriented dendritic trees in laminae III–VI showed a degree of correlation between the transverse extent of the tree and the size of the cutaneous receptive field—especially with the full extent of the field as revealed by intracellular recording. This is seen in Figs. 8.3–8.9, where it is obvious that this correlation depended on the depth of the cell in the dorsal horn as has been suggested by Proshansky and Egger (1977). In our sample of post-synaptic dorsal column cells, neurones with no input from glabrous skin did not have dendrites in laminae V or VI even though they had fields on hairy skin adjacent to the foot and toe pads.

II. Comparison with the spinocervical tract

A major difference in the information forwarded by the post-synaptic dorsal column system in comparison with the spinocervical tract is that the former carries some additional information. This is from slowly adapting Type I mechanoreceptors and sensitive mechanoreceptors in glabrous skin of the foot and toe pads, probably Pacinian corpuscles, rapidly adapting mechanoreceptors and slowly adapting Type I receptors. The projection for slowly adapting Type I receptors through the dorsal columns provides the only known pathway by which information from these receptors in the hind climb can reach thalamus and cortex: they do not project, as primary afferent fibres, through the dorsal columns and nor do they excite the neurones of the spinocervical tract.

The post-synaptic dorsal column pathway and the spinocervical tract between them carry information from all types of cutaneous afferent unit with myelinated axons and probably all with non-myelinated axons with the exception of sensitive thermoreceptor units. It might be a mistake, however, to assume that all the information is relayed to the thalamus and cortex. Non-primary axons ascending the dorsal columns terminate on a number of targets in addition to the dorsal column nuclei (see beginning of chapter). Also it is not inconceivable that some, at least, of the ascending non-primary axons have an inhibitory influence on their target neurones.

9 Other dorsal horn neurones

During the course of our extensive studies of the dorsal horn, we have made intracellular recordings from and injected horseradish peroxidase into many dorsal horn neurones. In the present chapter the anatomy of a representative sample of some of these neurones will be presented. In one aspect, however, these neurones differ from all others described in work from my laboratory: their axonal projections have not been defined. In this sense, therefore, the neurones are unidentified. But they provide important information about the histological organization of the dorsal horn, especially with regard to the arrangement of dendritic trees and the way these may collect information from different laminae of the horn. For these reasons the information will be presented here, even though the neurones form a heterogeneous collection.

A. Dorsal horn neurones with unidentified axonal projections

I. Neurones with somata in lamina III

Neurones in lamina III may send their axons into the spinocervical tract or into the dorsal columns (see Chapters 6 and 8). In addition there are many lamina III cells whose function is unknown. Indeed, until recently it was an assumption of many workers that recording from lamina III was difficult if not impossible (see Wall 1973). According to Wall et al. (1979) there is no difference between cells recorded in laminae II and III (see Chapter 10, Sect. B.II.2). Even the anatomy of lamina III neurones is little understood: Mannen and Sugiura (1976) show lamina III neurones with very extensive dendritic trees that ramify in laminae I–III or IV.

The cell shown in Fig. 9.1 represents a type we have seen in lamina III that is excited by cutaneous stimulation including noxious stimulation. The dendritic tree has a striking appearance: although the cell body is located in lamina III the dendritic development is mainly in laminae I and II dorsal to the soma and in laminae IV and V ventral to the soma. The dorsal dendritic arbor arises from two main dendrites and ramifies widely in the transverse plane across about half the width of the horn in lamina I and the outer parts of lamina II. The ventral dendritic arbor is also developed mainly in the transverse plane (more rostrally than the dorsal arbor, the complete dendritic tree being tilted so that the dorsal arbor is at and caudal to the cell body whereas the ventral arbor is at and rostral to the level of the soma) across one-third to one-half of the dorsal horn. Within lamina III itself the receptive area of the neurone consists of the soma and the four first-order dendrites.

The axon of the cell shown in Fig. 9.1 was also of considerable interest. It arose from one of the dorsally directed dendrites and gave numerous collaterals to the grey matter ventral to the soma in laminae IV, V and VI. In addition there were two main ascending axons, one ascending in the ipsilateral dorso-lateral funiculus and the other, after crossing the cord anterior to the central canal, in the contralateral ventral funiculus. Only the initial part of the axon is shown in Fig. 9.1.

Obviously cells such as these may have important roles to play in collecting information from wide areas of the dorsal horn. They bridge the barrier that seems to divide the areas of input for small myelinated and non-myelinated afferent fibres (laminae I and II: see Chapter 10) and those for the large myelinated fibres (see Chapters 2–5). This barrier, at the junction between laminae II and III, also marks off the boundary for the vast majority of dendrites from spinocervical

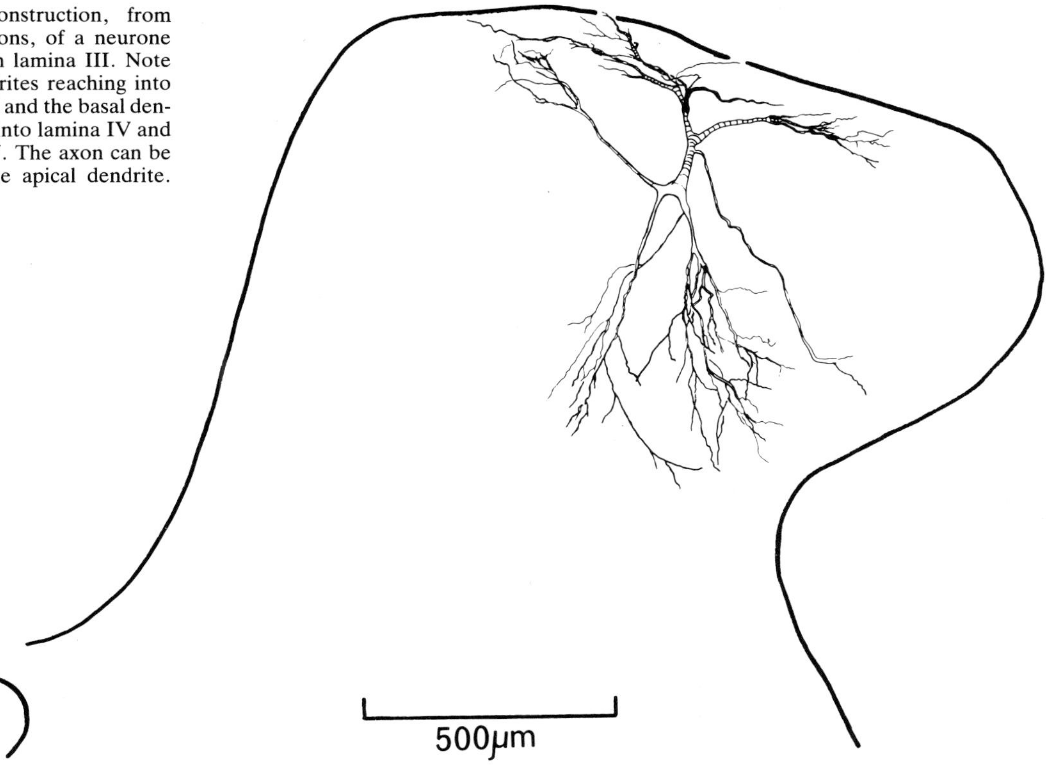

Fig. 9.1. Reconstruction, from transverse sections, of a neurone with its soma in lamina III. Note the apical dendrites reaching into laminae I and II and the basal dendrites reaching into lamina IV and dorsal lamina V. The axon can be seen leaving the apical dendrite.

500μm

tract neurones, even those with somata in lamina III (see Chapter 6).

II. Neurones with somata in lamina IV

In addition to neurones with axons projecting to the spinocervical tract and into the dorsal columns (already described in Chapters 6 and 8) there are many other neurones with their somata in lamina IV. A large number of these appear to have axons that project only for short distances from the cell and in our experience these have dendritic trees, in the majority of cases, that are similar to those of the lamina IV neurones of the spinocervical tract and the dorsal column pathway; that is, they have well-developed dorsally directed dendrites, although transverse and ventral dendrites are present. These cells are not illustrated here.

A further group of lamina IV neurones has been observed in our experiments. These have axons that ascend in the dorso-lateral funiculus to beyond the level of the lateral cervical nucleus. Their ultimate projection is unknown. Two cells of this type are illustrated in Fig. 9.2. That in

Fig. 9.2A is reconstructed from sagittal sections and has a dendritic tree architecture common for cells in this lamina—a dorsally directed set of dendrites. The cell of Fig. 9.2B, reconstructed from transverse sections, was located at the lateral edge of the lamina and had dendrites that always remained close to the lateral border of the grey matter, running dorsally into the white matter through the lateral curve of the most superficial three laminae and ventrally ramifying in lamina V. In addition to its ascending axon this neurone had a descending axon branch that crossed Lissauer's tract and descended in the most lateral part of the dorsal column (it is this descending branch that is shown in Fig. 9.2B).

In agreement with other workers (Scheibel and Scheibel 1968; Réthelyi and Szentágothai 1973; Mannen 1975; Proshansky and Egger 1977) our results have shown that cells with somata in lamina IV generally have dendritic trees that are restricted in the transverse plane. Dendrites are usually well developed dorsally and many do not penetrate into lamina II (again with the exception of cells having axons ascending the dorsal columns: see Chapter 8).

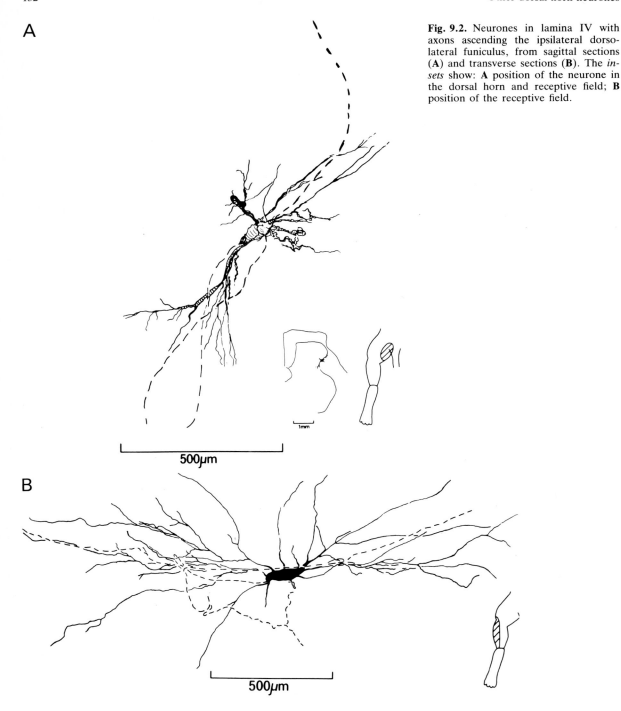

Fig. 9.2. Neurones in lamina IV with axons ascending the ipsilateral dorsolateral funiculus, from sagittal sections (**A**) and transverse sections (**B**). The *insets* show: **A** position of the neurone in the dorsal horn and receptive field; **B** position of the receptive field.

III. Neurones with somata ventral to lamina IV

Neurones with their cell bodies deeper than lamina IV all appear to have a common feature. This is that their dendritic trees are all essentially two-dimensional and restricted to the transverse plane of the cord; in the longitudinal axis of the cord they are rarely more than 300–400 μm in extent and yet they are usually very extensive in either the dorso-ventral or medio-lateral direction (or both).

The lamina V neurones shown in Figs. 9.3 and 9.4 illustrate the transverse development of the dendritic trees. Neither neurone had a rostro-caudal extent greater than 300 μm but both extended across the full width of the dorsal horn. In Fig. 9.3 the dendrites run mainly from the lateral parts of laminae III and IV to the medial parts of laminae V and VI. The axon projected through the ventral horn to the ventral funiculus. The neurone of Fig. 9.4, also situated in the lateral parts of lamina V, has a dendritic tree oriented roughly at right angles to that shown in Fig. 9.3, that is, the tree runs from the medial and mid parts of laminae IV and V to the lateral parts of laminae V, VI and VII.

The deeper neurones shown in Figs. 9.5–9.8 are all essentially bipolar with the main dendritic arborizations arising from either end of an elongated cell body. The neurone in Fig. 9.5, at the lamina V–VI border, has its dendrites running across the dorsal horn from medial to lateral, almost from edge to edge. Its axon entered the deepest parts of the ventral funiculus and ascended. Such a neurone is capable of collecting information from almost the complete extent of

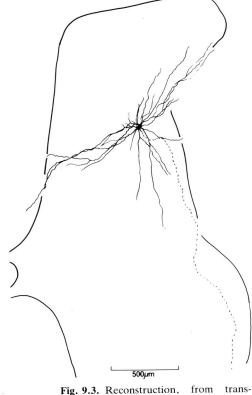

Fig. 9.3. Reconstruction, from transverse sections, of an interneurone with its soma in lamina V. Note the wide dendritic spread in the transverse plane.

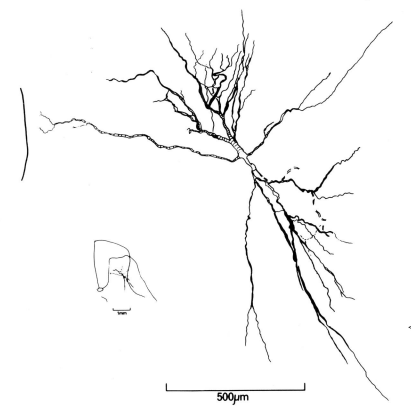

◁ **Fig. 9.4.** Reconstruction, from transverse sections, of an interneurone with soma in lamina V. Note the wide dendritic spread in the transverse plane. This neurone, and that shown in Fig. 9.3, has an essentially two-dimensional dendritic tree in the transverse plane.

the base of the dorsal horn. The neurones in Figs. 9.6 and 9.7 are similar and oriented dorso-ventrally, with dendrites running from lamina III dorsally to lamina VII ventrally. Both neurones have one or two dendrites that also project transversely (laterally or medially) and would obviously also be capable of collecting information from a wide area of cord. Finally, the deepest neurone of

and Egger (1977) from Golgi-stained preparations. Some conclusions may be drawn about the organization of the dendritic neuropil on the basis of these results and those presented earlier in Chapters 6 and 8. (1) Many neurones in laminae III and IV have well-developed dorsally directed dendrites restricted in the medio-lateral direction but extensive in the rostro-caudal direction. This

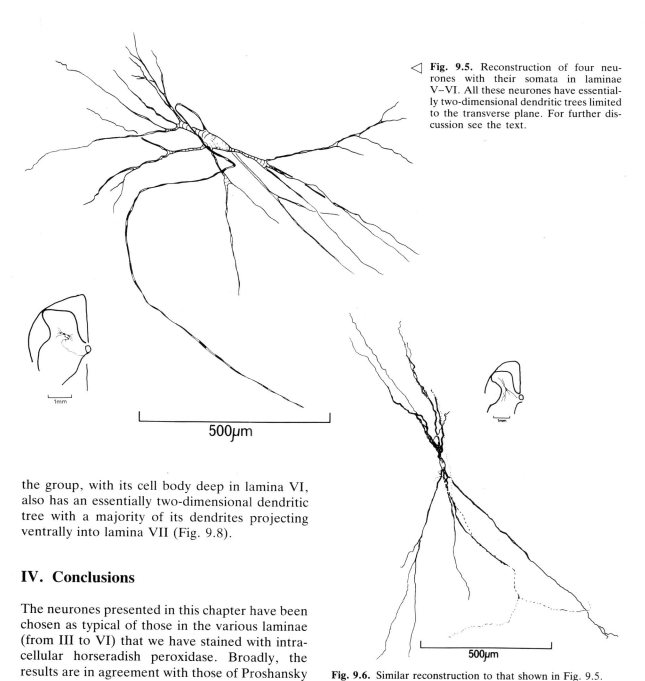

◁ **Fig. 9.5.** Reconstruction of four neurones with their somata in laminae V–VI. All these neurones have essentially two-dimensional dendritic trees limited to the transverse plane. For further discussion see the text.

500μm

the group, with its cell body deep in lamina VI, also has an essentially two-dimensional dendritic tree with a majority of its dendrites projecting ventrally into lamina VII (Fig. 9.8).

IV. Conclusions

The neurones presented in this chapter have been chosen as typical of those in the various laminae (from III to VI) that we have stained with intracellular horseradish peroxidase. Broadly, the results are in agreement with those of Proshansky

500μm

Fig. 9.6. Similar reconstruction to that shown in Fig. 9.5.

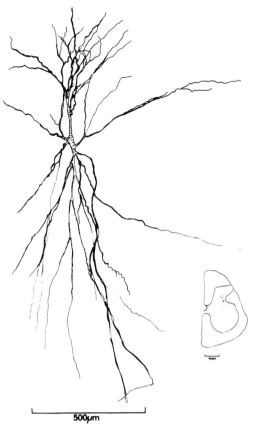

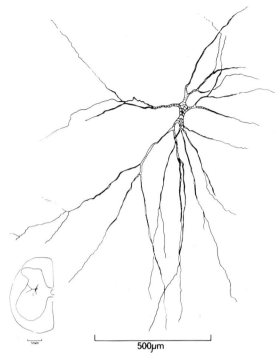

Fig. 9.8. Similar reconstruction to that shown in Fig. 9.5.

Fig. 9.7. Similar reconstruction to that shown in Fig. 9.5.

applies especially to spinocervical tract neurones and many cells with their somata in lamina IV. There are, however, exceptions, e.g. the neurones with axons ascending the dorsal columns may have dendritic trees restricted in all directions except dorso-ventrally (Chapter 8). (2) Many neurones with cell bodies in laminae III, IV, V and VI have dendrites in some or all of these laminae but rarely give dendritic branches to laminae II or I. Again there are exceptions, including the more dorsally located neurones with axons running into the dorsal columns. (3) Cells with somata in laminae V and VI often have bipolar dendritic trees running in the transverse plane of the cord. In this plane the tree can be very extensive and such a dendritic development may be responsible for the larger size of cutaneous receptive fields seen for the deeper dorsal horn neurones (Wall 1967). (4) Finally, there are strong correlations between the orientation of dendritic trees and the orientation of the terminal arborizations of primary cutaneous afferent fibres. This point will be discussed in more detail in the following chapter.

10   The organization of the dorsal horn

In Chapters 2 to 9 our results on the morphology of identified cutaneous afferent fibres and a variety of neurones in the dorsal horn have been described. In the individual chapters the relation of the morphology to the physiology has been discussed. In the present chapter this work, together with recently published results from other laboratories, will be brought together and an attempt made to place the data into perspective and to try to extract some guiding principles about the organization of the dorsal horn. In addition an appraisal will be made of the classification of dorsal horn neurones and the usefulness of the cytoarchitectonic scheme of Rexed.

To some extent the decision to attempt integration at this point, rather than at the end of the book, is arbitrary. It is certainly artificial to exclude the muscle afferent fibres and some of the neurones they contact, since they are partly situated in the dorsal horn. However, knowledge about muscle afferent connexions within the dorsal horn (laminae I–VI) is much less advanced than that concerning connexions made by cutaneous axons. Even less is known about the input from receptors in the joints and the viscera. It seems appropriate, though, to bring together the material so far presented, whilst bearing in mind the obvious omissions and hoping that the generalizations that are made will not be upset too drastically once new knowledge is acquired.

A. Organization of input from the skin

The intra-axonal injection of horseradish peroxidase has allowed the morphology of identified cutaneous afferent fibres to be studied for the first time. Other new and very powerful techniques, such as autoradiography, electron microscopy of degenerating terminals, immunohistochemistry, etc., have also provided much new information on primary afferent fibres. It is now possible to suggest a set of generalizations, or guiding principles, on the organization of cutaneous input to the lumbosacral dorsal horn. There will obviously be exceptions to these generalizing principles but a plan can be drawn up and it is hoped that it will provide a basis for discussion and quantitative work on the adult cord and for studies on the development of connexions within the cord.

I. Segregation of input according to axonal diameter and afferent unit type

There is now strong evidence for a segregation of cutaneous input to the dorsal horn according to diameters of peripheral axons. Axons of small diameter, the C and Aδ fibres, distribute their information to the upper two laminae of grey matter (the marginal cell layer, lamina I, and the substantia gelatinosa, lamina II, but not exclusively), whereas axons of larger diameter, the A$\alpha - \gamma$ fibres, send their input to deeper layers (laminae III–VI).

The evidence for the distribution from the smaller axons comes from a number of reports using quite diverse techniques. Réthelyi (1977) examined Golgi preparations from adult cats and concluded that the primary afferent input to lamina II came from fine, probably non-myelinated, axons. Degeneration and autoradiographic studies by Lamotte (1977) and Ralston and Ralston (1979) on the primate cord agree with Réthelyi and also with each other (but not for the same reason: see Ralston and Ralston 1979) that fine myelinated (Aδ) axons terminate in lamina I and non-myelinated axons project to lamina II.

According to Ralston and Ralston (1979) there is a certain amount of overlap but the general picture is as stated. Light and Perl (1977a, 1979a) combined lesions at the dorsal root entry zone with horseradish peroxidase uptake into cut dorsal root axons. They showed a clear differentiation of input, with the fine axons being distributed to the upper dorsal horn (laminae I and II) and the larger axons to deeper layers. Grant and Ygge (1978) and Grant et al. (1979) have used transganglionic degeneration and horseradish peroxidase transport from peripheral cutaneous nerves and obtained similar results. Light and Perl (1977b, 1979b) have injected horseradish peroxidase into single Aδ axons of high-threshold mechanoreceptors and showed a preferential distribution to lamina I (with some also to lamina V). Finally, substance P (the putative transmitter of fine axons) is localized, mainly, in laminae I and II (Hökfelt et al. 1975; Takahashi and Otsuka 1975; Chan-Palay and Palay 1977; Pickel et al. 1977).

The above evidence is impressive and leads to the conclusion that C fibres provide input to lamina II, Aδ fibres to lamina I and to the outer regions of lamina II (II$_o$, according to Ralston and Ralston 1979) and Aα–γ fibres to lamina III and deeper. In the experiments of Réthelyi (1977), Lamotte (1977), Ralston and Ralston (1979), Light and Perl (1977a, 1979a) and in the experiments localizing substance P, no differentiation into cutaneous, muscle, etc. afferent fibres was possible. Non-cutaneous axons were included in the studies and it is safe to conclude that the generalization about input in terms of axon diameter includes axons of all types. It will be shown that the generalization holds for the larger muscle afferent fibres (see Chapters 11–13) and that Group I muscle axons send most of their input to lamina V and deeper. Figure 10.1 illustrates the simplifying generalization.

The segregation of input may not, in fact, be so much according to peripheral axon diameter but more to the modality of the input. Axonal diameter and receptor modality are related to the extent that receptors responding to noxious stimuli are innervated by either C fibres or Aδ fibres, and it is these axons that provide input to laminae I and II. Very few axons conducting faster than the Aδ wave of the compound action potential innervate nociceptors. But C and Aδ axons do not innervate nociceptors exclusively:

many innervate sensitive mechanoreceptors and thermoreceptors. At present the distribution of input from fine fibres innervating sensitive receptors is not clear and the experiments described so far in this section provide little evidence on the distribution of fine axons to laminae other than I and II.

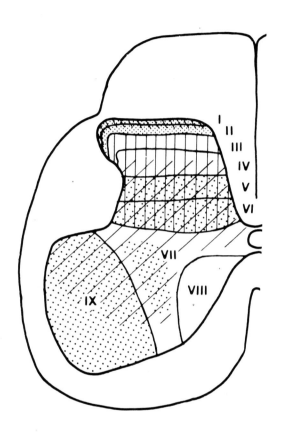

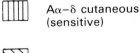 Aα–δ cutaneous (sensitive)

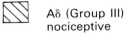 Aδ (Group III) nociceptive

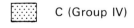 C (Group IV)

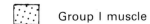 Group I muscle

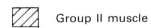 Group II muscle

Fig. 10.1. Diagrammatic representation of the distribution of cutaneous and muscle afferent fibres to the spinal grey matter.

That the organization may not be as simple as suggested in Fig. 10.1 is indicated by the results of Light and Perl (1977b, 1979b), who succeeded in injecting single Aδ axons with horseradish peroxidase. Aδ axons innervating high-threshold mechanoreceptors sent their collaterals to lamina I in accordance with the scheme but also to lamina V. Aδ axons innervating sensitive hair follicle receptors (Type D) supplied lamina III, that is they behaved like the large-diameter hair follicle afferent fibres. In view of the quite specific distribution of input from the large-diameter cutaneous and muscle afferent fibres it is quite possible that the specificity extends to the finer myelinated and non-myelinated axons and that they also distribute their input according to afferent unit type. If that is the case the principle of 'segregation of input according to axonal diameter' will not hold up. But it may be replaced with 'segregation according to afferent unit type', with nociceptor inputs and thermoreceptor inputs distributing to laminae I and II and the other afferent units to deeper laminae according to the detailed descriptions given in various chapters of this volume.

II. Specificity of the morphology of axon collateral arborizations according to afferent unit type

It is clearly established that for the larger cutaneous (and muscle: see Chapters 11–13) af-ferent fibres the morphological features of their collaterals at and near to their entrance to the spinal cord are (1) the same for each collateral from a single axon, (2) the same for all collaterals from axons innervating the same type of receptor, and (3) specific to the afferent unit type. This specificity extends to the branching pattern of the collaterals, the arrangement of the terminal arborizations, the laminar distribution of their synaptic boutons, the orientation of the terminal axons and the bouton arrangement on them. (Table 10.1) These points will be considered in turn.

With the exception of axons innervating hair follicle receptors, the majority of cutaneous axons (between 66% and 100% according to type: see Table 10.1) bifurcate into ascending and descending branches upon entering the cord. The axons from hair follicle receptors differ in that more than two-thirds do not bifurcate but turn and ascend the cord. The implications of this type of behaviour have been discussed in Chapter 2. Here it is sufficient to note the difference between one set of afferent fibres and the others. Muscle afferent fibres also behave like the majority of cutaneous axons and bifurcate upon entering the cord.

The collateral morphology of each type of large cutaneous axon has been described in previous chapters and it is obvious that the collaterals from each have quite specific morphologies. These differences are summarized in diagrammatic form in

Table 10.1. Summary of cutaneous primary afferent fibre organization in cat lumbosacral cord.

Type of afferent fibre	% of axons bifurcating	Collateral distribution[a] (μm)			Boutons	
		Transverse extent	Longitudinal extent	Dorso-ventral extent	Laminar distribution	Organization (main)
Hair follicle	27	150–400	100–1800	300–400	(II),III,(IV)	*En passant*
Rapidly adapting	66	50–300	400–600	300	III,(IV)	*En passant*
Pacinian corpuscle	100	170–350 (500)	400–750	700–800	III,IV / V,VI	*En passant* / *En passant* and *terminal* clusters
Slowly adapting Type I	92	250–500	100–700	250–650	III,IV,V,(VI)	*En passant* (hairy skin) *Terminal* (glabrous skin)
Slowly adapting Type II	100	500–600	100–300	400–650	III,IV,V,(VI)	*En passant*

[a] Collateral distribution refers to the area of the collateral containing boutons.

Fig. 10.2. The hair follicle afferent fibres and axons from Krause corpuscles give rise to the well-known 'flamed-shaped arbors' in transverse sections of the spinal cord. The other types of arborizations had not been described in detail before the introduction of intra-axonal injection of horseradish peroxidase. But the differences are so marked and produce such characteristic collaterals that the type of afferent unit may be identified from examination of the collateral morphology.

Associated with the morphology of the collaterals is the arrangement of their terminal axons. In general it may be said that terminal axons run in the longitudinal direction in the dorsal laminae and in the transverse plane in laminae V and particularly VI. The longitudinal arrangement in laminae I and II has been described by Réthelyi (1977) and its primary afferent fibre component shown to consist of C and Aδ fibres collaterals (see above). Within lamina III the longitudinal arrangement is especially marked and consists of branches from collaterals from myelinated cutaneous axons. As terminal branches of cutaneous collaterals pass deeper through lamina IV and into V their orientation changes so that

they tend to run both dorso-ventrally (or ventro-dorsally) and medio-laterally (or latero-medially), cutting across both the parasagittal and transverse planes. Within lamina VI and the deeper part of lamina V the orientation of terminal axons has changed again so that they lie in the transverse plane and run more or less in any direction within it. One afferent unit type has collaterals whose terminals cut across this pattern in its dorsal part—the collaterals from slowly adapting Type II units have terminals arranged within the transverse plane from lamina III down to lamina VI.

The distribution of synaptic boutons to particular laminae is also related to collateral morphology. The distribution of non-myelinated axons and high-threshold Aδ fibres to laminae I and II has been described. Most myelinated cutaneous axons have their boutons *terminaux* grouped together into a single region of the cord that may be limited essentially to a single lamina (hair follicle afferent fibres, lamina III) or spread over three to four laminae (slowly adapting Types I and II, laminae III–V and III–VI respectively). Collaterals from axons innervating Pacinian cor-

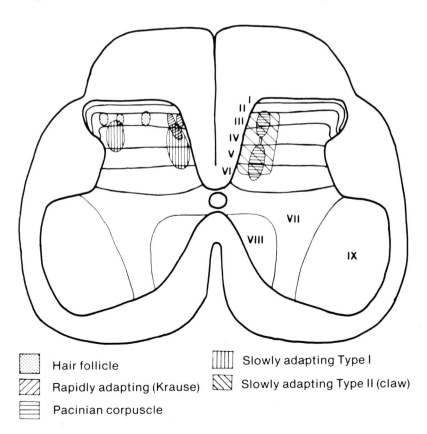

Fig. 10.2. Diagrammatic representation of the distribution of terminal arborizations of large myelinated cutaneous axons to the dorsal horn. Note the absence of input to the dorsal two laminae and the selective distributions of the different types of afferent units.

Hair follicle

Rapidly adapting (Krause)

Pacinian corpuscle

Slowly adapting Type I

Slowly adapting Type II (claw)

puscles generate two areas of termination, one in laminae III–V and the other in laminae V and VI.

Finally, the arrangement of the synaptic boutons on cutaneous axon collaterals also varies according to afferent unit type. Hair follicle afferent fibres have terminal axons with boutons *en passant*, whereas slowly adapting Type I units with receptors in glabrous skin have few such boutons. Collaterals from axons innervating Pacinian corpuscles have boutons *en passant* in their dorsal termination area whereas in the ventral region grape-like clusters of boutons make their appearance. Pacinian corpuscle axon collaterals also carry the largest boutons we have seen on any primary afferent fibre.

All of these differences in the morphology of collaterals from different types of afferent unit show that there must be great specificity in the organization of connexions between primary afferent fibres and spinal cord neurones. Hair follicle afferent fibres (Types G and T) can only make contact with neuronal somata and dendrites in and near lamina III. Axons from slowly adapting Type II units and Pacinian corpuscle units may contact neurones in laminae III, IV, V and VI, but they do so selectively and do not make contact with, for example, cells of the spinocervical tract in laminae III, IV and V. Furthermore, an important corollary of these results is that they provide independent, and overwhelming, support for the original electrophysiological classification of the afferent units. There is little reason to doubt, nowadays, that cutaneous receptors are highly specific in terms of the stimuli to which they respond. But to be able to predict the functional properties of the receptors from examination of the structure of the spinal cord collaterals from the axons that innervate them is remarkable. It demonstrates that the complete afferent unit (primary afferent neurone plus its receptors) is a specific entity, responding only to some forms of stimuli peripherally and making highly specified connexions centrally. The formation and maintenance of these central connexions are subjects that are just beginning to receive rigorous study. It is to be hoped that the precise information provided by combined electrophysiological and anatomical experiments such as those described in this book will provide a sound basis for future research on this important topic.

III. Receptive field transformation

It is not unreasonable to consider the skin as a two-dimensional sheet. The dorsal horn is a three-dimensional structure. Receptive fields of primary afferent units are transformed from the two-dimensional receptor sheet so that they may be represented in the three-dimensional spinal grey matter. These transformations are essentially the same for all cutaneous afferent units.

In the skin, receptive fields range from single spot-like areas (rapidly adapting mechanoreceptors in glabrous skin, some slowly adapting Type I units) to areas of from a few square millimetres to several square centimetres (hair follicle units, most slowly adapting Type I units). In addition the Pacinian corpuscles and the slowly adapting Type II receptors can be excited by stimulation of skin away from the receptor location. For all cutaneous afferent units, however, the information is distributed through the axon collaterals to a rostro-caudally running column of dorsal horn at least 10 mm and possibly up to several centimetres long (see Imai and Kusama 1969; Wall and Werman 1976; Devor et al. 1977). This column may be continuous (hair follicle afferent fibres) or interrupted, and varies from about 100 to 600 μm in width and about 200 to 800 μm in depth.

Therefore, peripheral receptive fields that are two-dimensional, and spot-like, round or oval are transformed into enormously elongated three-dimensional sheets or columns running through the dorsal horn. It is obvious, but perhaps worth stressing, that the whole of each receptive field is represented in each part of the column of terminal arborization, indeed is represented in each synaptic bouton. As trivial as this observation is, it is very important that one should be aware of its consequences. For a primary afferent unit with a very large receptive field, such as most of the lateral thigh, there is no way that spatial information *within* that field can be encoded in the input to the cord from that unit. Detailed spatial discrimination must be a function of assemblies of central neurones appropriately connected with primary afferent fibres. (Hair follicle units usually fire more vigorously when stimuli move against the hair than with the hair. But this phenomenon, per se, provides no information about direction of stimulus movement.) Also, where the primary afferent fibre innervates only a single receptor the central transformation is most extreme—from a point on the skin to a volume of spinal cord that demonstrates enormous amplification of relative space.

The organization of the primary afferent input into longitudinal columns stamps its effect on the somatotopic organization of the dorsal horn (see below). Neurones receiving the primary afferent input have receptive fields that are also arranged in longitudinally running columns.

IV. Somatotopic organization

There is a precise somatotopic organization of the cutaneous input to the dorsal horn that brings together, to the same dorso-ventral axis, information from different types of afferent unit that have receptors in the same skin area. The longitudinal columns, that are the terminal arborizations from individual cutaneous axons, overlap extensively in all directions. Nevertheless, if it were possible to record from the terminal arborizations with a microelectrode it would be apparent that in any

single dorso-ventral track through laminae III–VI of the dorsal horn receptive fields would all be on neighbouring parts of the skin. Primary afferent fibres do not all generate terminal arborizations of the same transverse extent (Fig. 10.2, Table 10.1). This will produce some smearing in the primary somatotopic map but will also probably provide continuity across adjacent skin areas, such as at the hairy/glabrous skin junctions.

V. Collateral spacing

A final generalization that can be made about primary afferent fibres in the spinal cord is that the spacing of their collaterals (within a centimetre or so of either side of their entrance to the cord) is correlated with the position of their terminal arborizations in the transverse plane. Fibres with terminations in the medial part of the dorsal horn have collaterals closer together than do axons with terminations in the lateral parts. This relationship is shown in Fig. 10.3.

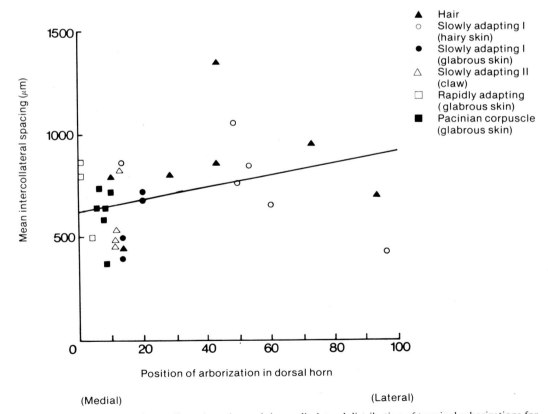

Fig. 10.3. The relationship between mean intercollateral spacing and the medio-lateral distribution of terminal arborizations for large myelinated cutaneous axons. The fitted regression line is shown and the correlation is significant at the 1% level.

This observation, that the spacing of collaterals from cutaneous axons in the lumbosacral cord is correlated with the position of their terminals in the transverse plane, raises many questions about spinal cord organization but provides few clues to their answers. Much more information is required before any satisfactory hypotheses may be set up; for example, it would be useful to know whether axons (of the same type) all give off about equal numbers of collaterals even though the spacing of these might vary. If that were the case then axons with terminals in the lateral parts of the cord would have a much greater rostro-caudal domain than those supplying the medial parts. In fact something of this sort may be taking place. Somatotopic maps generated by recording from dorsal horn neurones (see Chapter 6) do indeed show that in the lateral part of the horn a given location on the hind limb (usually lateral thigh or leg) is represented over a greater rostro-caudal distance than is the case for a single location (usually on a medial toe) represented in the medial horn. Another relevant observation in this context is that the dendritic trees of dorsal horn (spinocervical tract) neurones also have their greatest rostro-caudal spreads in the lateral horn and their shortest ones in the medial horn (Chapter 6). Perhaps these phenomena are simply due to differential growth (limited to the limb enlargements?) that causes individual segments to be wedge-shaped, being longer laterally than medially and therefore overlapping laterally much more than medially. The greater degree of overlap laterally has been shown to exist (P. B. Brown and Culberson 1981).

B. The neurones of the dorsal horn

In the past 10 to 15 years there has been a remarkable increase in interest in the anatomy, physiology and pharmacology of dorsal horn neurones. Detailed descriptions of some of the neuronal systems studied in my laboratory have been given in Chapters 6–9. But concurrently with our own studies there have been many anatomical and physiological experiments reported from other centres. Of special interest recently has been the most dorsal part of the dorsal horn, laminae I–III. The latest achievements have been the intracellular staining of small neurones in this region using the horseradish peroxidase technique (Bennett et al. 1979; Light et al. 1979).

Although there is a general consensus of opinion concerning the structure and function of the deeper parts of the dorsal horn, the literature on the more superficial laminae is not easy to sort out. An attempt will be made here to provide some major conceptual generalizations and to place the various disparate pieces of work into relationship with one another.

I. Lamina I (the postero-marginal cell layer)

Within Rexed's lamina I the large postero-marginal cells (Clarke 1859; Waldeyer 1888; Ramon y Cajal 1909) are the best characterized. It should be remembered, however (Rexed 1952), that lamina I contains other smaller neurones. Little is known about them.

1. Anatomy

a) *Dendritic organization.* Gobel (1978a) has examined the marginal cells in the trigeminal nucleus caudalis of adult cats. He divided them into four categories on the basis of their dendritic trees: spiny and smooth pyramidal cells and compact and loose multipolar cells. Whether this classification can be applied to marginal cells in the spinal cord remains to be seen. Gobel (1978a) states that all marginal cell dendrites in the adult cat are confined to lamina I or the regions immediately outside it. He considers that dendritic extensions into lamina II (e.g. as shown in Ramon y Cajal 1909, Fig. 380) are a feature of immature neurones. The view of Scheibel and Scheibel (1968), that the marginal cell dendritic tree is a flattened disc, is upheld, although in their neonatal material an occasional dendrite dipped down into lamina II. In an important series of experiments Light et al. (1979) have stained individual marginal cells with horseradish peroxidase. From their reconstructions (adult cats, caudal or lower sacral segments) dendritic trees have extents of about 150–200 μm in the transverse plane and about 500–1400 μm in the rostro-caudal direction: that is, the discs are ellipses with their longer diameter in the longitudinal axis. Rather similar measurements (500–680 μm for the rostro-caudal extent) have been made by Price et al. (1979)

from Golgi preparations of primate lumbosacral cord. There is also general agreement (Beal and Cooper 1978; Light et al. 1979; Price et al. 1979) that the great majority of marginal cell dendrites are confined to lamina I in the spinal cord of adult animals.

b) *Axonal projections.* Gobel (1978a) considered that most, if not all, marginal cells in the trigeminal nucleus caudalis are projection neurones, sending their axons out of the nucleus. Many marginal cells in the spinal cord also have axons that project to distant sites. Retrograde horseradish peroxidase studies have demonstrated projections to the lateral cervical nucleus (Craig 1978; Brown et al. 1980b), the medullary and mid-brain reticular formation and probably the dorsal column nuclei (Trevino 1976; Molenaar and Kuypers 1978), the thalamus (Trevino and Carstens 1975) and also to the cord a segment or two away from the cell body, including segments caudal to it (Burton and Loewy 1976).

Electrophysiological results suggest that many marginal cells do not project very far. Kumazawa et al. (1975) could only backfire 5 of 21 marginal cells in cat sacral and caudal segments from the contralateral cervical cord, and only 13 of 31 cells in the monkey. Cervero et al. (1979a) suggest that only about one-third of the marginal cells send their axons more than two segments away from the cell body. As has been discussed by Kumazawa et al. (1975), such negative results need cautious interpretation. Branching axons may not conduct antidromic impulses beyond branch points and deep axons may not be easily excited unless stimulating electrodes are very close to them.

Obviously the anatomical and physiological results show some disagreement. Golgi preparations are rarely examined as serial sections and observations from single thick sections reveal little about axonal projections. But the retrograde horseradish peroxidase studies indicate that marginal cells project to many different targets, through many different pathways. It is conceivable that some marginal cells have axons projecting through more than one pathway or give collaterals to many targets. In our own work (Brown et al. 1980b) a surprisingly large number of marginal cells were stained after horseradish peroxidase injections into the upper cervical cord. Counts of absolute numbers of marginal cells

have not been made but the present writer inclines to the view that probably a majority of marginal cells sends axons to sites more distant than neighbouring segments.

2. Physiological properties

All accounts of recordings from presumed marginal cells show they are excited by noxious stimulation of the skin. In the first report of their properties (Christensen and Perl 1970) three types were described: (1) excited by noxious mechanical stimuli with the input travelling in Aδ fibres, (2) excited by noxious mechanical and noxious thermal stimuli via Aδ and C fibres, (3) excited by noxious mechanical, noxious thermal and innocuous thermal stimuli via Aδ and C fibres. Subsequent studies have confirmed these observations (Willis et al. 1974; Handwerker et al. 1975; Kumazawa et al. 1975; Kumazawa and Perl 1978; Cervero et al. 1976; Menétrey et al. 1977; Mitchell and Hellon 1977; Necker and Hellon 1978; Price et al. 1979) although Handwerker et al. (1975) and Price et al. (1979) considered some cells to be excited by sensitive mechanoreceptors. In both monkey (Kumazawa and Perl 1978) and cat (Light et al. 1979) some cells in lamina I appear to be excited mainly by sensitive thermoreceptors (see also Iggo and Ramsey 1976). According to Light et al. (1979) these cells have many dendrites in lamina II.

The weight of the evidence therefore suggests that the three classes of marginal cell originally described by Christensen and Perl (1970) represent the majority of these neurones. In view of the evidence suggesting an exclusive high-threshold Aδ fibre input to lamina I, the C fibre evoked responses of marginal cells are presumably relayed through other neurones.

At present there is no evidence to suggest that the three physiological types of marginal cell can be correlated with anatomical types. Marginal neurones form a set of neurones excited by noxious stimuli that have wide-ranging projections through the neuraxis as far rostrally as the thalamus. Their effects will be widespread. How one thinks of these neurones in functional terms probably depends on preconceived notions about the nervous system. At one extreme it may be imagined that there are several subsets of neurones projecting through specific pathways such as the spinothalamic tract; at the other extreme marginal cells may be considered as a single population of neurones whose function might be to modulate activity at many sites in the nervous system, and this modulation could be either facilitatory or inhibitory. At the present time it is difficult to conceive of experiments that could differentiate between such ideas.

II. Lamina II (the substantia gelatinosa)

Lamina II is the substantia gelatinosa (Rolando 1824). Rexed (1952) in his original description of the cytoarchitectonics of the spinal grey matter noted that lamina II could be divided into an outer and an inner region. This division has been substantiated by recent work on the basis of afferent input to it (see Sect. A above) and also of the dendritic organization and axonal projections of its neurones.

1. Anatomy

Gobel (1975a, 1978b) has made an extensive Golgi study of the cells in the substantia gelatinosa of the cat's trigeminal nucleus caudalis. Unfortunately there are many contradictions in the de-

tailed descriptions of cells in the two papers. Also Gobel et al. (1977) and Gobel (1978a, b) divide the region into laminae II and III so that the layer equivalent to Rexed's lamina III becomes lamina IV etc. This is unnecessarily confusing; it would have been better to have divided II into II_o and II_i (for outer and inner respectively). This was done by Beal and Cooper (1978), although they include part of III in II_i, and Ralston (1979) and Ralston and Ralston (1979).

Several types of cells have been described by Gobel, including islet cells, stalked cells, spiny cells and arboreal cells. The islet cells (Ramon y Cajal's (1909) 'cellules centrales et antérieures': see his Fig. 380) are found mainly in the inner part of Rexed's lamina II (II_i or III in Gobel's terminology) (Fig. 10.4). They have their dendritic trees oriented in the longitudinal direction, within lamina II, and their axons ramify within the region of the dendritic tree, i.e. they are Golgi type II cells. The stalked cells (Ramon y Cajal's 'cellules limitrophes') (Fig. 10.4) have their cell bodies at the outer edge of lamina II near the border with lamina I. Their dendritic trees are directed mainly ventrally and to the medial and

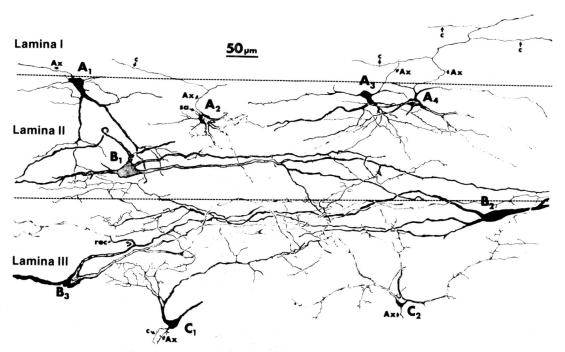

Fig. 10.4. Types of cells in laminae II and III. The figure is drawn from sagittal sections of Golgi-impregnated material. A_1–A_4, stalked cells of outer lamina II; B_1, B_2, islet cells of inner lamina II and the lamina II–III border; B_3, C_1, C_2, cells of lamina III. Ax, axons; c, collaterals; rec, recurving dendrite. (From Beal and Cooper 1978.)

lateral sides so that they form a cone with the apex at the soma. Dendrites are sometimes limited to the outer part of lamina II (II$_o$) and sometimes extend through the lamina into the outer part of (Rexed's) lamina III; occasional dendrites enter lamina I. The axons of stalked cells enter lamina I where they form an 'umbrella-like canopy' over the soma and dendrites of the parent cell. These two types of cells appear to be the most common neurones in the substantia gelatinosa. They have been described in the adult primate spinal cord (Beal and Cooper 1978; Price et al. 1979), where they have similar positions, dendritic trees and axonal projections (Fig. 10.4) as described above for the trigeminal nucleus caudalis.

In the descriptions of Gobel and of Beal and Cooper the axonal projections from the substantia gelatinosa are limited to those from stalked cells to lamina I and those from islet cells which remain within lamina II. The classical observations (see Ramon y Cajal 1909) that gelatinosa neurones project through Lissauer's tract were given modern support by Szentágothai (1964) and much recent work has been interpreted in the light of the latter report. The prevailing view is that the substantia gelatinosa is a closed system and axons of gelatinosa neurones only leave through Lissauer's tract to re-enter the gelatinosa a segment or two away. But it has been shown more recently (Willis et al. 1978) that some lumbosacral lamina II neurones are labelled after horseradish peroxidase injections into the primate thalamus. It is not safe to assume, therefore, that the only outputs from lamina II are (1) to lamina I from the limitrophe or stalked cells, and (2) via Lissauer's tract, the lateral propriospinal or the dorsal commissure pathway back to the ipsilateral or contralateral substantia gelatinosa (Ramon y Cajal 1909; Szentágothai 1964; see also Sugiura 1975).

2. Physiology

Until very recently there was no physiology of lamina II neurones. Advances in microelectrode techniques combined with greater care in maintaining the animal preparations have led to success in a number of laboratories. Unfortunately these new results have not provided a consensus of opinion on the functional properties of lamina II cells. Some of the reports are difficult to assess. The most clear-cut, and the most important, re-

sults have been obtained when it has been possible to combine electrophysiological recordings with intracellular horseradish peroxidase injections. The location and the morphology of the neurones have thus been defined and the only limitations to the experiments have been the sampling bias in intracellular studies (presumably against the smallest cells), the types of animal preparations used and the physiological tests for classifying neuronal responses.

Light et al. (1979) stained 17 cells in laminae I and II of unanaesthetized spinal cats. They noted that none of their cells really corresponded with Gobel's types and that the main correlation was between a cell's response properties and the region of its major dendritic arborization. As described above, cells with dendrites mainly in the marginal cell layer were dominated by input from Aδ axons innervating mechanoreceptive nociceptors. Neurones with most of their dendritic tree in lamina II$_o$ had inputs from C fibres innervating either mechanoreceptive nociceptors or sensitive thermoreceptors. Cells with dendrites in lamina I and lamina II$_o$ received input from nociceptors innervated by both Aδ and C fibres; those with dendrites in II$_i$ were excited by C fibres innervating sensitive receptors and responded to innocuous mechanical stimuli; those with dendrites limited to laminae II$_i$ and III were excited by Aδ fibres innervating sensitive mechanoreceptors. These results fit well with the scheme of Light and Perl (1979a, b) describing primary afferent fibre input to the most dorsal part of the spinal grey matter. Light et al. (1979) found no cells that had a soma in lamina I or II and a 'wide dynamic range' to natural stimuli, i.e. responded to stimuli from light touch through to heavy pressure and pinch. They did find neurones that showed marked habituation to repeated stimuli and these cells usually responded to innocuous mechanical stimulation.

Bennett et al. (1979) have stained 12 stalked (limitrophe) cells in the lumbosacral cord of cats anaesthetized with pentobarbitone. Six of these cells were excited only by noxious stimuli, the input being carried by Aδ or Aδ plus C fibres. They correspond with some of the neurones described by Light et al. (1979). The other six cells were 'wide dynamic range' neurones responding to myelinated low-threshold mechanoreceptive afferent fibres (Aα–γ) and nociceptive afferent fibres, including C fibres. It is of interest that of the two neurones illustrated by Bennett et al. the 'wide dynamic range' neurone had dendrites that reached just into lamina III, whereas the 'nociceptive-specific' neurone had a dendritic tree limited to lamina II_o. Bennett et al. (1979) also briefly mention that lamina II cells other than stalked cells sometimes receive an exclusive input from low-threshold mechanoreceptors.

It is the similarities between the results of Light et al. (1979) and Bennett et al. (1979) that should be stressed rather than the differences. The samples of stained lamina II neurones are exceedingly small and the variability of morphological types in lamina II great (Beal and Cooper 1979). It seems that some of the difficulty experienced by Light et al. in correlating the anatomy of their stained cells with the types of Gobel is due to the fact that they were working on lower sacral or caudal segments where lamina I is relatively thick (Rexed 1954). The major difference between the two sets of results is that Light et al. found no 'wide dynamic range' neurones whereas Bennett et al. did. The problem may be one of sampling. Neurones with dendrites entering lamina III should have ample opportunity to come into contact with primary afferent fibres conducting in the $A\alpha$–γ range and innervating sensitive mechanoreceptors. A pattern is beginning to emerge, however, and that pattern is in essential agreement with the scheme put forward by Perl's group.

If the evidence on the properties of lamina II neurones were limited to the above two sets of results the situation would be relatively clear-cut. There are a number of other reports, however, based almost solely on *extracellular* recordings and none including intracellular staining, that have thrown up conflicting results. Hentall (1977) used Wood's metal-filled microelectrodes in spinal cats and recorded units that responded 50–200 ms *after* an innocuous stimulus. Kumazawa and Perl (1978) found, in monkeys, responses in agreement with those of Light et al. (1979) described above. Wall et al. (1979) recorded, in decerebrate cats, 333 units 'in laminae II or III'. They used tungsten microelectrodes plated with platinum black. One-third of their cells had small receptive fields (less than 2 cm^2); one-half responded only to innocuous mechanical stimuli, with central latencies to electrical stimulation indicative of input from the larger myelinated axons; one-fifth of the sample responded over a 'wide dynamic range'; and one-fifth required

heavy pressure or pinching for excitation. Fourteen per cent of the sample of Wall et al. showed marked habituation to repeated mechanical stimulation and 20% responded to a single mechanical or electrical stimulus with a prolonged discharge lasting from 5 s to 3 min.

Price et al. (1979) have made a careful study (in monkey lumbosacral cord) in which they recorded a marginal cell and subsequently another unit within 200 μm deep to it, using platinum-coated tungsten microelectrodes. Most of the marginal cells projected to the thalamus. A majority of their units, including marginal cells, responded only to noxious stimuli and none of these were excited by afferent fibres conducting at greater than 45 m s^{-1}. The remainder of their units were either 'wide dynamic range' neurones or responded to innocuous mechanical stimulation; none of the latter were marginal cells. Both the 'wide dynamic range' neurones and those responding to innocuous stimulation included cells responding to input in fibres conducting at velocities greater than 45 m s^{-1}. An analysis of the pairs of units revealed that the dorsal (marginal) cell had a receptive field that contained or overlapped that of the ventral (putative lamina II) neurone and that the dorsal cell usually had a longer latency to electrical stimulation of the receptive field than did the ventral member of the pair, suggesting input to lamina I via lamina II.

Finally, Cervero et al. (1979b) recorded 110 neurones in the lumbosacral cord of chloralose-anaesthetized cats with high-impedance electrolyte-filled micropipettes. One of their criteria for accepting a unit as being located in the substantia gelatinosa was that it should show 'novel responses' to cutaneous stimuli. On the basis of the background activity and novel responses they introduced a new set of unit types into the literature ($\bar{1}$, $\bar{2}$, $\bar{3}$: see Chapter 1, Sect. C). These 'inverse classes' were inhibited by innocuous stimuli, noxious and innocuous stimuli, and noxious stimuli respectively.

Examination of all of the reports, including the intracellularly stained material, leads to the following conclusions:

1) The results of Kumazawa and Perl (1979) agree with those of Light et al. (1979).

2) The results of Price et al. (1979) agree with those of Bennett et al. (1979).

These agreements are not surprising. Each pair of

results emanates from the same laboratory.

3) The agreement between the results from Perl's laboratory and those of Dubner and Price is close, except for the absence of input from the faster conducting myelinated afferent fibres reported by Perl's group.

4) There are some areas of agreement between Wall et al. (1979) and the above: (a) about 20% of units recorded by Wall's group were nociceptor-specific compared with about 70% of the putative lamina II cells in the results of Price et al. (1979) and about 60% in Kumazawa and Perl (1979); (b) about 20% were 'wide dynamic range' neurones compared with 20%–25% in Price et al. (1979) and none in the study of Light et al. (1979). However, nearly 60% of units recorded by Wall et al. responded to innocuous stimulation and had latencies showing input from large myelinated axons, whereas Price et al. only found seven neurones (about 1%) of this type and Perl's group do not report any. It is possible that the $\bar{3}$ neurones of Cervero et al. (1979b), which constituted 33% of their 'inverse' neurones, are similar to or the same as Wall's units responding to innocuous stimuli.

5) It is difficult to place the inverse units of Cervero et al. (1979b) in relation to the other work. The $\bar{1}$ units accounted for 8% of their inverse group and were excited by noxious stimuli and inhibited by innocuous stimuli. If these units correspond with the nociceptor-specific types of Perl, Price et al. and Wall et al. then it is puzzling that they form such a small proportion of the sample. The $\bar{2}$ units were inhibited by noxious and innocuous stimuli and constituted 55% of the population. Price et al. (1979) found three neurones responding only with inhibition and Kumazawa and Perl (1979) showed that neurones responding to small temperature changes (20% of their sample) could be inhibited by noxious and innocuous mechanical stimuli to skin areas outside their receptive field for thermal stimuli. As discussed above the $\bar{3}$ units may correspond with units described by Wall et al. that responded to innocuous mechanoreceptive input travelling in large myelinated cutaneous axons. The restrictive criteria of Cervero et al. (1979b), including the necessity for the units to show 'novel responses' and to respond to stimulation of Lissauer's tract, may well be the cause of the disparities in relative numbers of different types of units recorded by this group in comparison with others. It is also

difficult to avoid the conclusion that some, at least, of their units were located in lamina III, as were those of Wall et al. (1979). Indeed Wall et al. state that they recorded from both II and III and there were no differences between the two—a surprising observation. In the final analysis extracellular recording methods are never going to provide accurate data about cellular localization.

6) All groups have reported some cells with what might be termed unusual properties. These include habituation, prolonged discharges and 'off' responses. It is not clear, yet, what contribution such cells make to the total population of recordable neurones in lamina II nor what their functional roles are.

7) Major differences in the results between the various groups of workers could well be due to the use of different species, different microelectrodes, different anaesthetics or different preparations (spinal, decerebrate).

8) Finally it should be kept in mind that the substantia gelatinosa is a very complicated neuropil. As well as its neurones playing the standard roles of excitatory or inhibitory cells (and none of the above electrophysiological experiments could differentiate between the two) lamina II contains axo-axonic (Ralston 1971, 1979; Kerr 1975a, b), dendro-dendritic (Coimbra et al. 1974; Gobel 1974, 1976; Ralston 1979) and dendro-axonic (Gobel 1976) synapses. The possibilities for neuronal interaction are numerous.

Figure 10.5 is an attempt to present a diagrammatic scheme for the anatomical and functional organization of laminae I and II. It incorporates the evidence presented earlier on the primary afferent fibres input to these laminae and also the neurone types for which the best evidence exists. Laminae I and II cannot be considered in isolation and the figure also includes some aspects of lamina III. This latter lamina seems, in some respects, to be a transition or connecting zone between the first two laminae and the more ventral laminae IV, V and VI. Lamina III will, however, be considered together with laminae IV–VI in the following section.

III. Laminae III–VI

The remaining laminae of the dorsal horn, laminae III–VI, will be considered together. With these laminae we move on to apparently firmer ground. There are a number of reasons why it seems reasonable to discuss laminae III–VI in a single section. (1) Myelinated cutaneous afferent fibres innervating sensitive mechanoreceptors distribute their input to these laminae, some axons to all four layers. (2) The laminae contain many large neurones, in addition to smaller ones, and a majority of them have dendritic trees limited to these laminae. (3) Most of the cells of origin of the spinocervical and post-synaptic dorsal column pathways, and the spinothalamic tract in primates, are situated within this part of the cord. (4) There is a gradual shift in the orientations of dendritic trees from lamina III through to lamina VI and the anatomical picture is relatively clear, at least for the dorsal part of the region. (5) Physiological results are also less contradictory for laminae III–VI in comparison with laminae I and II.

1. Anatomy

a) *Dendritic trees.* Many neurones with cell bodies in laminae III–VI have dendritic trees limited to these laminae and lamina VII. Some neurones, and these may be very important in the operation of the dorsal horn mechanisms, have dendritic trees that link laminae I and II with the deeper layers. The general organization of laminae III–VI will be considered first.

In laminae III and IV many neurones, including some of those with the largest cell bodies, have dorsally directed dendrites, sometimes to the exclusion of any others. Cells of this type have been illustrated earlier (see Figs. 6.24–6.27, Fig. 8.3) and described by many authors. Even cells with dendrites projecting in other directions usually have prominent dorsal dendrites. The dendrites of spinocervical tract cells are mainly oriented in the longitudinal axis of the cord so that the dendritic tree is narrow in the transverse plane, as recognized by Scheibel and Scheibel (1968). Such neurones, even those in lamina III, tend to limit their dendritic trees to laminae III and IV (and V where they have ventral dendrites). Only rarely do spinocervical tract cells' dendrites penetrate into lamina II and then they remain in II$_i$; this is a striking observation when the trees are viewed in parasagittal sections (see Fig. 6.16A), for dendrites can be seen ap-

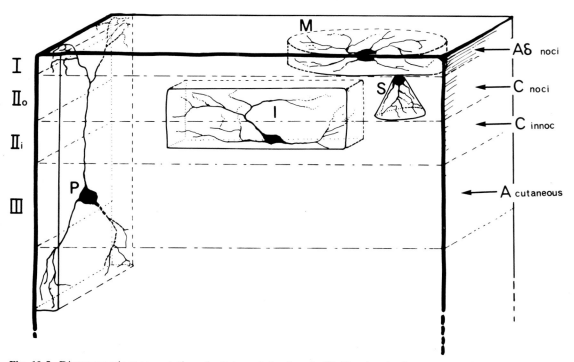

Fig. 10.5. Diagrammatic representation of cell types in laminae I–III. The drawing is meant to show the dendritic trees of cells viewed in a parasagittally cut block of cord. I, islet cell of lamina II; M, marginal cell of lamina I; P, 'pyramidal' cell of lamina III with dendrites bridging laminae I to IV. S, stalked cell of lamina II. The terminations of cutaneous axons are indicated to the right.

proaching lamina II and then running along the lamina II–III border. The dendritic extensions of post-synaptic dorsal column neurones into lamina II and I (Brown and Fyffe 1981b; see Chapter 8) may be important for the reception of input from non-myelinated and fine myelinated afferent fibres, but this input will be limited to distal dendritic branches.

At the other extreme, neurones deep in lamina V and in VI have dendritic trees that radiate from the cell body but which are confined to the transverse plane, thus forming a disc-like tree (Scheibel and Scheibel 1968). The dendrites may penetrate as far dorsally as lamina III and as far ventrally as VII (or VIII). Many trees are very extensive within the transverse plane, linking many laminae and also extending across one-half to two-thirds of the dorsal horn. Between these two extremes there is a region of transition; neurones with cell bodies in lamina V and the adjacent parts of IV and VI show intermediate patterns of dendritic tree development. In general, dendritic trees of lamina VI neurones are simpler than those of lamina V cells (Proshansky and Egger 1977).

The basic pattern of dendritic tree organization is as described by Scheibel and Scheibel (1968) on the basis of Golgi studies of immature animals (see Fig. 1.2). But some trees cut across this organization. A typical neurone type ('pyramidal neurone') seems to be that illustrated in Fig. 9.1. The cell body is in lamina III and there are one or two apical dendrites running dorsally through laminae III and II to break up into terminal branches in the marginal layer. Other dendrites emerge from the basal part of the soma to distribute in laminae IV and V. The trees are developed essentially in the transverse plane and can obviously link up the dorsal four or five laminae of the cord (their axonal arborizations are also extensive: see below). Similar neurones with small somata also exist (see Mannen and Sugiura 1976). The dendritic tree organization of the dorsal horn is presented schematically in Fig. 10.6, which is based on the scheme of the Scheibels modified in the light of more recent work.

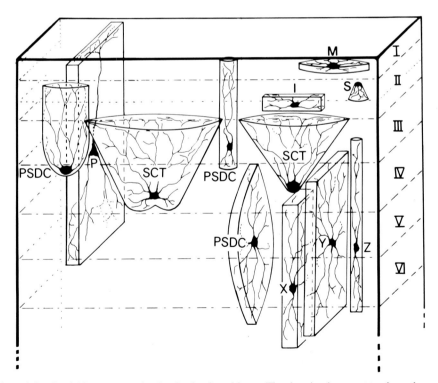

Fig. 10.6. Diagrammatic representation of the dendritic tree organization in the dorsal horn. The drawing is meant to show the organization as viewed in a parasagittal block of tissue. I, islet cell of lamina II; M, marginal cell of lamina I; P, pyramidal cell of lamina III; PSDC, the three main types of neurones sending axons through the dorsal columns; S, stalked cell of lamina II; SCT, spinocervical tract cells; X, Y, Z interneurones of laminae V and VI.

b) *Axonal projections.* Several ascending pathways take origin from cells in laminae III–VI. These include the spinocervical tract, the spino-thalamic tract (in primates mainly; a few cells of this tract are in laminae III–VI in cat) and the post-synaptic pathways to the dorsal column nuclei, via both the dorsal columns and dorso-lateral funiculi, and spinoreticular paths (for references see Chapters 1, 6 and 8). Cells of the spinocervical tract are situated in laminae III–VI (and possibly I) with the vast majority in III and IV (Chapter 6). Cells of the post-synaptic pathway to the dorsal column nuclei are in laminae III and IV and the medial part of V (and VI in cervical cord) (Chapters 1 and 8; Rustioni and Kaufman 1977). There are a few spinothalamic neurones in laminae III–VI in the cat, mainly V and VI (Trevino et al. 1972), but most are in laminae I, VII and VIII in this species, whereas the monkey has a large contribution from lateral parts of laminae IV and V. Other dorsal horn neurones have propriospinal connexions, and some of these neurones receive group I muscle inputs (Czarkowska et al. 1976).

A characteristic feature of most neurones in laminae III–VI is that they have axon collateral arborizations near the cell body. These axon collaterals ramify ventral to the cell's dendritic tree (and within it), so that the preferential direction of conduction of information at the segmental level must be from III to IV, from IV to V, etc. The recent Golgi and horseradish peroxidase data have provided morphological evidence in support of Wall's (1967) cascade arrangement of dorsal horn neurones. It should be stressed, however, that the local axon collaterals are usually distributed more widely in the dorso-ventral direction than expected from Wall's electrophysiological results—usually to at least two and often three laminae. Furthermore, Wall's (1967) latency results were not confirmed by P. B. Brown et al. (1975). The local axon collaterals of neurones in laminae III–VI usually terminate over regions that are longer rostro-caudally and wider medio-laterally than the parent cell's dendritic tree, thus contributing to the expansion of receptive fields that does exist as one records cells more ventrally in the horn.

The 'pyramidal neurones' of lamina III have very extensive axonal projections. That illustrated in Fig. 9.1 had two major axonal branches, one ascending in the ipsilateral dorso-lateral funiculus and the other in the contralateral ventral cord. In addition they have local axonal arborizations in laminae III–V or III–VI (see also Matsushita 1969; Sugiura 1975).

There seem to be few axonal projections in the dorsal direction; the flow of information is essentially from lamina III to VI and from II to I where the main dorsally directed axons are. In adult animals there is also little in the way of connexions across the dorsal horn in the transverse direction. The dorsal horn may be considered as a laminated structure arranged in columns. This scheme is illustrated in Fig. 10.7, but does not differentiate between possible excitatory and inhibitory neurones; as a working hypothesis it might be expected that neurones with axons projecting through ascending pathways are excitatory, though this assumption may not be warranted. Some neurones in the scheme are shown projecting out of the dorsal and into the ventral horn (to motor nuclei) to provide the continuation of information transmission to the output side of the nervous system. Interneurones with connexions to motoneurones, with the notable exception of those receiving Group I muscle excitation, have not yet been identified.

c) *Somatotopic organization.* The precise somatotopic organization of cutaneous primary afferent fibre collaterals described above (Sect. A.IV) is reflected in the organization of receptive fields of neurones in laminae III–VI. Receptive field size increases from lamina III through to VI and is presumably due to both the increasing transverse spread of dendritic trees in the deeper laminae and the fact that the neurones' axonal projections generally spread more widely in the transverse plan than do the dendrites. Both of these features of organization cut across the essentially dorso-ventrally arranged sagittal sheets of primary afferent fibre terminals.

C. Descending input to the dorsal horn

The spinal cord dorsal horn is under the influence of numerous neuronal pathways that arise in the brain. Indeed, at least since the time of Sherrington (see 1906) it has been known that spinal reflexes initiated by cutaneous stimulation are

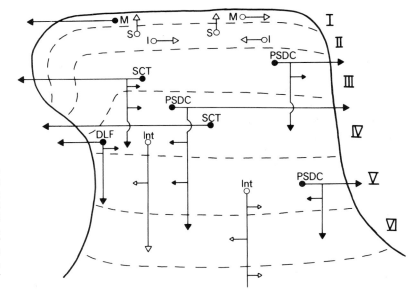

Fig. 10.7. Diagrammatic representation of the axonal projections of dorsal horn neurones. DLF, neurone sending its axon through the dorso-lateral funiculus but not terminating at the lateral cervical nucleus; I, islet cells of lamina II; Int, interneurones with short axons; M, marginal cells of lamina I; PSDC, cells of the post-synaptic dorsal column pathway; S, stalked cells of lamina II; SCT, spino-cervical tract neurones.

under a tonic inhibitory control in decerebrate preparations. Modern studies may be considered to have started with Magoun and Rhines (1946) and Hagbarth and Kerr (1954). Descending influences on spinal cord are carried by a number of well-known pathways including corticospinal, rubrospinal, vestibulospinal and reticulospinal tracts, the latter having been well-characterized recently.

The effects of activity in these descending pathways include actions on primary afferent fibres, on neurones giving rise to ascending pathways and on interneurones of many different types, including those mediating the actions on primary afferent fibres and tract cells. It is beyond the scope of this chapter to review the very extensive literature on descending pathways and their actions; the reader is referred to Lundberg (1964b), various articles in the *Handbook of Sensory Physiology*, vol. 2 (Iggo 1973) and the recent book by Willis and Coggeshall (1978). The aim of the present section is to indicate the sites of termination of descending systems within the dorsal horn and relate them to the scheme of its organization.

I. Descending pathways: actions and terminations

1. Corticospinal tract

Electrical stimulation of wide areas of the cerebral cortex may produce effects on the spinal cord, including primary afferent depolarization (Andersen et al. 1962, 1964; Carpenter et al. 1962, 1963b) and inhibition or excitation of dorsal horn neurones including ascending tract cells (Wall 1967; Fetz 1968; Maillard et al. 1971; Brown and Short, 1974; Coulter et al. 1974, 1976; Brown et al. 1977a). Some of the actions studied in the reports referred to above probably involved relays from cerebral cortex to spinal cord via other central nuclei, such as the red nucleus or cells in the reticular formation. But some of the actions are due to activity in corticospinal neurones (see Phillips and Porter 1977 for a thorough account of corticospinal actions).

Corticospinal axons terminate in the dorsal horn (Nyberg-Hansen and Brodal 1963; Liu and Chambers 1964; Petras 1967; Coulter and Jones 1977). Degeneration methods and methods based on retrograde transport of horseradish peroxidase show that the terminations are in laminae III–VI or III–VII and that laminae I and II are free from corticospinal endings. Coulter and Jones (1977) showed that projections to discrete regions of the horn arise in cortical cytoarchitectonic areas 4, 3a, 3b, 1, 2 and 5, with classical sensory areas projecting more dorsally than motor areas. Most reports suggest that corticospinal terminals are concentrated in the lateral parts of the dorsal horn. Scheibel and Scheibel (1966b, 1968) go as far as to suggest that for neurones in lamina IV, corticospinal axons make synaptic contact on laterally directed dendrites and not on dorsally or medially directed ones, which are supposed to receive inputs from cutaneous afferent fibres and axons entering the dorsal horn from the dorsal columns, respectively. So far there has been no direct evidence in support of the Scheibels' scheme. Jankowska et al. (1979) describe excitatory post-synaptic potentials in neurones of the post-synaptic dorsal column pathway, the spino-cervical tract and a few other interneurones in the dorsal horn; these are attributed to activity in the corticospinal (pyramidal) tract.

2. Raphe-spinal system

The importance of the raphe-spinal system has become apparent in recent years. It has been known, since the description by Brodal et al. (1960), that the raphe nuclei project to the spinal cord via the dorso-lateral funiculus. Raphe neurones contain serotonin (5-hydroxytryptamine) (Dahlström and Fuxe 1965) and ionophoresis of serotonin onto dorsal horn neurones generally depresses their activity (Engberg and Ryall 1966; Randic and Yu 1976). The evidence therefore suggests a role for the raphe-spinal system in descending inhibitory control of dorsal horn neurones. Electrical stimulation of the nucleus raphe magnus (or near to it) produces inhibition of many types of dorsal horn cells: interneurones of uncertain identity (Basbaum et al. 1976; Fields et al. 1977; Guilbaud et al. 1977; Willis et al. 1977), and spinothalamic tract cells in primates (Beall et al. 1976; Willis et al. 1977). In addition electrical stimulation of this region produces primary afferent depolarization, presumably via the excitation of dorsal horn interneurones (Proudfit and Anderson 1974).

The descending pathway from nucleus raphe magnus to spinal cord has been shown to be bilateral and to descend in the dorso-lateral funiculi (Basbaum and Fields 1977; Basbaum et al. 1978). Of particular interest is the demonstration by Basbaum et al. (1978) that in the cat this pathway terminates in lamina I and the subjacent lamina II and also deeper in lamina V and medial parts of laminae VI and VII. Laminae III and IV are spared. In the opossum Goode (1976) has shown degenerating terminals in lamina I and adjoining grey matter after lesions of the nucleus raphe magnus. It is significant that those parts of the cord receiving this serotonergic descending input are those parts now considered to be concerned with nociception and to give rise to spinothalamic (and spinoreticular) tracts.

3. Reticulospinal pathways

In addition to the raphe-spinal pathway other descending tracts take origin from the brain stem. One such system has been the subject of numerous studies by Lundberg and his collaborators. Indeed the pathway (the dorsal reticulospinal system) was described on the basis of electrophysiological and neuropharmacological experiments even though anatomical methods had failed to recognize it. The system arises in the medial medulla and descends in the dorso-lateral funiculus of the cord (Holmqvist and Lundberg 1959, 1961; Engberg et al. 1968b, c, d). It is tonically active in the decerebrate preparation and produces inhibition of various spinal reflexes, interneurones and ascending tract cells, as well as producing primary afferent depolarization (Holmqvist and Lundberg 1959, 1961; Holmqvist et al. 1960; Carpenter et al. 1963a; Engberg et al. 1968a, b, c, d). It is likely that the tonic inhibition of dorsal horn interneurones activated by cutaneous stimulation, and of spinocervical tract cells, is also produced by this system (Wall 1967; Brown and Franz 1969; Brown 1971; Besson et al. 1975; Handwerker et al. 1975; Cervero et al. 1976, 1977).

The dorsal reticulospinal system appears to include, but also be more than, the raphe-spinal system. Engberg et al. (1968b) showed that destruction of most, if not all, of the raphe nuclei reduced but did not remove the tonic descending inhibition. Recently, on the basis of autoradiographic studies, Basbaum et al. (1978) have demonstrated a dorsal pathway originating in the nucleus reticularis magnocellularis. This pathway is ipsilateral and terminates in similar regions of the cord to the raphe-spinal system, that is, in laminae I, II, V, VI and VII. Part of this system also descends in the ipsilateral ventral and ventro-lateral funiculi. It could obviously be responsible for some of the inhibitory effects seen on spinocervical tract neurones (Brown et al. 1973).

A further component of reticulospinal control has also been demonstrated by Basbaum et al. (1978). In confirmation of earlier studies (Nyberg-Hansen 1965; Petras 1967) Basbaum et al. have shown that the nucleus reticularis gigantocellularis gives origin to bilateral pathways running in the ventral and ventro-lateral funiculi. These pathways terminate in more ventral regions than the dorsally located systems (raphe-spinal and dorsal reticulospinal systems), mainly in laminae VII and VIII but also in the lateral parts of lamina V. Stimulation of this pathway is probably responsible for the inhibition described by Jankowska et al. (1968).

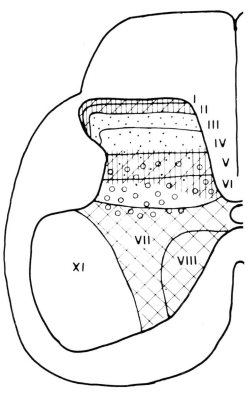

Corticospinal
(sensory cortex)

Corticospinal
(motor cortex)

Raphe-spinal

Reticulospinal
(N. reticularis magnocellularis)

Reticulospinal
(N. reticularis gigantocellularis)

Fig. 10.8. Diagrammatic representation of the termination areas of various descending systems in the lumbosacral spinal cord of the cat.

4. Other descending systems

Many other pathways are able to influence neurones in the dorsal horn, either directly or indirectly. These include rubrospinal and vestibulospinal tracts and possibly reticulospinal pathways other than those described above. Most research on the rubro- and vestibulospinal tracts has been concerned with motor mechanisms, but there is sufficent evidence of involvement with primary afferent transmission and dorsal horn neurones (Erulkar et al. 1966; Cook et al. 1969a, b; Carpenter et al. 1963b; Hongo and Jankowska 1967) to make several new studies quite reasonable propositions.

II. Summary

Figure 10.8 summarizes the locations of some of the descending systems and their termination sites in the spinal grey matter. A major conclusion that may be drawn is that some of the terminations respect the lamination pattern of the horn. This is especially marked for the dorsal two laminae, which receive raphe-spinal and some reticulospinal (from the nucleus reticularis magnocellularis) terminations but none from the corticospinal tracts. Furthermore there appears to be some selective distribution of the corticospinal fibres in that those from somatic sensory cortex tend to end in laminae III–V whereas those from classical motor cortex go to laminae V–VII. At present, however, most descending systems appear to terminate rather widely in the dorsal horn in several (three to five) laminae and often end in the ventral horn as well. Further research may show a greater degree of selectivity in the connexions made by descending systems. An important line in present (and future) research is the identification of transmitters used by various descending systems and individual components of the systems. The demonstration of the distribution of serotonin-containing fibres to those parts of the cord dealing with noxious inputs indicates the importance of this approach.

11 Afferent fibres from primary endings in muscle spindles

In this and the following two chapters the morphology of afferent fibres from the receptors in muscle spindles and the Golgi tendon organs will be described. These receptors, especially those in muscle spindles, have been studied in detail by both anatomists and physiologists for many years. It is outside the scope of this book to review the enormous amount of information now available on the structure and function of muscle spindles and tendon organs. The reader is referred to the excellent monograph by Matthews (1972), and to the reviews by Barker (1974), Hunt (1974) and McIntyre (1974) all in the *Handbook of Sensory Physiology*, vol. III/2, *Muscle Receptors*. A very brief introduction will, however, be provided here, together with a somewhat more detailed account of the central projections of the afferent fibres.

Spindles in cat hind limb muscles contain two types of sensory endings: the primary (annulospiral) ending and the secondary (flower-spray or annulospiral) ending. Both endings are located at the equatorial region of the spindle, the secondary ending on either one or both sides of the primary ending. The two types of receptors are innervated by afferent nerve fibres of different conduction velocities and have different properties.

In general, the axons innervating primary endings are, in Lloyd's (1943b) classification, of Group I diameter and those innervating secondary endings of Group II diameter. It is, perhaps, unfortunate that the use of the words primary and secondary for muscle spindle receptors and of Group I and Group II for muscle afferent fibres leads to the (albeit unconscious) association of primary with Group I and secondary with Group II. This point, and the more important one of relating elevations in a compound action potential from muscle nerve to particular receptors in muscle and tendon, has been discussed in a scholarly

way by McIntyre (1974) (see also Chapter 13).

In Lloyd's classification, as originally proposed (1943b), axons 12 to 20 μm or more in diameter were called Group I, those between 6 and 12 μm were designated Group II and those less than 6 μm comprised Group III. By using the conversion factor of 6 (Hursh 1939) these diameters may be related to axonal conduction velocities of 72–120 m s^{-1}, 36–72 m s^{-1} and less than 36 m s^{-1} respectively. It should be noted that Group III fibres are myelinated; the non-myelinated axons that conduct at less than 2 m s^{-1} came to be called Group IV.

There is no doubt that primary endings are usually innervated by Group I fibres and secondary endings by Group II fibres (Merton 1953; Hunt 1954). Group I fibres also innervate Golgi tendon organs (Hunt and Kuffler 1951; Hunt 1954; Laporte and Bessou 1957; Hunt and McIntyre 1960a; Coppin et al. 1969). However, within the set of axons innervating spindle receptors (both primary and secondary endings) the division between Group I and Group II fibres, which at 72 m s^{-1} indicates the trough between the two population peaks, does not necessarily indicate a clean separation into axons innervating primary and secondary endings respectively. According to Matthews (1963) afferent fibres from muscle spindles in the cat's hind limb are from primary endings if they have conduction velocities of 80 m s^{-1} or more. This conclusion has been substantiated (Hunt 1954; Hunt and McIntyre 1960a; Sumner 1961; Coppin et al. 1969; MacLennan 1972; Matthews 1972).

Both primary and secondary muscle spindle receptors produce a regular sustained discharge in their nerve fibres when the length of the muscle is maintained above a certain threshold value, the discharge frequency being related to muscle length in an approximately linear fashion over a particular range of muscle length (Eldred et al.

1953; Harvey and Matthews 1961). Primary endings have a much greater dynamic sensitivity (response during increasing extension) than secondary endings (Cooper 1961; Hunt and Ottoson 1973). Because of this the primary endings respond to vibration, applied either to the muscle (Kuffler et al. 1951; Granit and Henatsch 1956; Bianconi and Van der Meulen 1963; Crowe and Matthews 1964) or to the tendon in longitudinal direction (M. C. Brown et al. 1967). Primary endings will follow, in a 1:1 way, vibration applied to the tendon at frequencies of 200–500 Hz and less than 10 μm displacement. Secondary endings and tendon organ receptors are much less sensitive to vibration and only rarely follow vibration in a 1:1 fashion and then only at high amplitudes and low frequencies (M. C. Brown et al. 1967). Vibration applied to the tendon may therefore be used to differentiate primary from secondary spindle endings.

A. Central projections of muscle spindle primary endings

Following accepted practice, the axons innervating muscle spindle primary endings will be called Ia. The central effects of impulses in the Ia fibres are better known than those of any other primary afferent fibres. This knowledge is of both reflex actions at the segmental level and actions on various ascending pathways. Anatomical knowledge of the morphological organization underlying the physiological effects is less well advanced.

Group Ia afferent fibres make monosynaptic excitatory connexions with α-motoneurones. These contacts are made both with motoneurones supplying the muscle that contains the primary endings (homonymous muscle) and with those supplying synergists (heteronymous muscles). They provide, therefore, the afferent limb of the monosynaptic reflex much studied by electrophysiologists from Eccles and Pritchard (1937), Renshaw (1940) and Lloyd (1943a) onwards. This monosynaptic, or more correctly myotatic, reflex has been shown unequivocally to be produced by activity of spindle primary endings. Thus Lundberg and Winsbury (1960a), using brief weak muscle stretch that only excited primary endings,

showed that a pure Ia input produces monosynaptic excitatory post-synaptic potentials in the homonymous motoneurones.

Anatomical evidence for the presence of monosynaptic connexions between the largest primary afferent fibres and α-motoneurones is plentiful but indirect (Sprague 1958; Szentagothai 1958; Illis 1967; Sterling and Kuypers 1967a; Conradi 1969; Iles 1976). Electron microscope studies have indicated that such afferent fibres make both axosomatic and axodendritic contacts with motoneurones (Conradi 1969; McLaughlin 1972a, b). Unfortunately there is no way, using anatomical techniques, that the Ia fibres can be identified with certainty. The assumption is made that the axons of largest diameter are Ia fibres. This is a reasonable assumption but, of course, depends on electrophysiological evidence.

For many years it was accepted that only Ia fibres make monosynaptic connexions with motoneurones. Recently electrophysiological evidence has been presented showing that Group II afferent fibres from spindle secondary endings terminate in the ventral horn close to the motor nuclei (Fu et al. 1974; Fu and Schomburg 1974). Furthermore, Kirkwood and Sears (1974) and Stauffer et al. (1976) have shown that Group II afferent fibres may make monosynaptic excitatory connexions with motoneurones. Obviously great care is necessary in the interpretation of anatomical material purporting to show Ia afferent fibre collaterals. Only when the anatomical technique is combined with the electrophysiological identification of the primary afferent fibre is it possible to be sure that Ia fibres have been stained; such a technique is the intra-axonal injection of horseradish peroxidase.

Most of our knowledge of the anatomical organization of the monosynaptic reflex pathway between Ia fibres and motoneurones derives from electrophysiological studies. This is because of the problems of identification referred to above, together with the fact that motoneurones, being the largest neurones in the mammalian nervous system, are relatively easy to record from intracellularly. The development of methods that allow the limitation of the afferent input to a single Ia fibre (Kuno 1964a, b) heralded a series of investigations on the Ia–motoneurone connexions by many groups of workers.

Mendell and Henneman (1971) have shown that a single Ia fibre innervating the medial gastrocnemius muscle will excite all, or nearly all, of the approximately 300 motoneurones innervating the same muscle. These authors have also calculated that each medial gastrocnemius motoneurone will receive monosynaptic excitation from all or nearly all of the 60 or so Ia fibres from the homonymous muscle. On the basis of the numbers of motoneurones supplying medial gastrocnemius/soleus (Boyd and Davey 1968) and lateral gastrocnemius, Iles (1976) has estimated that a single Ia afferent fibre from triceps surae gives monosynaptic connexions to about 550 motoneurones. This figure has been revised downwards (see Scott and Mendell 1976; and Chapter 13) but is still of the order of 450–500 motoneurones.

Electrophysiological analysis, in agreement with the anatomical data, has shown that the monosynaptic connexions are probably distributed over both soma and dendrites of the motoneurones (Terzuolo and Llinas 1966; Burke 1967; Rall et al. 1967; Jack et al. 1971). The evidence, essentially, is that excitatory post-synaptic potentials produced by activity in single Ia fibres have a variety of shapes, both shorter and longer than the composite potential produced by electrical excitation of a peripheral nerve (Brock et al. 1952), suggesting that the synapses are distributed over the soma and proximal and distal dendrites of the motoneurones (see for example Rall 1967). Such analyses, although suggesting the mean positions, in electrotonic terms, of synapses from a single Ia afferent fibre upon the receptive surface of a motoneurone (Barrett and Crill 1974a, b; Jack and Redman 1971), do not provide any direct evidence for the numbers and locations of such synapses. This problem will be taken up in Chapter 14.

In addition to their connexions with motoneurones, Group Ia axons excite other neurones (interneurones) at the segmental level of entry. These are neurones in and around the intermediate region of the dorsal horn (lamina VI and dorsal VII) and the interneurones responsible for the Ia-evoked 'direct' inhibition of motoneurones. For many years it was believed that the interneurones interposed on the Ia inhibitory pathway were located in the intermediate region (the story of the controversy surrounding the idea that an inhibitory interneurone was interposed has been told many times: see e.g. McIntyre 1974). Recently the location of the Ia inhibitory interneurones has been established beyond doubt by a superb series of experiments carried out by Jankowska and her colleagues that culminated in the intracellular staining of the neurones with Procion Yellow (Hultborn et al. 1971a, b, c; Jankowska and Roberts 1972a, b; Jankowska and Lindström 1972). The Ia inhibitory interneurones are located in lamina VII just dorsal and dorso-medial to the motor nuclei.

The identification of the Ia inhibitory interneurones raises the question of the identity of the monosynaptically excited interneurones in lamina VI. Examination of the original data (Eccles et al. 1954a, c, 1956) reveals that the evidence depended upon electrical stimulation of muscle nerves (see McIntyre 1974). A later study (Eccles et al. 1960) using similar techniques was interpreted in a similar way. However, R. M. Eccles (1965) concluded that 41 of 45 interneurones in this region could be excited by Ib afferents, and Hongo et al. (1966) could not differentiate between Ia and Ib effects. The problem has been re-investigated by Lucas and Willis (1974) using adequate stimulation of the receptors. Only 4 of 46 neurones in the intermediate region could be excited monosynaptically by Ia fibres whereas at least 42 of them could be activated monosynaptically by Ib fibres. In conclusion, therefore, it is likely that some interneurones in lamina VI receive monosynaptic excitation from Ia afferent fibres, but that many more receive monosynaptic excitation from Ib afferent fibres. Among the candidates for interneurones receiving Ia excitation will be those on the pathway producing primary afferent depolarization of the Ia terminals themselves (Eccles et al. 1961a, c, 1962, 1963; Voorhoeve and Verhey 1963; Cook et al. 1965; Barnes and Pompeiano 1970a, b; see review by Schmidt 1973).

From the electrophysiological data it may be concluded that, at the segmental level, Ia afferent fibres should give collaterals to at least three main regions: the intermediate region (lamina VI and possibly the dorsal part of lamina VII), the region where Ia inhibitory neurones are located (lamina VII, dorsal and dorso-medial to the motor nuclei), and the motor nuclei (lamina IX). These three regions are where the somata of neurones known to receive monosynaptic excitation from Ia afferent fibres are located. Obviously the synaptic contacts may not be limited to the somata, but may be on dendrites. Therefore, the positions of the Ia boutons could be shifted considerably depending on the morphology of the neurones' dendritic trees. In fact Szentágothai (1967a) has shown that collaterals from presumed Ia fibres give off side branches that arborize precisely in the above regions—that is in the medial third of lamina VI and in a half-moon-shaped area in lamina VII immediately adjacent to the medial border of the motoneurone pool—before entering the motor nuclei. As will be described below, the intra-axonal injection of horseradish peroxidase has confirmed these conclusions.

Of the extrasegmental projections of the Ia fibres the best known is that to Clarke's column, the origin of the dorsal spinocerebellar tract. There are very secure monosynaptic excitatory connexions between Ia afferent fibres and neurones of the dorsal spinocerebellar tract (Lundberg 1964a; Oscarsson 1973). Clarke's column terminates caudally at L-4 in the cat and therefore collaterals to it arise from Ia fibres as they ascend the dorsal columns. The organization of collaterals to Clarke's column has been the subject of detailed study by Réthelyi (1968, 1970). Collaterals tentatively identified on anatomical grounds as belonging to Ia fibres give rise to very large climbing-type terminals on the somata and dendrites of dorsal spinocerebellar tract neurones.

Little is known of other projections of Ia fibres. The spinal border cell component of the ventral spinocerebellar tracts receives both excitatory and inhibitory actions from spindle primary endings (Lundberg and Weight 1971) and some of the excitatory input is monosynaptic. Collaterals to the spinal border cells in segments rostral to L-7 would therefore be expected.

B. Morphology of Group Ia afferent fibres

In our studies (Brown and Fyffe 1978a, b, 1979; Fyffe 1981; and the present work) Group Ia fibres have been identified as follows: all axons were contained within muscle nerves (usually the nerves to lateral gastrocnemius/soleus, medial gastrocnemius or muscles innervated by the posterior tibial nerve), had conduction velocities of more than 80 m s^{-1} (measured from the point of stimulation in the distal popliteal fossa to the spinal cord) and had a regular discharge when isolated. The sample was not, therefore, contaminated with Group II fibres, which conduct at less than 80 m s^{-1} (Matthews 1963) and which have a completely different collateral morphology (see Chapter 13). No systematic tests were carried out to differentiate Ia from Ib (Golgi tendon organ) afferents. But all axons classed as Ia had their receptors located in muscle. The final differentiation was made on the basis of collateral morphology: Ia fibres had collaterals reaching the motor nuclei whereas Ib fibres had collaterals that arborized widely in the intermediate region (see Chapter 12). Tentative classifications were made during the electrophysiological recording; Ib fibres usually had no continuing activity when isolated and nearly always required noticeable muscle stretch (manual extension or flexion of joints) to excite them. The tentative classification always agreed with the histological results.

In spite of their large diameter and the relative ease with which they could be impaled with microelectrodes, Ia afferent fibres were more difficult to stain with horseradish peroxidase than the smaller cutaneous axons. Using our standard technique it was necessary to pass about 200 nA min of charge through the electrode in order to achieve staining to the level of the terminal boutons in the motor nuclei. Burke et al. (1979), who have also stained identified Ia fibres, treated their tissue with cobalt chloride to intensify the reaction product (Adams 1977). Hongo et al. (1978) and Ishizuka et al. (1979) have also stained Group Ia fibres with horseradish peroxidase, using a pressure injection technique. The results from the laboratories of Burke and Hongo are essentially the same as ours—any differences will be noted in the following account.

I. Entry of axons into the spinal cord, branching and collateral distribution

Figure 11.1 shows the main features of Ia fibres: the total lengths of axons stained, whether they could be traced into the dorsal root, whether they bifurcated, and the number and points of origin of their collaterals. Between 4 and 11 mm of axons were stained. In the total sample of 23 Ia fibres 20 could be traced into the dorsal root and all of these bifurcated into ascending and descending branches shortly after entering the spinal cord. As noted by Hongo et al. (1978) the caudally projecting branches are often of smaller diameter than the rostrally projecting ones. In our material the caudal branches did not terminate as a collateral, but rather the intensity of staining became less until the branch could not be followed further. In other words, the total extent of the caudal branches remains unknown. The longest caudal branch was about 7 mm.

The rostral and caudal branches of Ia afferent fibres move medially within 1–2 mm of the bifurcation and ascend or descend the cord in the dorsal columns, giving of collaterals as they do so. Collaterals are given off, on average, about every millimetre. In our material the intercollateral spacings varied from 100 to 2600 μm (1040 ± 513 μm; mean ± s.d., $n = 73$). Similar mean values were observed by Hongo et al. (1978) for a pooled sample of Ia and Ib axons although Ib fibre give off collaterals at significantly closer intervals (see Chapter 12).

In our material the spacing of collaterals on the ascending and descending branches of the axon did not differ significantly. Hongo et al. (1978) state that collaterals are spaced further apart on the ascending branch. Again, this is probably due to the pooling of Ia and Ib fibres, since Ib fibres have collaterals spaced significantly closer together on their descending branches (Brown and Fyffe 1979; see Chapter 12).

The important point is that Group Ia fibres, within a centimetre or so either side of their entrance into the cord, give off collaterals about every millimetre. There is no suggestion that the frequency varies over this region, and in particular the frequency is not higher close to the position of entrance, as it is with the hair follicle afferent fibres. Scheibel and Scheibel (1969) in a Golgi study of presumed Ia fibres in the kitten's cord have shown that collaterals arise at intervals of 100–200 μm. These figures have been applied to the adult cat, (1) in estimations of the numbers of collaterals from a single Ia axon that supply a single motoneurone (Mendell and Henneman 1971), and (2) in estimations of the number of motoneurones supplied by a single collateral (Iles 1976). Unfortunately for these estimates kittens grow. This point will be discussed further below (see Sect. B.V and also Chapter 14).

Collaterals were given off over total lengths of axon (rostral plus caudal branches) of up to 8.2 mm (5.0 ± 2.16 mm; mean ± s.d.). These values obviously do not represent anything other than a lower limit. It is to be expected that collaterals will arise over the length of the relevant motor nuclei; the triceps motor nucleus is about 10 mm in length in the adult cat (Romanes 1951; Sprague 1958) and according to Sprague monosynaptic connexions from Ia fibres to motoneurones spread over five segments, a distance of some 30 mm. In addition further collaterals will be given off to neurones of the ventral and dorsal spinocerebellar tracts in more rostral segments.

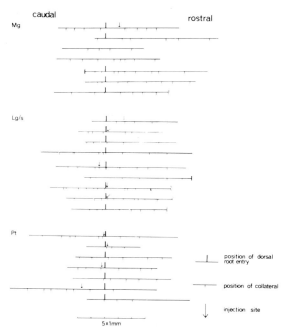

Fig. 11.1. Diagrammatic representation of the branching pattern of Ia afferent fibres in the spinal cord. The total length of each axon stained is shown, together with (where possible) the position of its entry into the cord through the dorsal root, the position of the origin of each stained collateral and the site of injection of horseradish peroxidase. All axons that could be traced into the dorsal root bifurcated upon entering the cord. Axons ran in the medial gastrocnemius (Mg), lateral gastrocnemius/soleus (Lg/s) and posterior tibial (Pt) nerves. (From Fyffe 1981.)

II. Morphology of collaterals

Group Ia muscle afferent fibre collaterals near the position of entry of the axon into the cord illustrate, in a striking fashion, the general rule that all collaterals from the same type of primary afferent fibre have a similar morphology. As may be seen from Figs. 11.2–11.5, not only are Ia collaterals from the same axon very similar but the similarity extends to collaterals from other axons from the same muscle in different cats, and to collaterals from muscles of the same functional group such as triceps surae.

Ia collaterals enter the dorsal horn through its dorsal or medial border. They descend through the dorsal laminae of the grey matter (laminae I–V) usually without branching, although they may give off branches occasionally at the level of lamina IV or V. When viewed as reconstructions from serial transverse sections the collaterals entering the horn at its dorsal border usually drop almost vertically, although collaterals arising close to the bifurcation of the parent axon often run medially along the dorsal border of the grey matter before descending. When viewed as reconstructions from serial sagittal sections, however, it can be seen (Fig. 11.6) that the collaterals move rostrally as they descend. When they enter the grey matter from deep in the dorsal columns, as they do for example when the ascending branch

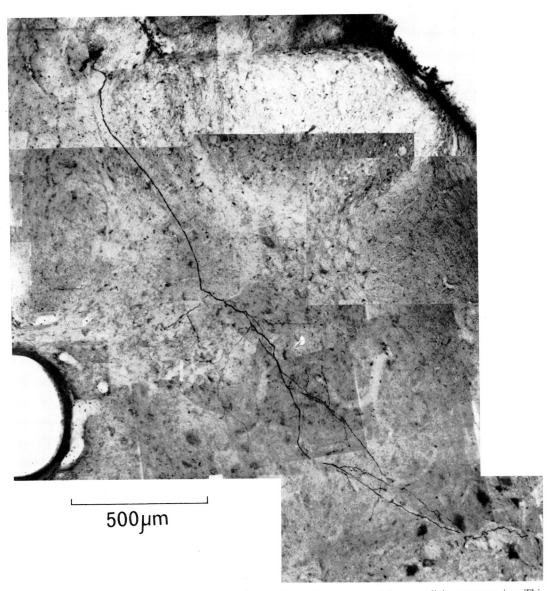

Fig. 11.2. Photomontage, from 100-μm transverse sections, of a Ia afferent fibre collateral from medial gastrocnemius. This collateral is reconstructed in Fig. 11.3A. (From Brown and Fyffe 1978a.)

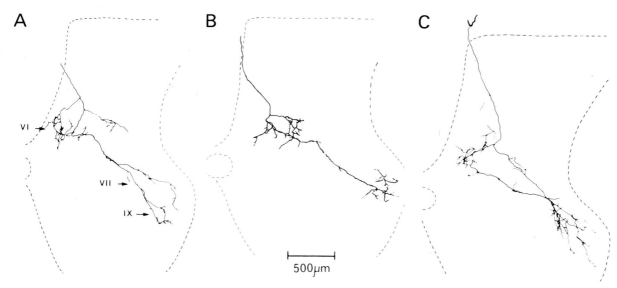

Fig. 11.3. Reconstructions, from transverse sections, of three adjacent collaterals from a Ia afferent fibre from medial gastrocnemius. **A** is the most caudal and **C** the most rostral of the three. Similarities among the three collaterals are striking. Each collateral gives branches which arborize in the medial intermediary region (lamina VI), then moves laterally across the cord to break up into arborizations in the Ia inhibitory interneurone region (lamina VII) and the motor nucleus (lamina IX). (From Brown and Fyffe 1978a.)

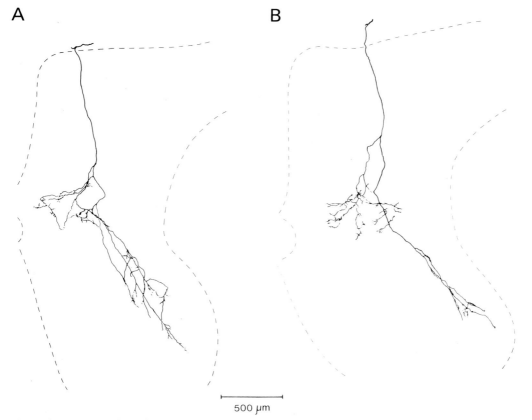

Fig. 11.4. Reconstructions, from transverse sections, of two adjacent Ia afferent collaterals from lateral gastrocnemius/soleus. Compare this figure with 11.3—the similarities are obvious. (From Brown and Fyffe 1978a.)

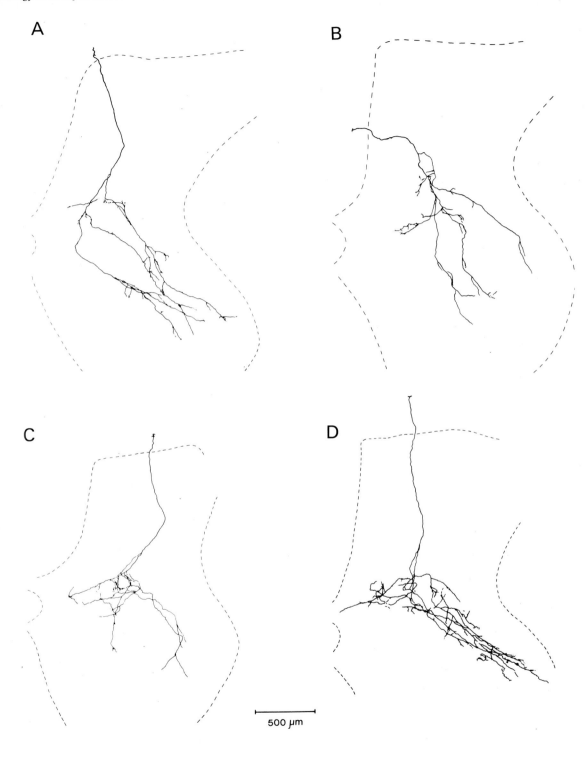

Fig. 11.5. Reconstructions, in the transverse plane, of Ia afferent fibre collaterals from medial gastrocnemius (**A**), lateral gastrocnemius/soleus (**B**), and muscles innervated by the posterior tibial nerve (**C** and **D**). (From Brown and Fyffe 1978a.)

moves rostrally towards Clarke's column, then
they may run more or less directly to lamina V or
VI (Fig. 11.5B).

The first set of daughter branches arises from
the collateral at or near lamina VI and this gives
rise to a fairly rich arborization at this level. Collaterals from triceps surae and muscles innervated
by the posterior tibial nerve provide arborizations
to the medial or middle third of lamina VI. The
main collateral, after giving off its branches to
lamina VI, changes direction and heads towards
the appropriate motor nuclei. In the case of collaterals from afferents innervating the afore-
mentioned muscles this involves a trajectory towards the ventro-lateral part of the ventral horn.
Collaterals often divide into two to four branches
as they move towards the motor nuclei and during
this part of their course, just dorsal and dorso-
medial to their motor nuclei, they give off fine
branches which provide the arborizations to the
inhibitory interneurones in lamina VII (Fig.
11.3A). Finally the collaterals terminate, after
relatively little further branching, in the motor
nuclei. The horseradish peroxidase injection experiments have, therefore, confirmed Szentágothai's (1967a) predictions about the morphology of Ia collaterals.

As mentioned above and shown in Fig. 11.6, Ia
collaterals run rostrally from their point of origin
from the parent axon to their termination in the
motor nuclei. This is presumably not the situation
found in the kitten. Scheibel and Scheibel (1969)
examined sagittal sections of lumbosacral cord in
the kitten and observed that collaterals dropped
vertically to the motor nuclei (see their Figs. 6,
8, 9, 12). The rostral trajectory is a common
feature of all primary afferent fibre collaterals but
is most easily observed in Ia collaterals because of
the long distance they travel from the dorsal columns superficial to the dorsal horn to the motor
nuclei deep in the ventral horn. It seems likely
that the rostral trajectory of the collaterals de-
velops as the kitten grows.

When viewed in reconstructions from sagittal
sections, Ia collaterals have an overall inverted-
V-shaped outline, albeit tilted because of the rostral trajectory described above (Fig. 11.6). This
results in the terminal arborizations occupying
greater rostro-caudal lengths of cord in the motor
nuclei than in the lamina VI region. The arborization in lamina VI rarely reaches as far rostrally as
the arborization in the motor nuclei, but does

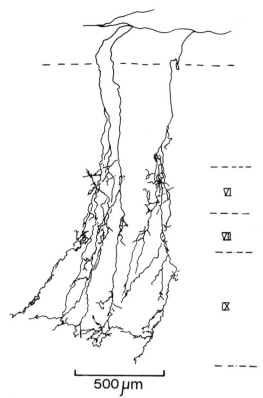

Fig. 11.6. Reconstructions, from sagittal sections, of adjacent
collaterals from a Ia afferent fibre innervating lateral
gastrocnemius/soleus. The collaterals clearly follow a rostral
trajectory as they run ventrally, and the inverted-V-shaped
outline of the collaterals and their branches can be seen.

usually reach as far caudally and may extend
farther.

III. Terminal arborizations

1. In the intermediate region (lamina VI)

When viewed in transverse sections or reconstructions from such sections (Figs. 11.3, 11.4A) the
terminal arborization in the intermediate region is
seen to be strictly limited to lamina VI near the
point of entry of the parent axon into the spinal
cord. Collaterals given off more rostrally as the
parent axon runs deep in the dorsal columns often
give terminals to the most dorsal part of lamina
VII as well (Fig. 11.5B).

In transverse sections and reconstructions this
arborization appears as a thin transversely
oriented sheet of terminal branches. But it may
be well-developed in the sagittal plane, although
it is the shortest of the three sets of terminal

arborizations due to the inverted-V-shape arrangement of the individual collaterals and their branches. In spite of this, where collaterals arise fairly close together (at or less than the average spacing) the arborizations from adjacent collaterals may form a continuous sheet, or almost a continuous sheet with gaps between individual arborizations from adjacent collaterals of only 100–200 μm, in the sagittal plane. Thus for the three collaterals reconstructed in Fig. 11.3 the sheet extended (in lamina VI) for 1300 μm continuously in the sagittal plane, and for the two collaterals of Fig. 11.4 for 1100 μm with a gap of only 150 μm between the two. Obviously, where collaterals are given off far apart (more than 1.5 mm) there are larger gaps between arborizations.

The arborizations in the intermediate region are the most complex of the three sets arising from Ia collaterals near the level of their dorsal root entry. But they fail to reach the complexity of most terminal arborizations of cutaneous afferent fibres or of Group Ib and II muscle afferent fibres.

2. In the Ia inhibitory interneurone region (lamina VII)

Terminal arborizations in this region of lamina VII, just dorsal and dorso-medial to the motor nuclei, are the simplest of all the Ia collateral arborizations at the segmental level. The arborization consists of fine individual branches given off the main collateral branches as they descend towards the motor nuclei. These fine branches are usually 100–200 μm in length and run predominantly in the transverse plane. At this level the sagittal extent of the complete collateral is usually of the order of 400–1000 μm (due to the inverted-V-shape). Therefore, the arborization in the inhibitory interneurone region tends to form a continuous column where adjacent collaterals arise within 500–1000 μm of each other.

3. In the motor nuclei (lamina IX)

Terminal arborizations in the motor nuclei (lamina IX) are intermediate in complexity in their terminal branching pattern and bouton organization (see below) between the arborizations in lamina VI and those in lamina VII. The terminal parts of the main collateral branches divide a number of times to produce daughter branches of the third to fifth (or more) order before carrying synaptic boutons. At this level the sagittal extent of a single Ia collateral varies from 300 μm (usually at least 750 μm) to 1200 μm and the arborizations of adjacent collaterals from the same Ia fibre often form continuous columns of terminals within the motor nuclei, particularly where adjacent collaterals arise within 500–1000 μm of each other. Even when collaterals arise at the upper limits of the range of intercollateral spacings (2.0–2.5 mm) the gaps between their terminal arborizations are considerably less than this and rarely as much as 1 mm, when the collaterals are well stained.

There are two major differences between our results and those reported by Burke et al. (1980). First, Burke et al. state that each collateral is oriented mainly across the cord (transversely) with little or no rostro-caudal spread, in agreement with the results of Iles (1976). As described above, we find a well-developed rostro-caudal organization at all levels, but particularly in the motor nuclei. Secondly, Burke et al. (1980) describe Ia collaterals that do not penetrate to the motor nuclei. All of our well-stained collaterals penetrated into the nuclei.

The most reasonable explanation for the differences between the two sets of results is that the degree of staining varied. With the horseradish peroxidase technique only collaterals arising near the injection site can usually be traced to the level of boutons in the motor nuclei. This is so whether the injection is made near the dorsal root entrance of the axon or considerably further away. When we have injected axons 4–7 mm away from the entrance site, well-stained collaterals still reach the motor nuclei. We have no case of a well-stained Ia collateral that does not reach the motor nuclei, nor have we any well-stained Ia collaterals oriented across the cord as a plate of arborizations (as the Ib collaterals tend to form).

IV. Synaptic boutons

1. In the intermediate region (lamina VI)

Camera lucida drawings of Ia endings in lamina VI are shown in Fig. 11.7, and photomicrographs in Fig. 11.10A–C. These figures should be compared with Figs. 11.8, 11.9 and 11.10D–H, which show boutons in laminae VII and IX respectively.

The morphology and organization of boutons in lamina VI differs from that in the other regions

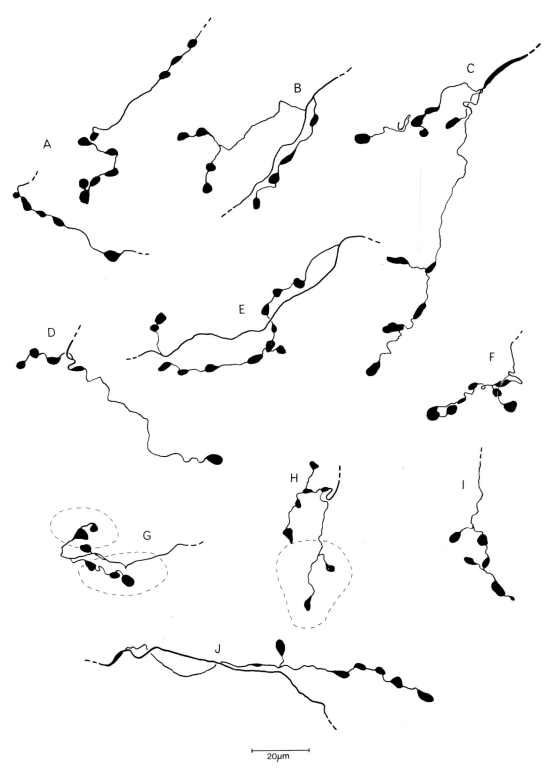

20μm

Fig. 11.7. Camera lucida drawings of terminal arborizations and synaptic boutons of Ia afferent fibre in lamina VI. The somata and proximal dendrites of neurones with which the boutons appear to make contact in counterstained sections are indicated by *dashed lines*. This figure should be compared with Figs. 11.8 and 11.9. Note the boutons *en passant* and the clusters of boutons on neurones. (From Brown and Fyffe 1978a.)

of termination of Ia collaterals. Usually the terminal axon branches carry boutons *en passant* along their last 20–100 μm. Four to five boutons are commonly carried but sometimes there are as many as eight before the final bouton *terminal* (Fig. 11.7B, E, J). These *en passant* arrangements are oriented mainly in the transverse plane of the cord.

In addition to the boutons *de passage*, which are not as well-developed in Ia collaterals as in many cutaneous afferent fibres, another characteristic feature of the terminals in lamina VI, not seen in lamina VII or often in lamina IX, is the presence of small clusters of five to eight boutons carried on two or three short branches of a terminal axon. These clusters are contained within small volumes of cord (areas of 20 μm × 20 μm in 100-μm thick sections), and in sections counterstained to show Nissl substance (cresyl violet stain) may be seen to be arranged in close association with the somata and proximal dendrites of lamina VI neurones (see Fig. 11.7G, H, Fig. 11.10C). These clusters may form the anatomical basis for the well-known secure transmission between Ia afferent fibres and neurones in the intermediate region (Eccles et al. 1956). But the boutons *en passant* could well form climbing-type synapses on individual dendrites and this could also lead to secure transmission. Further analysis will have to await ultrastructural studies.

Single collaterals give rise to more boutons in lamina VI than in the other two areas of termination. Between 29 and 112 boutons were carried on individual collaterals 65 ± 23.4 mean ± s.d., $n = 20$); similar numbers were observed by Ishizuka et al. 1979).

Boutons in this region range in size from 2.5 μm × 2.5 μm to 6.5 μm × 3.5 μm (4.5 ± 1.18 × 2.76 ± 0.69; mean ± s.d., $n = 62$). There was no significant difference between the sizes of boutons in lamina VI and those in the other two regions.

2. In the Ia inhibitory interneurone region (lamina VII)

As shown in the camera lucida drawings of Fig. 11.8 and the photomicrographs of Fig. 11.10D–F, boutons in this region are more simply organized and the terminal axon carries fewer of them than in the other two regions of terminal arborization (compare with Figs. 11.7, 11.9). Because of the close proximity of this region to the

motor nuclei, and of the dorsal projections of motoneuronal dendrites through the region (through lamina VII and into lamina IV: see Fig. 14.1 and also Fig. 1 in Cullheim and Kellerth 1976), it is not possible to be sure of the termination sites of this type of ending. When both Ia fibres and motoneurones are stained however (see Chapter 14), these simple endings are not found on motoneurone dendrites.

In many Ia collaterals two distinct terminal arborizations may be seen—in lamina VII and in the motor nuclei. Each has its own type of bouton arrangement. In fact the double-staining experiments (Chapter 14) suggest that all Ia–motoneurone contacts are made within the confines of the motor nuclei.

The terminal axonal branches in lamina VII usually arise directly from the main collateral branches as they descend to the motor nuclei, without the intervention of other daughter branches. These fine terminal branches of 1 μm or less in diameter follow a more or less direct path to their termination as a bouton *terminal*. Over the last 100 μm or so of their path they may carry one to three boutons *de passage*. Occasionally the terminal axon bifurcates into two daughter branches each carrying one or two boutons (Fig. 11.8C). Sometimes single boutons are offset from the terminal axon on very short (1–2-μm) stalks (Fig. 11.8B). In counterstained sections the boutons may be seen to lie over the cell bodies of neurones that are often spindle-shaped and about 20–30 μm in their long axis. These neurones are presumably Ia inhibitory interneurones (Jankowska and Lindström 1972).

Single Ia collaterals give rise to fewer boutons in lamina VII than in either lamina VI or lamina IX. Between 10 and 42 boutons are carried on individual collaterals (19 ± 7.5; mean ± s.d., $n = 10$): Ishizuka et al. (979) counted 10 to 40. The boutons in this region are of similar size to those in the other termination regions (3 μm × 2.5 μm– 75 μm × 3.5 μm; 4.71 ± 1.53 × 3.03 ± 0.77, means ± s.d., $n = 29$).

3. In the motor nuclei (lamina IX)

Camera lucida drawings and photomicrographs of boutons in lamina IX are shown in Figs. 11.9 and 11.10G, H respectively. Their complexity of organization is intermediate between that in lamina VI and that in lamina VII. At one extreme

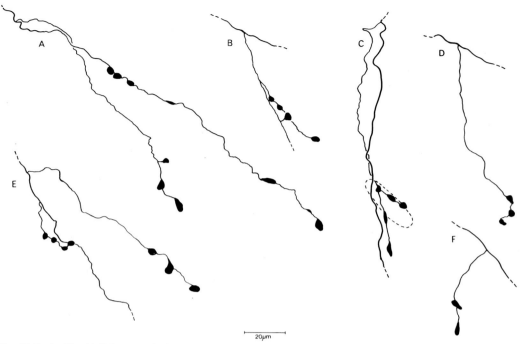

20μm

Fig. 11.8. As Fig. 11.7, but terminal arborizations are in lamina VII. To be compared with Figs. 11.7 and 11.9. Note the simple types of terminals. (From Brown and Fyffe 1978a.)

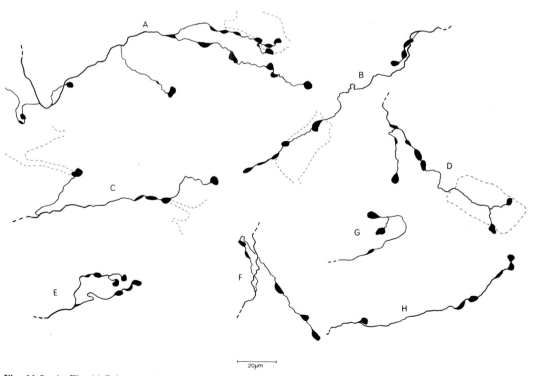

20μm

Fig. 11.9. As Fig. 11.7, but terminal arborizations are in the motor nuclei (lamina IX). To be compared with Figs. 11.7 and 11.8. Note the boutons on somata and proximal dendrites of motoneurones. (From Brown and Fyffe 1978a.)

some terminals are very simple, carrying isolated boutons at the end of, or in the course of, terminal axons. These terminal axons do not arise directly from large-diameter branches, as the terminals in lamina VII do, but from finer third-to fifth-order daughter branches of the collaterals reaching the motor nuclei. They were sometimes on or closely adjacent to motoneurones (in counterstained sections). At the other extreme some terminals are more complex, including some with four or five boutons *en passant* plus a bouton *terminal* (Fig. 11.9D, H), and some arranged in clusters similar to those in the lamina VI region (Fig. 11.9E). But clusters of boutons are not a common feature in the motor nuclei.

Single collaterals usually carry about 130 boutons within the motor nuclei (63–192; 127 ± 43.6, mean ± s.d., $n = 20$). A similar figure has been reported by Ishizuka et al. (1979), who counted 135 on average.

The number of boutons carried on single Ia collaterals within the motor nuclei is of some importance. It provides indirect evidence, for the possible numbers of motoneurones contacted by a single collateral, that supports the direct evidence provided by staining experiments on Ia–motoneurone pairs (Chapter 14). These latter experiments indicate that on average a single collateral gives about three to four boutons to a motoneurone and that motoneurones rarely, if ever, receive boutons from other collaterals of the same Ia fibre. Therefore, each Ia collateral should supply between about 20 and 50 motoneurones. On the basis of other evidence (see Sect. B.V below; and Chapter 14) the upper value should be nearer the real state of affairs. Bouton counts obviously depend on the assumption that all boutons are stained, which may not be the case. Furthermore, synaptic contact may be made at sites other than axonal swellings (boutons), again leading to an under-estimate of the number of contacts made.

Boutons in the motor nuclei range in size from 3.5 μm × 3 μm to 7 μm × 3.5 μm (5 ± 1.06 × 2.76 ± 0.63; means ± s.d., $n = 49$). These values are not significantly different from those in the two other regions of termination.

V. The organization of collaterals

An attempt is made in Fig. 11.11 to show, in diagrammatic form, the organization of Ia collaterals from a single axon (specifically a triceps surae axon) at and near its point of entry into the lumbosacral cord. It is worth stressing, in view of the many difficulties of identification presented by purely anatomical studies, that the morphology as revealed by the intra-axonal injection of horseradish peroxidase is essentially the same as revealed in the Golgi studies of Szentágothai (1967a). However, horseradish peroxidase undoubtedly provides much more detail than the silver stains and than cobalt chloride as used by Iles (1976).

Group Ia afferent fibres enter the cord and immediately bifurcate into ascending and descending branches: very few Ia fibres do not bifurcate. Collaterals arise from the ascending and descending branches of Ia axons at an average spacing of about 1 mm over distances of up to rather more than 8 mm in our material. The horseradish peroxidase method does not stain more than about 10 mm of axon and according to Sprague (1958) monosynaptic connexions to motoneurones spread over five segments in the cat's lumbosacral cord. Triceps surae motoneurones occupy a length of about 10 mm in the adult cat (Romanes 1951) so our values represent a lower limit: Sprague's (1958) figures would give a length of up to 30 mm of axon to provide collaterals to motoneurones.

These recent results on Ia collaterals in adult cats are at variance with those reported from a Golgi study in kittens by Scheibel and Scheibel (1969). These authors state that collaterals arise within 2–10 mm of the dorsal root entrance at intervals of 100–200 μm, each axon giving rise to between 10 and 100 collaterals. Obviously, allowances have to be made for growth but it seems that the Scheibels overestimated the number of collaterals arising from a single axon. It is extremely difficult to follow individual axons through material stained by the Golgi method. It is possible, however, that an axon produces a large number of collaterals initially and that only those that make sufficient functional contacts are retained.

The number of collaterals given off from a single Ia fibre bears on the question of how many motoneurones receive connexions from a single collateral. As discussed above, an estimate of 20–50 motoneurones per Ia collateral may be derived from (1) the number of boutons carried by single

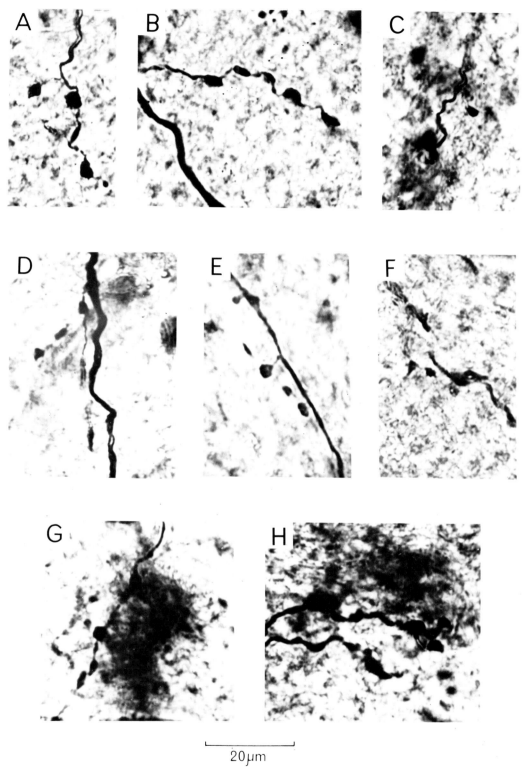

Fig. 11.10. Photomicrographs from 100-µm thick transverse sections, of terminal arborizations and synaptic boutons of Ia afferent fibre collaterals in lamina VI (**A–C**), in lamina VII (**D–F**), and in lamina IX (**G** and **H**). Sections **C, D, G** and **H** were counterstained with cresyl violet. In all photographs dorsal is at the top. (From Brown and Fyffe 1978a.)

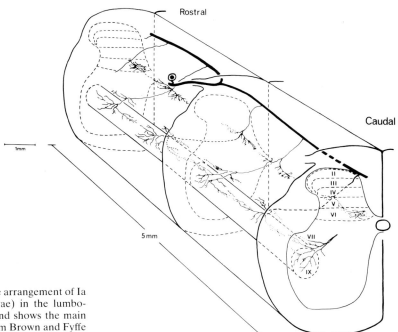

Fig. 11.11. Schematic representation of the arrangement of Ia afferent fibre collaterals (from triceps surae) in the lumbosacral cord. The figure is drawn to scale and shows the main features of the collateral morphology. (From Brown and Fyffe 1978a.)

collaterals in the motor nuclei, and (2) the average number of boutons contacting a single motoneurone from an individual collateral. Scheibel and Scheibel (1969) and Iles (1976) have estimated 9 and 11 motoneurones per Ia collateral respectively. As pointed out above, however, these estimates were based on the intercollateral spacing in kittens.

Given that Ia collaterals arise about every millimetre from the ascending and descending branches of the axon in the region of the appropriate motor nuclei, then triceps surae motor nucleus, which is some 10 mm long, would be supplied by about 10 collaterals. The triceps surae motor pool contains about 725 motoneurones (Boyd and Davey 1968; Iles 1976) and each triceps Ia afferent fibre should contact about 550 of these (nearly all motoneurones of the homonymous muscle and about two-thirds of those of the heteronymous muscles), as calculated by Iles (1976) from the observations of Mendell and Henneman (1971). These figures may have to be modified in view of the more recent results of Scott and Mendell (1976) showing that homonymous projections range from 70% to 100% and heteronymous projections from 40% to 75%. These figures give values of 375–595 motoneurones contacted by a triceps surae Ia afferent fibre and an average of about 475 rather

than 550. Therefore each Ia collateral should have monosynaptic contacts with some 45–50 motoneurones—a value about five times higher than the estimates of Scheibel and Scheibel (1969) and Iles (1976) and at the upper end of the estimates made on the basis of numbers of boutons per collateral and per motoneurone. Obviously the numbers will be different for different muscle groups.

The estimates of 45–50 motoneurones per Ia collateral are likely to be more accurate than the lower estimates based on bouton counts, due to the uncertainties about whether all boutons are stained and whether contacts are limited to boutons. Certainly the value of 1 mm for the average spacing of Ia collaterals is probably accurate as it is unlikely that the horseradish peroxidase method stains collaterals in an all-or-none manner. Further support for these estimates may be derived from a consideration of the motoneurones' receptive surface. In a 100 μm thick transverse section through the triceps surae motor pool stained with cresyl violet about 10 large motoneuronal somata are seen. The sagittal extent of the terminal arborization of a single Ia collateral from triceps occupies from 300 to 1200 μm, usually about 750 μm. Therefore a single Ia collateral has ample opportunity to come into contact with the somata and proximal dendrites of 50 or so motoneurones, and with the more distal dendrites of many more. Further consideration is given to these problems in Chapter 14.

Scheibel and Scheibel (1969) described three kinds of collaterals running to the motor nuclei; they called these 'simple', 'compound' and 'complex'. 'Simple' collaterals projected only to a single motoneurone pool, 'compound' collaterals to more than one motoneurone pool of synergistic function, and 'complex' collaterals to motoneurone pools of apparently antagonistic function. As pointed out by Réthelyi and Szentágothai (1973) interpretation of 'motor' and 'non-motor' branches of Ia collaterals is important here. In our material the vast majority of Ia collaterals projected to circumscribed regions of the ventral horn clearly associated with the appropriate motor cell column. Occasionally, however (Fig. 11.5B, C), branches of the same collateral were distributed to more than one motor cell column, but whether the columns belonged to synergistic or antagonistic muscles is unknown. Examination of this point will have to await combined structural and functional studies.

On the basis of degeneration studies Sterling and Kuypers (1967b) concluded that, in the brachial cord, the terminal branches of Ia collaterals in the motor nuclei run in the sagittal plane making climbing-type synapses with the motoneurone dendrites. At brachial levels the motoneurone dendrites run mainly in the sagittal plane. Scheibel and Scheibel (1969) deny this from a study of their Golgi material of the lumbosacral cord, concluding that the Ia terminal arborization in the motor nuclei is developed only in the transverse plane of the cord and is essentially two-dimensional. A clear differentiation must be made between the total longitudinal extent of the terminal arborization of a single Ia collateral in the motor nuclei and the orientation of the last 100 μm or so of the terminal branches of the arborization that carry the synaptic boutons. As our material clearly shows, Ia collaterals in the lumbosacral cord are organized like an inverted V in the sagittal plane and the longitudinal extent of the arborization in the motor nuclei may be more than 1 mm. The general orientation of the terminal parts of the collaterals, however, is dorsoventral, more or less at right angles to the motoneurone dendrites (see Chapter 14). There are relatively few synaptic arrangements of the

climbing type; most are of the crossing-over type. This point will be discussed fully in Chapter 14.

All well-stained Ia collaterals in our material projected to the motor nuclei. We have no evidence that collaterals within 8 mm or so of the dorsal root entrance may project only to the intermediate and/or inhibitory interneurone region. Burke et al. (1980) appear to conclude that collaterals may not project to the motor nuclei. This point has been discussed above (Sect. B.III.3) and the opinion expressed that collaterals not projecting to the motor nuclei are probably incompletely stained.

In addition to their projection to motoneurones, all Ia collaterals also had terminal arborizations in lamina VI and in the region of lamina VII containing the Ia inhibitory interneurones. At and near the point of entry of the Ia axon into the cord all collaterals have all three areas of termination. This means that, in general, monosynaptic action of Ia fibres is made at the segment of entry (except monosynaptic excitation of spinocerebellar tract neurones). Any actions mediated through one or more interneurones on motoneurones or ascending tract neurones more than one or two segments away from the point of entry will, in all likelihood, involve interneurones having axons linking the two levels of the cord. Hultborn et al. (1971b) noted that Ia inhibitory interneurones are located in the same spinal segments as contain the motoneurones with the same peripheral monosynaptic input, and predicted that the interneurones would have axons travelling longitudinally for some distance. This prediction has been confirmed both electrophysiologically (Jankowska and Roberts 1972a, b) and by intracellular dye injection (Jankowska and Lindström 1972). That there may be monosynaptic connexions to interneurones as far as three segments away from the point of entry is likely, however. Eccles et al. (1956) found interneurones in the intermediate region of lower L-7 that were excited monosynaptically from Ia fibres from quadriceps.

In the intermediate region of the cord there are many neurones that receive monosynaptic excitation from low-threshold (Group I) muscle afferent fibres (Eccles et al. 1956, 1960; R. M. Eccles 1965; Hongo et al. 1966; Lucas and Willis 1974). According to a recent study by Czarkowska et al. (1976), using intracellular injection of horseradish peroxidase into cells in the intermediate region, there are at least six types of neurones receiving monosynaptic Group I excitation. The six types were differentiated on the basis of their axonal projection rather than on their location, soma size or shape, or their dendritic tree morphology. Two types projected to the motor nuclei, two to the ipsilateral funiculus, one to the contralateral ventral funiculus and one widely within laminae VI and VII. From the point of view of their input none of the groups constituted a uniform population; most were excited by both Ia and Ib fibres as far as could be shown, and most cells that were apparently only excited from Ia afferents projected either to the motor nuclei or to the ipsilateral lateral funiculus.

On the basis of the morphology of the terminal arborizations of Ia axon collaterals in lamina VI it might be expected that there would be a heterogeneous population of interneurones receiving Ia input. The terminal arborizatons of Ia collaterals in this region exhibit a wide range of synaptic arrangements, from single boutons (rare) to boutons *en passant* and also cluster formations of boutons. In counterstained preparations the clusters of boutons are seen to be arranged on cell bodies, obviously providing the possibility for fairly secure synaptic transmission. Boutons *en passant* have not, in counterstained sections, been seen on or near neuronal somata. Presumably they are organized along dendrites as climbing-type synapses. In lamina VI the dendritic orientation is mainly dorso-ventral (Scheibel and Scheibel 1968), as is the *en passant* arrangement of boutons on Ia collaterals.

In the Ia inhibitory interneurone region of lamina VII the Ia terminal arborizations are extremely simple. Few boutons are carried by the terminal axon: sometimes a single bouton, often two to three and sometimes four boutons. In counterstained material the boutons often appear to lie on neuronal somata—of the presumed inhibitory interneurones. It is, however, surprising that a single collateral gives so few boutons to individual neurones.

Electrophysiological evidence appears to show a strong linkage between Ia fibres and the inhibitory interneurones (Hultborn et al. 1971b), since the interneurones are able to follow peripheral Group I stimulation at more than 300 Hz whereas motoneurones (with an average of about four boutons from each Ia collateral) can only follow stimulation at 50–100 Hz (Eccles and Rall 1951; Eccles 1953; Hultborn et al. 1971b). Obviously, electrical stimulation of muscle nerves, even at stimulus strengths close to threshold, will excite a considerable number of afferent fibres and a somatic location for the synapses will provide the anatomical substrate for secure synaptic linkage. A somatic (or proximal dendritic) location of Ia synapses on Ia inhibitory interneurones would be expected from the fast rise time and short duration of the excitatory post-synaptic potentials evoked in the interneurones by the monosynaptic Ia input (see text-figure 1 in Jankowska and Lindström 1972). It seems highly unlikely that activity of a single Ia afferent would lead to firing of a Ia inhibitory interneurone and considerable summation would be required (see R. M. Eccles and Lundberg 1958a, b). The degree of convergence onto single Ia inhibitory interneurones is unknown; it is likely to be high.

12   Afferent fibres from Golgi tendon organs

Tendon organs are relatively simple structures in comparison with muscle spindles, and the anatomy of Golgi tendon organs has aroused considerably less interest than that of muscle spindles. For structural details the reader is referred to Matthews (1972) and, especially, Barker (1974). In physiological studies also, the tendon organ has been overshadowed by the muscle spindle receptors. Again the reader should refer to Matthews's book, and the reviews of Hunt (1974) and McIntyre (1974). Only the briefest introduction will be presented here on the physiology of tendon organs.

Golgi tendon organs are slowly adapting mechanoreceptors and respond to stretch of the muscle in whose tendon they are situated. They have little sensitivity to the rate of change of tension in the tendon (Matthews 1933). In early electrophysiological studies it was noted (Matthews 1933; Hunt and Kuffler 1951) that tendon organs generally had higher mechanical thresholds to stretch than muscle spindle receptors. They behaved as though they were in series with the extrafusal muscle fibres, discharging during muscle contraction. This was in contrast to the spindle receptors, which behaved as though they were in parallel with the muscle fibres. Tendon organs usually had no continuing activity when first isolated. It was on the basis of results such as these that the generally accepted view arose that tendon organs were responsible for the 'clasp-knife reaction' (part of the 'lengthening reaction' of Sherrington 1909) and also the 'autogenetic inhibition' of the electrophysiologists (Granit 1950; Hunt 1952; Laporte and Lloyd 1952; Eccles et al. 1957a, c; R. M. Eccles and Lundberg 1959a, b).

More recent studies have led to a questioning of the early results on the properties of tendon organs, and as a consequence there has been a change in emphasis in the interpretation of the central role of impulses in tendon organ afferent fibres. Thus Jansen and Rudjord (1964) showed that tendon organs of soleus muscle were often excited by quite small twitches of the muscle producing less than 50 g tension, and that even as little as 10 g or less was effective for some receptors. But Jansen and Rudjord also showed that some tendon organs in soleus did not discharge within the normal range of passive extension. Alnaes (1967) found that, for tendon organs in tibialis anterior muscle, passive stretch within the normal range was always effective and the passive and twitch thresholds were similar: but these thresholds were often less than 50 g.

Houk and Henneman (1967) studied the responses of tendon organs of soleus muscle during extrafusal contraction produced by stimulation of single motor fibres. They found that contraction of a single motor unit was sufficient to activate a tendon organ and in any one experiment between 4 and 15 different soleus α-motor fibres were capable of eliciting such activation.

The important point is that these more recent experiments establish tendon organs as low-threshold mechanoreceptors capable of being excited by contraction of a single motor unit, which points to a regulatory, rather than an emergency, function for tendon organs in motor control. This point of view is one with which recent studies on the spinal cord have much in sympathy.

A. Central projections of afferent fibres from tendon organs

I. Afferent fibres from tendon organs

Golgi tendon organs are innervated by afferent fibres running in muscle nerves. The fibres have a large diameter and conduct impulses at 70–120 m s^{-1} in cat hind limb nerves (Hunt 1954; Hunt and McIntyre 1960a). Only a few conduct at below this range. They are therefore within Group I of Lloyd's (1943b) nomenclature. As described in Chapter 1, Group I contains nerve fibres innervating muscle spindle primary endings as well as tendon organs. In addition, many muscle nerves contain a few axons conducting at Group I speeds but with receptors outside muscle, such as Pacinian corpuscles (see McIntyre 1974). Group I fibres may, however, be classified *functionally* into Ia fibres from muscle spindle primary endings and Ib fibres from tendon organs. It needs to be stressed that this classification is a functional one (see Matthews 1972).

In some cat hind limb nerves Ib fibres have, on average, a lower conduction velocity (diameter) than Ia fibres. Bradley and Eccles (1953) and Eccles et al. (1957a) noted that the Group I wave in the compound action potential from quadriceps, the flexor hamstrings and also triceps surae may be split, in some cats, into two components. They called these components 'Ia' and 'Ib'. The central actions of the lower threshold 'Ia' component were those expected for input from spindle primary endings. The central actions of the higher threshold 'Ib' component were those expected (at that time) for input from tendon organs. These early interpretations of electrophysiological results have been most persuasive and have led to an enormous amount of experimental work in which electrical stimulation of muscle nerves has been used to investigate the central effects of 'Ia' and 'Ib' inputs ('Ia' and 'Ib' in the Eccles sense).

This body of experimental work has been interpreted on the assumption that there is equivalence between (1) 'Ia' and 'Ib' inflexions in a compound action potential and (2) activity in Ia and Ib nerve fibres from muscle spindle primary endings and Golgi tendon organs respectively. If this were indeed the case then an ideal ex-

perimental model would be available for the study of central actions of the two sorts of afferent units. In reality it depends upon which muscle nerves are being utilized.

In the nerve to semitendinosus (Coppin et al. 1969) about 50%, or rather more, of the Ia fibres may be recruited by electrical stimulation before any Ib fibres are brought into the volley. But the remaining 50% or so of the Ia fibres have electrical thresholds that completely overlap those of the Ib fibres. Therefore, although a pure Ia volley may be evoked by electrical stimulation of this nerve it is not possible to elicit a pure Ib volley, nor is it correct to assume that when the 'Ib' inflexion appears a completely new population of afferent units is being excited. According to McIntyre (1974) similar conditions could be expected in the nerves to quadriceps, posterior biceps and semimembranosus, at least in those cats where a split Group I compound potential occurs.

In the nerves to soleus and tibialis anterior (MacLennan 1971) electrical stimulation sufficient to activate about 50% of the Ia fibres will also activate 10%–20% of the Ib population. In the nerve to peroneus longus there is very little difference between the electrical thresholds of the afferent fibres innervating the two sets of receptors (Jack and MacLennan 1971; MacLennan 1971). Furthermore, Ia–Ib separation by electrical stimulation does not appear to be possible for cat forelimb muscle nerves nor for any muscle nerves in primate species.

It must be admitted, however, that although the situation is far from ideal the very careful use of graded electrical stimulation of muscle nerves (especially by Lundberg and his co-workers) has been important in sorting out the organization of the segmental motor apparatus and the ascending projections of receptors with afferent fibres in muscle nerves. But much less is known of the central actions of Ib fibres (and Group II fibres) than of Ia fibres.

II. Central effects of Ib input: autogenetic inhibition

Autogenetic inhibition (that is, inhibition of motoneurones by stretch of the muscle they innervate) has been recognized for many years (e.g. Sherrington 1909). It is generally accepted that tendon organs play a part in this reflex effect. Whether they play an exclusive role is unknown but appears unlikely. Undoubtedly, massive tendon organ discharge, such as occurs during a fused tetanus of a muscle, will powerfully inhibit motoneurones of that muscle, as Hunt (1952) demonstrated using monosynaptic testing. But Hunt also showed that autogenetic inhibition was elicited by spindle afferent discharges evoked by fusimotor stimulation. In both of these cases Hunt also showed that the antagonistic muscles were facilitated. Obviously neither a fused tetanus nor fusimotor activation provides a pure input to the central nervous system.

On the assumption that autogenetic inhibition is due, at least in part, to the activity of tendon organ afferents the central pathways may be analysed. Laporte and Lloyd (1952) showed that electrically evoked Group I muscle afferent volleys could inhibit the monosynaptic reflex of synergistic motoneurones. The central latency of the effect was such as to require at least one interneurone to be interpolated in the pathway between the afferents and the motoneurones. Direct intracellular recording of Group I inhibitory actions on homonymous and synergistic motoneurones has been provided by many workers (e.g. Eccles et al. 1957c; R. M. Eccles and Lundberg 1959a, b). These results may also be interpreted as showing that at least one interneurone is present in the pathway.

These early experimental results were not all in complete agreement (see Matthews 1972, pp. 342–346). Some of the differences were probably due to the different levels of excitability (or biasses) of motoneuronal pools in preparations with and without long propriospinal reflexes functioning or with different anaesthetic conditions.

III. Location of interneurones excited by Ib afferent fibres

The early work was all interpreted, correctly, as showing no direct tendon organ action on motoneurones. Interneurones were necessary on the pathway from Ib afferent fibres to motoneurones. Examination of field potentials in the spinal cord, evoked by electrical stimulation of muscle nerves, showed that 'Ib' fibres made synaptic contacts in a rather wide transverse region of the intermediate zone (laminae VI and VII and possibly V: Eccles

et al. 1954c; Coombs et al. 1956). Later work using intracellular recording methods (Eccles et al. 1960; Hongo et al. 1966) demonstrated that interneurones in this region did indeed receive Group I muscle input, some of which was thought to be due to activity in tendon organ afferent fibres. But the experiments are open to the criticism of interpretation of all such work using electrical stimulation.

Lucas and Willis (1974) used adequate stimulation of receptors to avoid the pitfalls of electrical nerve stimulation. Forty-two of 46 interneurones in laminae VI and VII were excited monosynaptically by tendon organ afferent fibres. Only four of the 46 interneurones received monosynaptic excitation from Ia afferent fibres.

Lundberg and his collaborators have made a sustained attack on the problems of convergence onto interneurones activated monosynaptically by Group I muscle afferents. All of this work is based on electrical stimulation of nerves and, over the years and with the most careful use of techniques, a picture has emerged that must be correct in its broad outline at least. Many interneurones in the dorsal horn and intermediary region (laminae IV–VII) receive monosynaptic excitation from Group I muscle afferent fibres. Most of this excitation is from Ib afferents (R. M. Eccles 1965; Lucas and Willis 1974).

A subset of these interneurones receiving monosynaptic excitation from tendon organ afferents consists of inhibitory interneurones projecting to motoneurones. In addition to their input from Ib fibres they also receive monosynaptic excitation from the rubrospinal tract (Hongo et al. 1969) and the corticospinal tract (Illert et al. 1976). Inhibitory effects are received from the dorsal reticulospinal system (Anden et al. 1966; Engberg et al. 1968a), and this inhibitory input may also be monosynaptic. Recent indirect evidence (recording from motoneurones) shows that cutaneous and joint afferent fibres also excite these interneurones, disynaptically, and therefore facilitate the inhibitory effects of the Ib input to motoneurones (Lundberg et al. 1977, 1978). Lundberg et al. (1978) discuss their results in terms of feedback from the periphery controlling the central command programme for movement. Such modern views on the central role of Ib afferent fibres necessitate much more sophisticated functions for the tendon organs than simply autogenetic inhibition.

The interneurones that receive monosynaptic excitation from Ib afferent fibres and, in turn, inhibit homonymous and synergistic motoneurones must form only a part of the total population of interneurones at the segmental level receiving monosynaptic Ib excitation. Interneurones on the excitatory path from tendon organ afferents to antagonistic motoneurones will also be present (Hunt 1952; Eccles et al. 1957b; Lundberg et al. 1977). Doubtless there are many more interneurones also receiving monosynaptic tendon organ activation, including neurones on pathways responsible for pre-synaptic inhibitory action evoked by input in tendon organ afferent fibres (see Schmidt 1973). But at present little is known about the convergence patterns onto these neurones, or their projections to other neurones. A start on the problem has been made by Jankowska and her colleagues (Czarkowska et al. 1976); they have described six types of interneurones within the intermediary region (laminae V–VII) on the basis of horseradish peroxidase injections. The neurones received input from Group I muscle afferent fibres; as far as could be shown by the electrical stimulation techniques used, this input was from both Ia and Ib afferents.

In summary, therefore, the electrophysiological evidence predicts that Golgi tendon organ afferent fibres near their entrance to the spinal cord should arborize rather widely in the transverse plane in laminae V–VIII. On the basis of this evidence Réthelyi and Szentágothai (1973) have suggested that some coarse collaterals with wide areas of termination in laminae VI and VII are indeed the collaterals of tendon organ afferent fibres. We shall see that this prediction is correct. The extrasegmental projections of tendon organ afferent fibres have been less well worked out. Like the projections of the spindle primary endings, the best known ones are those to the dorsal and ventral spinocerebellar tracts. Dorsal spinocerebellar tract neurones excited monosynaptically by Group I muscle afferents seem to be excited either by Ia fibres or by Ib fibres but not by both (Lundberg and Winsbury 1960b; McIntyre and Mark 1960; Jansen and Rudjord 1965). On the basis of a Golgi study Réthelyi (1968) has made a tentative identification of the tendon organ collaterals to Clarke's column as those giving branches to the ventro-lateral portion of the column, with the neurones they contact separate from, and fewer than, those receiving presumed Ia terminations.

The ventral spinocerebellar tract receives strong excitatory actions from tendon organ afferents, and those cells of origin of the tract located in laminae V–VII of the cord (Hubbard and Oscarsson 1962) receive monosynaptic excitation from Ib afferents (see Oscarsson 1973). However, the spinal border cell component of the tract (Burke et al. 1971b; Lundberg and Weight 1971) receives mainly Ia excitation and few cells appear to be monosynaptically activated by tendon organ afferent fibres.

B. Morphology of axons innervating Golgi tendon organs

As described in the introduction to Sect. C in Chapter 1, all fibres classified as Group I in our experiments had peripheral conduction velocities of more than 80 m s^{-1}. Group Ia and Ib axons were differentiated according to the presence or absence of continuing activity when first isolated and their sensitivity to muscle stretch. Final allocations to the Ia or Ib categories were based on the morphology of their collaterals. The morphology always agreed with the tentative classification made during the electrophysiological recording session.

Our results on the morphology of Ib afferent fibres (Brown and Fyffe 1978b, 1979; Fyffe 1981; and the present work) are in essential agreement with the preliminary report of Hongo et al. (1978). Any differences will be noted in the following account.

I. Entry of axons into the spinal cord, branching and collateral distribution

The main features of the Ib axonal branching pattern and collateral spacing are shown in Fig. 12.1. Of 11 Ib axons stained (7 from lateral gastrocnemius/soleus, 1 from medial gastrocnemius and 3 from muscles innervated by the posterior tibial nerve) 10 could be traced back from the point of injection into the dorsal root. Nine of these bifurcated shortly after entering the spinal cord. Between 5.1 and 9.9 mm of axon were stained, ascending branches for distances of

5.0–9.6 mm and descending branches for 0.0–3.8 mm. None of the branches terminated as a collateral so, as with nearly all our afferent fibre material, the axons must have been longer than indicated by the peroxidase method.

The ascending branches of Ib axons are thicker than the descending branches and both give off collaterals. The collateral spacings on Ib fibres are unusual in that collaterals are more closely spaced on descending branches than on the ascending branches. For 84 collaterals spaced out on 11 axon lengths of 3.4–8.0 mm the mean spacing was 890 ± 506 μm (mean ± s.d.; range 100–2600 μm), a value not significantly different from that for Ia afferent fibre collateral spacings. But when the spacings on ascending and descending branches are compared marked differences may be observed. For 50 collateral spacings on ascending branches the values were 100–2600 μm (1080 ± 524 μm, mean ± s.d.), whereas for 27 collateral spacings on descending branches they were 200–1500 μm (690 ± 331 μm, mean ± s.d.). The difference between the mean spacings

on ascending and descending branches is highly significant ($P < 0.001$) and not correlated with distance from the dorsal root entrance zone. The implications of this difference are not immediately apparent. Larger samples of Ib axons from different muscles will be necessary before speculation is justified. It is worth noting, however, that Hongo et al. (1978) observed a similar difference in their pooled sample of Group I axons. It will be recalled (Chapter 11) that Ia fibres do not show this difference in collateral spacings on their ascending versus their descending branch. The results of Hongo et al. are presumably a reflexion of the spacings on the Ib component of their sample (seven Ia axons and four Ib axons).

II. Morphology of Ib collaterals

The general morphological features of collaterals from Golgi tendon organ afferents are shown in the photomontage of Fig. 12.2 and the camera lucida reconstructions of Figs. 12.3–12.6. These

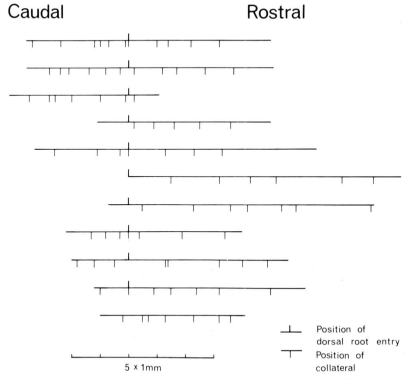

Fig. 12.1. Diagrammatic representation of the branching pattern of Ib afferent fibres in the spinal cord. The total length of each axon stained is shown, together with (where possible) the position of its entry into the cord through the dorsal root and the position of origin of stained collaterals. All but one of the axons that could be traced into the dorsal root can be seen to bifurcate upon entering the cord. For further description see the text. (From Brown and Fyffe 1979.)

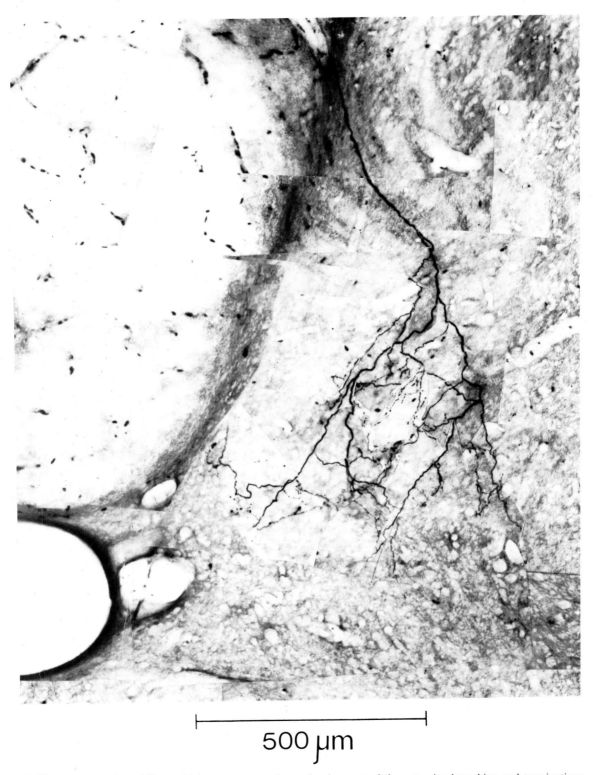

Fig. 12.2. Photomontage, from 100-μm thick transverse sections, showing part of the extensive branching and terminations in lamina VI of a Ib afferent fibre collateral. This collateral is reconstructed in Fig. 12.4A. (From Brown and Fyffe 1979.)

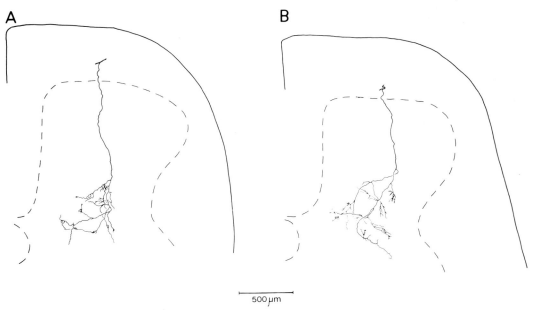

Fig. 12.3. Reconstructions, in the transverse plane, of two adjacent collaterals from the descending branch of a fibre from medial gastrocnemius Ib afferent. Collateral A was caudal to collateral B. The collaterals enter the dorsal horn at its dorsal edge and run ventrally to lamina V before branching into the characteristic fan-shaped arborizations in lamina VI and the dorsal part of lamina VII. The outline of the grey matter is indicated by the *dashed line*. (From Brown and Fyffe 1979.)

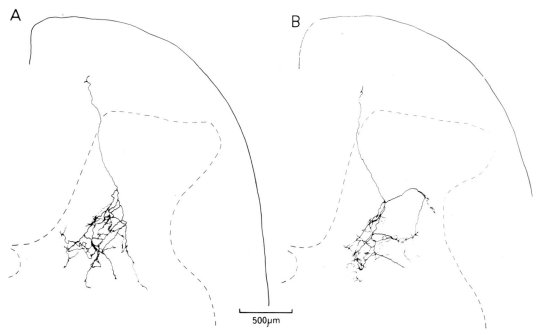

Fig. 12.4. Reconstructions, in the transverse plane, of two adjacent collaterals from the ascending branch of a Ib afferent fibre from lateral gastrocnemius/soleus. The main arborizations in medial and central lamina VI are similar to those in Fig. 12.3. The more rostral collateral (**B**) also projects to the lateral parts of laminae V and VI. (From Brown and Fyffe 1979.)

Fig. 12.5. Reconstructions, in the sagittal plane, of two adjacent collaterals from the ascending branch of a Ib afferent fibre from lateral gastrocnemius/soleus. This view shows the cranial trajectory of the collaterals towards their terminal arborizations. Although the collaterals arise close to each other on the parent axon there is no overlap between the two arborizations. The rostro-caudal extent of each arborization is restricted to less than 400 μm, in contrast to the wide transverse spread seen in Figs. 12.3, 12.4 and 12.6. The *dashed line* indicates the dorsal border of the dorsal horn. (From Brown and Fyffe 1979.)

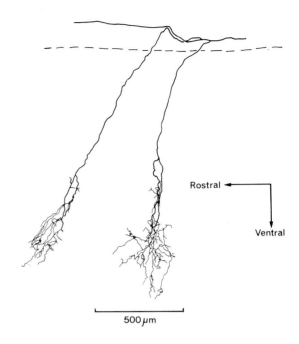

Fig. 12.6. Reconstructions, in the transverse plane, of two collaterals from different Ib axons. Collateral A is from the descending branch of an afferent fibre from lateral gastrocnemius/soleus and has a small arborization in lamina IV as well as the major zone of termination in central lamina VI and the dorsal part of lamina VII. Collateral B is from an afferent from lateral gastrocnemius/soleus ascending the cord. The collateral arises about 7 mm from the dorsal root entry. The main arborization is in the medial half of laminae V and VI. There are also prominent projections to the lateral part of lamina VI, and to dorso-lateral lamina VII. (From Brown and Fyffe 1979.)

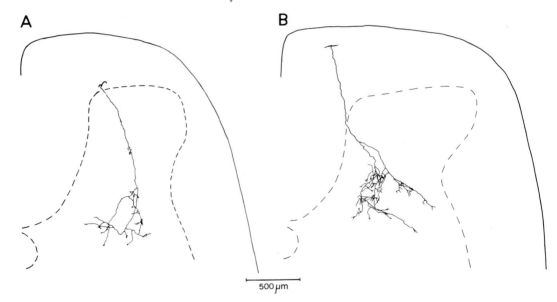

all represent collaterals from within 10 mm of either side of the point of entry of the parent axon into the lumbosacral cord. As with all other types of primary afferent fibres the morphology is characteristic of the type, and the homogeneity of the morphology within the type is striking.

Collaterals of Ib afferent fibres usually enter the dorsal horn at its dorsal (Figs. 12.3, 12.6A) or medial (Figs. 12.2, 12.4, 12.6B) border and run ventrally in a fairly direct course to lamina IV or

V before branching. In reconstructions from sagittal sections (Fig. 12.5) it can be seen that the collaterals also project rostrally as they run through the dorsal horn, so that the terminal arborizations are rostral of the point of origin of the collateral.

Usually the collateral begins to branch at the level of lamina V. Branching is normally profuse and quickly gives rise to second-, third- and fourth-order branches, producing a wide triangular (or fan-shaped: Hongo et al. 1978) arborization in laminae V–VII. This arbor is some 400–800 μm wide in the transverse plane and situated in the medial and central parts of the laminae (Figs. 12.2, 12.3, 12.5, 12.6A).

In contrast to the wide arborization of Ib collaterals in the transverse plane the rostro-caudal extents of the individual collaterals are restricted. In the sagittal plane (Fig. 12.5) the arborization usually measures between 200 and 400 μm. There is no overlap between the arborizations of adjacent collaterals from the same axon, even when they arise as close together as 100 μm or so, as in the example of Fig. 12.5. It can be seen from Fig. 12.5 that although the collaterals arise very close together they separate soon after leaving the parent axon and their terminal arborizations are some 300–400 μm apart in the sagittal plane. Each collateral of a Ib afferent fibre has an arborization that occupies its own private volume of spinal cord. In our sample of Ib fibres there was never any overlap of the terminal arborizations from adjacent collaterals. The Ib fibres differ markedly from the Ia afferents, therefore, since the latter form sagittal columns of terminals up and down the cord. Ia collaterals, however, are much more restricted in the transverse plane (lamina VI) than Ib collaterals.

On the descending branch of one Ib axon three collaterals gave off fine branches in lamina IV (Fig. 12.6A). These fine branches formed their terminal arborizations almost immediately after their origin and they carried bouton arrangements different from those in more ventral laminae (see below).

Within about 7–8 mm of either side of the dorsal root entrance of the Ib axons the collaterals do not penetrate ventral to the level of the central canal. In other words their deepest terminations are in the dorsal part of lamina VII.

The limitation of most of the arborization of Ib collaterals to the medial and central parts of laminae V–VII that is seen near the dorsal root entrance of the axon is, however, characteristic only of this area. The more rostral collaterals in our sample, even in axons stained near the dorsal root entrance and therefore less than 1 cm from it, often displayed projections to the lateral grey matter in addition to the usual projections. Two such collaterals are shown Figs. 12.4B and 12.6B. Figure 12.4 shows two adjacent collaterals from an ascending branch of a Ib afferent fibre from lateral gastrocnemius/soleus. The collateral in Fig. 12.4A is the more caudal of the pair and has the characteristic fan-shaped arborization. The more rostral member (Fig. 12.4B) sends a branch across lamina V to terminate near its lateral border and there are also other branches to the lateral third of lamina VI. Figure 12.6B shows another collateral from a Ib afferent from lateral gastrocnemius/soleus arising about 10 mm rostral to the entrance of the parent axon. It sends branches to the lateral parts of lamina VI in addition to the usual arborization in the medial part of the grey matter.

Hongo et al. (1978) noted that collaterals in the rostral parts of L-7 may project to the lateral grey matter (to the dorso-lateral corner of lamina IX according to them). These authors also proposed that Ib collaterals may be tentatively classified into two types according to whether they formed fan-shaped arborizations limited to lamina VI (in their material) or had terminal distributions to laminae VI and IX. It is here that our results and those of Hongo et al. are in disagreement. It seems premature to classify Ib collaterals into two types on the basis of only four stained afferent fibres. Our own work is more extensive but still limited as regards sample size. But it seems obvious that Ib collateral morphology (collaterals of axons from hind limb muscle nerves in cat) depends upon the position of the collateral in the lumbosacral cord. In caudal and middle regions of L-7 and in S-1 the fan-shaped type of arborization is usual and is generally limited to the medial and central parts of the grey matter in lamina VI and dorsal lamina VII. Occasional terminals are also given to lamina IV. Towards the rostral parts of the L-7 segment and in L-6, Ib collaterals still provide arborizations to the medial and central parts of lamina VI and dorsal VII, but in addition send branches across the cord to the lateral grey matter where they terminate in lateral laminae V–VII. In none of our material do we consider there are terminations in the dorso-lateral corner of lamina IX as suggested by Hongo et al. (1978). It seems likely (as suggested by Hongo et al.) that some of the branches projecting to the lateral grey matter in L-6 are supplying spinal border cells that project into the ventral spinocerebellar tract. Obviously the story is far from complete; collaterals of Ib afferents to Clarke's columns will show further differences in morphology.

III. Terminal arborizations and synaptic boutons of collaterals

A characteristic feature of the branching pattern of Ib collaterals within lamina VI is that axons (about 3–4 μm in diameter) often branch into three finer axons, that is, they trifurcate. An ex-ample of such a trifurcation is shown in Fig. 12.7A. Although occasional examples of trifurcations have been seen in other primary afferent fibre collaterals only Pacinian corpuscle afferents have anywhere near the number of tri-furcations seen in Ib collaterals.

The photomicrographs of Fig. 12.7B–F and the

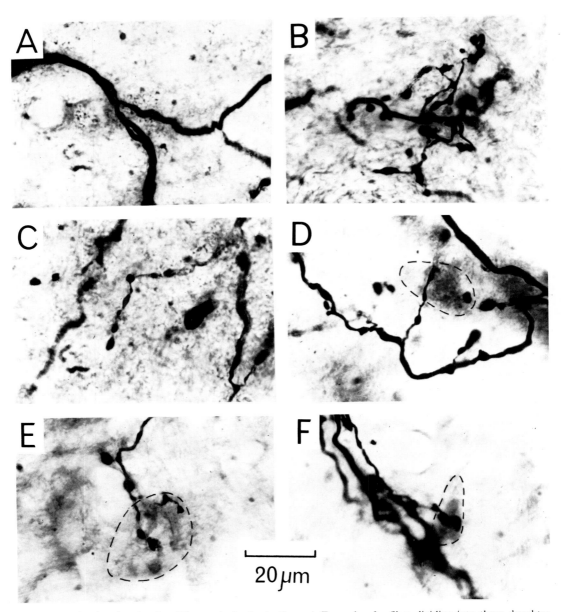

Fig. 12.7. Photomicrographs showing details of Ib terminal arborizations. **A** Example of a fibre dividing into three daughter branches in lamina VI. **B** Complex clustering of boutons observed in the central part of lamina IV, dorsal to the main arborization. **C–F** Boutons in lamina VI. **D–F** are from counterstained sections. Somal profiles are outlined. **C** Branch carrying several boutons *en passant*. **D** Two boutons *en passant* contacting a stained cell body. **E** Four contacts on a medium-sized lamina VI neurone. **F** Two or three contacts on a cell near the lateral border of lamina VI. (From Brown and Fyffe 1979.)

camera lucida drawings of Fig. 12.8 illustrate some of the terminal patterns and bouton arrangements seen on Ib collaterals. Within the fan-shaped arborization in lamina VI and dorsal lamina VII the fine terminal axons run in the transverse plane and are usually oriented dorso-ventrally or medio-laterally even though the thicker pre-terminal axons run more often at about 45° to these directions within the fan-shaped arrangement. Boutons are arranged predominantly *en passant* along the terminal branches and up to ten boutons (commonly five to eight) are carried before the bouton *terminal* (Fig. 12.8A–E). In lamina VI another common feature is that boutons are often offset from terminal axons on short, fine stalks (Fig. 12.8C).

Some terminal branches within lamina VI divide several times and produce quite complex clusters of boutons (Fig. 12.8B, D), particularly in the central parts of the lamina. In counter-stained sections these clusters may often be seen in close association with the profiles of neuronal somata (Fig. 12.7E). Occasionally boutons *de passage* are also seen in close association with somata (Fig. 12.7D). Only a small proportion of Ib boutons in lamina VI seems to be involved in possible somatic contacts. The predominant boutons *en passant* along the final 20–25 μm of the terminal branches may be expected to be involved in climbing-type or crossing-over-type contacts with dendrites. Terminal branches from the fan-shaped arborization projecting into dorsal lamina VII usually have rather simpler arrangements and carry a few boutons *en passant*.

Outside the fan-shaped area of termination in laminae VI and VII more variable bouton arrangements are present. The most dorsal terminations in lamina IV are quite different from any other Ib arborizations. The branches given off the main collateral are fine and almost immediately break up into their terminal arborizations, which form complex clusters of boutons within a small area of about 30 μm × 40 μm (Fig. 12.7B). Terminals in lateral lamina V give rise to a high density of boutons, mainly of the *en passant* type, oriented dorso-ventrally in line with the lateral border of the lamina (Fig. 12.8H). In the lateral parts of laminae VI and VII the terminals are often arranged transversely across the cord and carry a few boutons *en passant* with single boutons offset from the main terminal branch.

Ib collaterals carry a large number of boutons. Between 56 and 384 have been counted on single collaterals (179 ± 114; mean ± s.d.). This is similar to the number carried by Pacinian corpuscle afferent fibre collaterals and some cutaneous afferent collaterals, and much greater than the number carried by single Ia collaterals in the lamina VI arborization (see Chapter 10). The boutons vary in size from about 1.0 μm × 1.0 μm to 5.0 μm × 3.0 μm with a mean of 3.1 ± 0.97 μm × 1.7 ± 0.53 μm (±s.d., $n = 170$).

IV. Organization of collaterals

Figure 12.9 is a summary diagram of the organization of collaterals from a Ib afferent fibre at and near its point of entry into the lumbosacral spinal cord (at about L-7). Attempts have been made to present the main features as revealed by intra-axonal injection of horseradish peroxidase.

Group Ib axons behave like nearly all other large primary afferent fibres after entering the cord—they bifurcate into ascending and descending branches. The descending branch is usually obviously thinner than the ascending branch. Collaterals arise from the branches at an average separation of about 890 μm, a value similar to that for Ia fibres. However, Ib axons are unusual in that the collaterals are given off closer together on the descending branch than on the ascending branch. Although the difference between the spacings on the two branches was highly significant in our sample it is probably wise to wait until a large sample of Ib afferent fibres from a wide range of hind limb muscles has been obtained before considering any possible functional significance of the observation.

The morphology of Ib collaterals is in agreement with the general principle that all primary afferent fibres have collaterals with morphologies specific to the afferent unit type. Furthermore, experiments using intra-axonal injection of horseradish peroxidase have confirmed that predictions made by Réthelyi and Szentágothai (1973) concerning the morphology of Ib collaterals are correct. Also, as was to be expected, the morphology agrees with the electrophysiological data.

Near their entrance to the spinal cord Ib collaterals form wide fan-shaped arborizations in laminae V–VII. In the transverse plane these

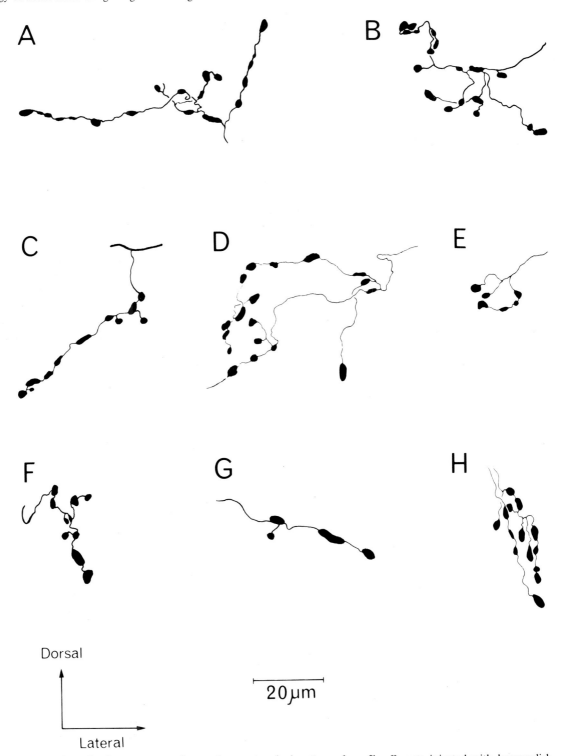

Fig. 12.8. Reconstructions, in the transverse plane, of some terminal patterns from Ib afferents injected with horseradish peroxidase. The terminals in **A–E** were located in the medial and central parts of lamina VI and illustrate examples of boutons *en passant* along the fine terminal branches. More complex branching and clustering of boutons is also evident. Single boutons are often offset from the terminal branch on short, fine stalks. In **F–H** are reconstructed some terminals in lateral parts of lamina VI. Boutons were fewer in this region, but even close to the lateral border of the neck of the dorsal horn (e.g. in **H**) complex arrangements could be seen. (From Brown and Fyffe 1979.)

arborizations are within the medial and central parts of the spinal grey matter and are 400–800 μm wide. In the sagittal plane they are restricted to a rostro-caudal spread of 200–400 μm, so the Ib collaterals essentially form transverse plates of arborizations across the spinal cord rather similar to those formed by slowly adapting Type II cutaneous afferent fibres. Terminal arborizations of adjacent collaterals from the same axon do not overlap in the sagittal plane of the cord. Each collateral from a single Ib axon provides boutons to its own private volume of cord. Presumably terminal arborizations of collaterals from different Ib axons converge onto the same volume of cord to provide the convergence onto neurones receiving Ib input (see for example Hongo et al. 1966).

Within the fan-shaped arborization of Ib collaterals in laminae V–VII, terminal boutons are restricted to lamina VI and the dorsal part of lamina VII. There are three main types of terminal axon arrangement, which may reflect at least three types of contacts on different classes of interneurones. Boutons *de passage* are common and in general arranged either medio-laterally or dorso-ventrally. They are particularly well-developed in medial parts of lamina VI and conceivably reflect climbing or crossing-over types of synaptic arrangements on dendrites of interneurones. Until the dendritic tree morphology of cells receiving such monosynaptic input from Ib afferents has been determined it is not possible to know whether the medio-lateral and dorso-ventral arrangements do, or do not, reflect any real differences. In the middle parts of lamina VI boutons are often arranged in cluster formations suggestive of somatic contacts. Indeed in counterstained preparations (Fig. 12.8E) these clusters of boutons may be seen in close association with stained nerve cell bodies. Depending upon the degree of convergence from other Ib afferent fibres onto these neurones such contacts may be very powerful in exciting the cells.

The presence of Ib boutons within lamina IV was expected from previous electrophysiological reports (Hongo et al. 1966). However, such endings were uncommon, and have been found on only three (10%) well-stained collaterals so far. But all three collaterals showed a similar picture, of very fine branches given off the collateral as it descended through lamina IV. At this level the axis cylinder was about 7 μm in diameter and the fine branches were about 1 μm. Almost immediately the fine branches broke up into their terminal arborizations and produced clusters of boutons located in the middle of the dorsal horn in the ventral half of the lamina. The clusters of boutons could be seen, in counterstained sections, to be in close association with neuronal somata. Most lamina IV neurones receive excitatory input from cutaneous afferent fibres (e.g. neurones of the spinocervical tract and the postsynaptic dorsal column pathway: see Chapters 6 and 8). These neurones may also receive excitation from high-threshold muscle afferent fibres but there appear to be no reports of monosynaptic excitation from Group I muscle afferents. Obviously if our sample is representative only a few Ib collaterals will project to lamina IV neurones, but such a projection undoubtedly exists (Hongo et al. 1966).

At rostral levels in L-7 and caudal L-6, Ib collaterals, in addition to their arborization in laminae V–VII, also send branches more laterally to the lateral parts of laminae V, VI and VII. At this level a set or sets of contacts are made that are different from those in the medial and central parts of laminae VI and VII. Cells that are prime candidates to receive such Ib input are the spinal border cells, now known to give rise to axons running in the ventral spinocerebellar tract (Cooper and Sherrington 1940; Burke et al. 1971b). According to Burke et al. (1971b) spinal border cells receiving monosynaptic Ib input (based on electrical nerve stimulation) are in a minority, and most receive monosynaptic Ia input or monosynaptic excitation from Group I muscle afferent fibres (Lundberg and Weight 1971). Furthermore, very few cells discharged impulses in response to electrical stimulation of nerves.

In lumbar segments L-3–L-5 spinal border cells are clearly situated within lamina IX and they were recorded in this region by Burke et al. (1971b). These authors showed, however, that in L-6 some of the recording sites were in the most lateral parts of laminae VI and VII. This is where Ib collaterals send branches in our material. According to Burke et al. (1971b) no ventral spinocerebellar tract neurones (spinal border cells) could be found in the L-7 segment with their electrophysiological techniques. Furthermore, G. Grant (personal communication) in a recent retrograde horseradish peroxidase study has shown that there are many spinocerebellar neurones in

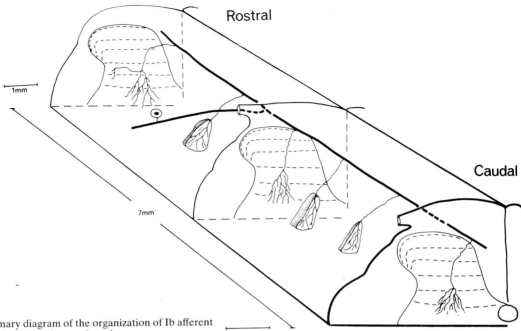

Rostral

Caudal

1mm

7mm

1mm

Fig. 12.9. Summary diagram of the organization of Ib afferent fibre collaterals in the lumbosacral cord.

the L-5 and L-6 segments in the cat, but he could find none in L-7. Obviously it is difficult to determine the precise border between two adjacent spinal cord segments (if such a thing exists at all) and whether some of our material is from caudal L-6 or rostral L-7 is perhaps debatable. It is certainly premature, however, to assume that all Ib collateral branches to the lateral parts of laminae V–VII are destined to contact spinal border cells. In counterstained sections, though, boutons have been seen in close proximity to large neuronal

somata which may well have belonged to spinal border cells. Most boutons in these regions were of the *en passant* type and therefore more likely to be in contact with dendrites.

In order to complete the picture of Ib afferent fibres from hind limb muscles in the cat injections of horseradish peroxidase will need to be made in more rostral segments. By so doing the collaterals to the spinal border cells in L-3–L-5 will be revealed, as will the collaterals to Clarke's column.

13   Afferent fibres from secondary endings in muscle spindles

The structure and function of the secondary endings in muscle spindles have been well reviewed recently (Matthews 1972; Barker 1974; Hunt 1974; McIntyre 1974). The reader should refer to these accounts for a detailed treatment, and also to Chapters 11 and 12 of the present work for an introduction to muscle spindle and tendon organ receptors and the problems of selective activation of their afferent fibres (see Sects. 11A, 12A, 12B).

Secondary endings in muscle spindles of cat hind limb muscles are innervated by axons conducting in the Group II range of Lloyd (1943b), that is at 24–72 m s^{-1}, and they have a diameter of 4–12 μm (Hunt 1954). It is reasonable to assume that most Group II muscle afferent fibres innervate muscle spindle secondary endings, but there is overlap with other axons at both ends of the range—at the upper end with small Group I fibres from Golgi tendon organs or even spindle primary receptors and at the lower end with axons from various mechanoreceptors (Paintal 1960). In fact a small minority of axons within the Group II range innervate receptors other than muscle spindle secondary endings (Paintal 1960; Bessou and Laporte 1960, 1961). However, according to Matthews (1963) afferent fibres from muscle spindles conducting at less than 60 m s^{-1} are almost certainly from secondary endings.

A. Central projections of axons from muscle spindle secondary endings

I. Terminations of Group II fibres

For convenience in the following account, axons from secondary endings in muscle spindles will be called Group II. Where the terminology is misleading, or where axons other than those from spindle secondaries are referred to, this will be clarified.

Coombs et al. (1956) used electrical stimulation of muscle nerves in an attempt to localize spinal cord neurones excited by volleys in Group II fibres. The evoked focal synaptic potential extended from the dorsal horn to the ventral part of the intermediate region (approximately from lamina IV to VI). Recently a well-controlled series of experiments by Fu et al. (1974) and Fu and Schomburg (1974) has provided detailed electrophysiological evidence on the termination of Group II axons in the cat's lumbosacral cord.

Fu et al. (1974) used a double-shock technique to provide a pure Group II input and averaged the focal synaptic potentials generated in the cord. They observed three such potentials: a dorsal potential with a latency appropriate for monosynaptic excitation, a ventral potential about 0.6–1.5 ms later than the dorsal potential and a late potential found over a wide region of the cord. The monosynaptically evoked dorsal potential from the nerve to gastrocnemius/soleus was observed in caudal L-6 to cranial S-1 and was localized to lamina IV dorso-lateral to the dorsal Group I potential in lamina VI. The ventral Group II focal synaptic potential was seen in only some 50%–70% of microelectrode tracks in which the dorsal potential was recorded. It was located between the positions of the Group-I-evoked potentials in laminae VI and IX and also often extended, itself, into lamina IX (the motor nuclei). In the longitudinal axis of the cord the ventral potential extended from caudal L-5 to cranial S-1, that is it was more extensive in this direction than the dorsal focal synaptic potential. The late Group II potential was less well defined than the other two.

In order to (1) control the possibility that some

of the effects observed by Fu et al. (1974) were due to excitation of axons from receptors other than spindle secondaries, and (2) check whether the responses in the ventral region could be monosynaptically evoked, Fu and Schomburg (1974) adopted a different approach. Single identified Group II (spindle secondary) axons were prepared in continuity and their antidromic responses recorded upon microelectrode stimulation in the spinal cord grey matter using well-controlled microstimulation. Low-threshold areas were found in the dorsal horn and the ventral horn (corresponding with the areas of maximal focal synaptic potential found by Fu et al.) and in the spinal grey matter in between. The ventral area extended into the motor nuclei as well as being medial or dorso-medial to it. The experiments showed, therefore, that Group II axons project not only to the dorsal horn but also to the motor nuclei in the ventral horn. Furthermore, it was shown that the conduction velocities of the collateral branches to the ventral horn were much slower than those of the parent axons and that this accounted for the 0.6–1.5 ms between the onset of the focal synaptic potential in the dorsal horn and that in the ventral horn.

II. Location of neurones activated by Group II axons

The results of Fu and his co-workers provide a firm basis for experiments aimed at localizing and recording from neurones excited by Group II axons. Most of these experiments remain to be performed, using stimuli as well-controlled as those of Fu et al. (1974).

According to presently accepted views activity in Group II afferent fibres evokes, both ipsilaterally and contralaterally, pre-synaptic inhibition in Golgi tendon organ (Ib) axons (see Schmidt 1973). It is unlikely that this effect accounts for all of the dorsal horn terminations of Group II fibres. Many neurones in the dorsal horn are excited by activity in muscle afferent fibres with electrical thresholds within the Group II range (and higher). Unfortunately these afferent fibres, along with those from cutaneous and joint receptors, were lumped together by Holmqvist and Lundberg (1961) as the 'flexor reflex afferents', a concept which has had, if anything,

a confusing rather than a clarifying influence upon contemporary neurophysiological thought. Although flexion reflexes, and nocifensor responses generally, undoubtedly take precedence over other responses in many circumstances it seems naive to consider all muscle afferent fibres (other than those with Group I conduction velocities) and all cutaneous and joint afferent fibres to have similar functions, even in the restricted area of spinal reflexology.

The observation that Group II fibres reach as far as the motor nuclei leads to the question of whether they excite motoneurones. It has been shown that they do (Kirkwood and Sears 1974; Stauffer et al. 1976), albeit weakly. Therefore some, at least, of the ventral horn terminations of Group II axons are likely to be on motoneurones. But the dendrites of motoneurones extend dorsally well into lamina V (see Chapter 14). Contacts made by Group II fibres upon motoneurones are not necessarily made within the motor nuclei and all terminals within the motor nuclei are not necessarily upon motoneurones.

Group II axons excite neurones of the spinocerebellar tracts. Some dorsal spinocerebellar tract cells receive input, probably monosynaptic, from Group II fibres (Laporte et al. 1956; McIntyre and Mark 1960; Eccles et al. 1961c). There will, therefore, be projections of Group II collaterals to Clarke's column. Neurones of the ventral spinocerebellar tract are also affected by input from spindle secondary endings. The spino-olivary pathway also receives excitation from Group II afferent fibres (Armstrong et al. 1968; Oscarsson 1968).

III. Central effects of impulses in Group II fibres

The generally accepted role for spindle secondary endings in spinal reflex mechanisms is one of excitation of flexor muscles with concurrent inhibition of extensors (Lloyd 1943b, 1946, 1952). This effect is usually observed as a facilitation of the monosynaptic test reflex or as excitatory post-synaptic potentials in flexor motoneurones and inhibitory post-synaptic potentials in extensors (Lloyd 1946; Brock et al. 1951; Eccles 1962; R. M. Eccles and Lundberg 1959a). But this is not their only action. Flexor inhibition and extensor excitation have been reported following electrical stimulation of muscle nerves at Group II strength (R. M. Eccles and Lundberg 1959a; Holmqvist and Lundberg 1961; Wilson and Kato 1965). Some of these effects may be accounted for by the admixture of axons other than those from spindle secondary endings in the Group II volley.

A further role for spindle secondary endings has been suggested by Matthews (1969, 1972), that of autogenetic excitation: that is, excitation of α-motoneurones belonging to the muscle containing the receptors and also the motoneurones of synergistic muscle. It is suggested that the excitation is via polysynaptic pathways in the cord and is additional to the well-known monosynaptic autogenetic excitation from the spindle primary endings. Support for this idea has been obtained by Westbury (1972), but see Grillner (1970) and Cangliano and Lutzemberger (1972). The recognition of a monosynaptic connexion between Group II afferent fibres and motoneurones (Kirkwood and Sears 1974; Stauffer et al. 1976) provides compelling evidence in support of autogenetic excitation and demonstrates that some component of the excitation, at least, is monosynaptic.

There are few other known or suggested actions for spindle secondary endings. They appear to be involved in various long spinal reflexes linking the forelimbs and hind limbs with each other (see McIntyre 1974).

B. Morphology of axons innervating muscle spindle secondary endings

The results to be described are taken from the work of Fyffe (1979, 1981). Group II axons from muscle were relatively more difficult to stain satisfactorily with horseradish peroxidase than either the Group I muscle or the cutaneous afferent fibres. The reported sample is small and consists of only three axons. Enough information is provided, however, from the 17 collaterals that they gave off to allow useful generalizations to be made about them.

The axons all ran in the nerve to lateral gastrocnemius/soleus and they had conduction velocities of 54, 59 and 61 m s^{-1}, that is, well within the Group II range. The axons carried a very regular

discharge at resting muscle length, responded with an increased discharge to muscle stretch and the receptors were located within the muscle belly. There can be no doubt that axons from spindle secondary endings were being studied.

I. Entry of axons into the spinal cord, branching and collateral distribution

All three axons from spindle secondary endings in lateral gastrocnemius/soleus bifurcated into an ascending and a descending branch upon entering the cord. Seventeen collaterals were given off the branches, one at the point of bifurcation so that for that particular axon there was a trifurcation into ascending and descending branches and a collateral. The average intercollateral spacing for Group II fibres was 800 μm (range 100–1400 μm), a value similar to those for other primary afferent fibres.

II. Morphology of collaterals

Figures 13.1–13.3 show the morphology of collaterals from axons innervating spindle secondary endings of lateral gastrocnemius/soleus, as seen in reconstructions from transverse sections. In each figure an adjacent pair of collaterals from the same axon is shown. Compared with collaterals from other muscle and cutaneous afferent fibres, collaterals from Group II axons show more variability in the detail of their branching and terminal arborizations. But there are still great similarities between all the collaterals in the sample. All but one collateral (shown in Fig. 13.3B) had three main areas of arborization: in the dorsal horn, in the intermediate region and in the ventral horn. Like other collaterals of primary afferent fibres the Group II collaterals pursue, from their origin in the dorsal columns to their termination in the ventral horn, a rostral trajectory, so that their dorsal arborizations originate caudal to their ventral terminals.

The collaterals usually descend to the level of lamina IV before branching: occasionally a branch arises more dorsal than this (Fig. 13.2A). The dorsal region of arborization extends, in toto, from lamina IV at its border with lamina III to the dorsal half of lamina VI. In any single collateral,

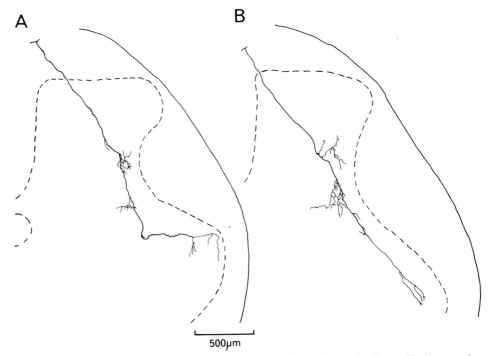

Fig. 13.1. Reconstructions, from transverse sections, of two adjacent collaterals from a Group II muscle afferent fibre innervating lateral gastrocnemius/soleus. Note the three areas of terminal arborization in laminae V, VI–VII and IX. The *dashed line* indicates line border of grey matter. (From Fyffe 1979.)

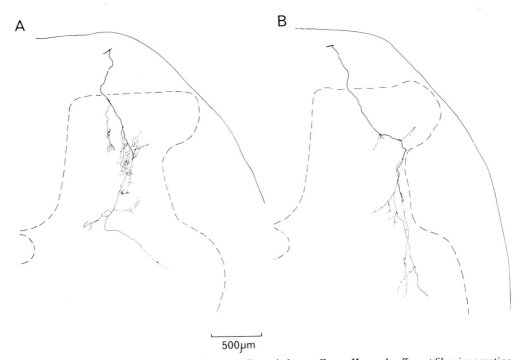

Fig. 13.2. Reconstructions, from transverse sections, of two adjacent collaterals from a Group II muscle afferent fibre innervating lateral gastrocnemius/soleus. Note the branch giving an arborization to lamina IV in **A**. (From Fyffe 1981.)

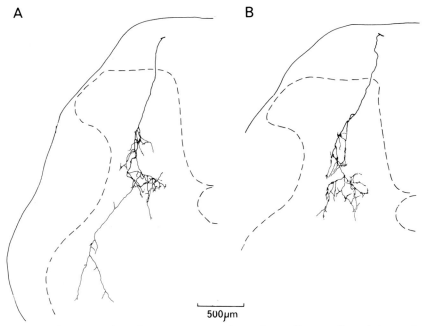

Fig. 13.3. Reconstructions, from transverse sections, of two adjacent collaterals from a Group II muscle afferent fibre innervating lateral gastrocnemius/soleus. Note the absence of an arborization to the motor nuclei in **B**. (From Fyffe 1981.)

however, the dorsal arborization is less extensive than this and is usually limited to lamina V. It is normally generated by three to six branches from the collateral as it descends through laminae IV and V. In the collateral shown in Fig. 13.2A a branch arose in lamina II and provided an arborization exclusively to lamina IV. In other collaterals the dorsal arborization varied from being only weakly developed with little branching of the axons supplying it (Figs. 13.1, 13.2B) to being more extensive (Fig. 13.3). The dorsal region, in the present sample of collaterals from axons to lateral gastrocnemius/soleus, was situated in the middle or the lateral part of the dorsal horn. Even in adjacent collaterals the dorsal regions of arborization were not necessarily lined up rostrocaudally as they generally are in other types of collaterals.

The second region of terminal arborization is developed in lamina VI and the dorsal part of lamina VII. It is nearly always clearly separated from the dorsal region (and the ventral region) by cord containing no terminations. This intermediate arborization is located lateral to the lamina VI arborization of Group Ia axon collaterals from the same lateral gastrocnemius/soleus spindles (see Fig. 11.4) and lateral to the arborization of Ib

collaterals from the same muscle group near the entrance of the parent axon into the spinal cord (see Figs. 12.3, 12.4). Like the dorsal arborization, that in laminae VI and VII is variably developed. At one extreme some collaterals have only one (Fig. 13.1A) or two to three (Fig. 13.2) branches at this level, giving rise to a rather scant arborization, whereas other collaterals (Fig. 13.3) generate much more extensive terminal regions.

The terminations of Group II collaterals in the ventral horn usually arise from a single axonal branch that is the continuation of the main collateral after it has given off its branches to laminae VI and VII. The collateral is considerably thinner here than it was in the dorsal horn (0.8–1.2 μm compared with 2–2.5 μm within lamina IV and 4–5 μm before giving off the dorsal branches). The branch to the ventral horn was not always present (Fig. 13.3B) and sometimes there were two branches running to the ventral horn (Fig. 13.2B). The ventral termination is never strongly developed, however, and consists of a few branches to lamina VII dorsal and dorsomedial or dorso-lateral to the motor nuclei (cf. the lamina VII arborization of Group Ia muscle afferent fibre collaterals) and also to the motor nuclei themselves.

The arborizations of the collaterals of Group II fibres are essentially two-dimensional. There is very little development in the rostro-caudal plane; even in lamina IV, where longitudinal extension might be expected.

III. Terminal arborizations and synaptic boutons

As mentioned above, the terminal arborizations of Group II collaterals are developed essentially in the transverse plane of the cord. Within the three regions of termination there are differences in the organization of the terminal axons and in the bouton arrangements.

In the dorsal region the terminal axons typically carry boutons *en passant* (Figs. 13.4, 13.5A). Up to about ten boutons are carried on the final 50–60 μm of axon. This is the characteristic pattern in the dorsal region although occasional single boutons, offset from the axon on short stalks, are also seen (Fig. 13.4B).

In the lamina VI–VII termination region boutons *de passage* are again common but terminal axons usually only carry about five boutons before the bouton *terminal* (Figs. 13.5B, 13.6, 13.7). A much more common feature in this region is the occurrence of boutons offset from the axon on short stalks. These are usually single (Fig. 13.5B) but sometimes the stalk carries a bouton *de passage* as well as the bouton *terminal*. The offset type of bouton is common enough in this region to be called characteristic and is more obviously developed in the lamina VI–VII termination of Group II collaterals than in any other primary afferent termination we have studied. In this region too there are occasional clusters of boutons—five or six boutons found close together and arising from three of four short terminal axons (Fig. 13.4B). In the present material the terminations in the ventral horn were too faint to allow generalizations to be made about their synaptic boutons.

IV. Organization of collaterals

The organization of Group II collaterals is illustrated in Fig. 13.6. Essentially, the morphology has not provided any major surprises and agrees well with expectations from electrophysiological results, especially those of Fu et al. (1974) and Fu and Schomburg (1974).

Group II collaterals have a more variable morphology than those of other primary afferent fibres we have studied but the general pattern is clear. The variable morphology between individual collaterals possibly accounts for some of the difficulty experienced by Fu and his colleagues in localizing the intermediate region of termination and for the variability of some of their results.

Group II muscle spindle afferent fibres provide direct input to three regions of the cord near their dorsal root entrance. These regions are: the dorsal horn (laminae IV to dorsal VI), the intermediate region (lamina VI and dorsal VII) and the ventral horn (laminae VII and IX). Neurones with somata and dendrites in these regions may receive monosynaptic excitation from axons of spindle secondaries.

The results of Fyffe (1979, 1981) described in this chapter provide direct morphological evidence that information from spindle secondary endings can reach the motor nuclei directly. Group II synapses may be located on the soma and proximal dendrites of α-motoneurones and this seems likely in view of the rapid rise times (1 ms) of Group II monosynaptic excitatory postsynaptic potentials observed by Stauffer et al. (1976). However, the monosynaptic connexions between Group II axons and motoneurones may also be made more dorsal to this in laminae VII, VI or even V, as motoneuronal dendrites reach as far as this into the dorsal horn (see Fig. 14.1). The results also provide direct support for the observations (Fu and Schomburg 1974; Stauffer et al. 1976) of a slower central conduction velocity to the ventral horn for Group II impulses in comparison with Group Ia impulses: the Group II axonal branches to the ventral horn are much thinner than those of Group Ia collaterals (about 1 μm compared with 2–3 μm).

It is of interest to compare the areas of terminal arborization of the Group Ia, Ib and II muscle afferent fibres near their entry into the spinal cord. Figure 13.7 represents an attempt at such a comparison for axons from lateral gastrocnemius/soleus. It should be realized that average, rather than maximal, extents of the arborizations are represented. At the level of entry the Group Ib arborization pattern is the simplest, being generally a single area in laminae V, VI and

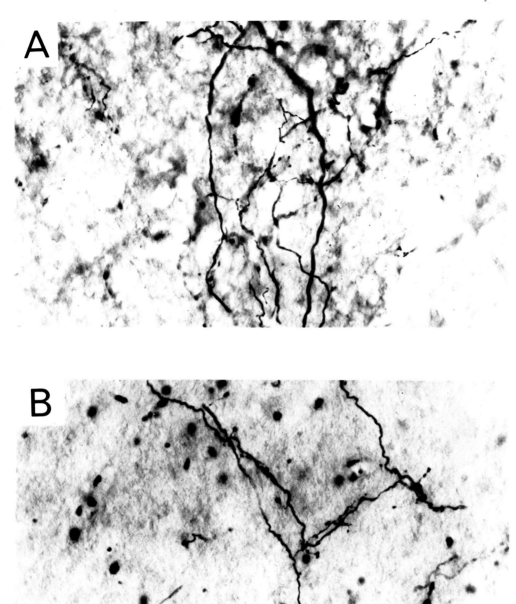

Fig. 13.4. Photomicrographs, from 100-μm sections, of terminal arborizations of Group II muscle afferent collaterals. **A** Terminals in laminae III–IV where boutons *en passant* are common. **B** Terminals in laminae VI–VII. Note the boutons *en passant* dorsally (VI) and the clusters of boutons ventrally (VII). The faint axon branch passing ventrally and to the left is heading for the motor nuclei. (From Fyffe 1981.)

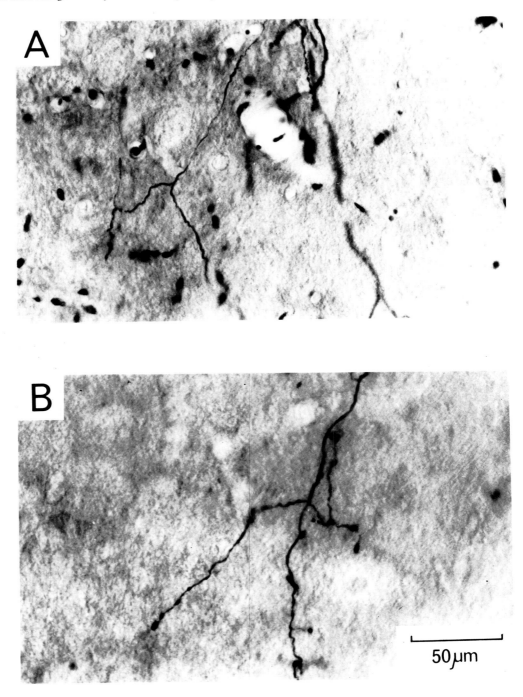

Fig. 13.5. Photomicrographs, from 100-μm sections, of terminal arborizations of Group II muscle afferent collaterals, **A** from laminae V–VI. Note the boutons *en passant* dorsally (lamina V). **B** from lateral lamina VI. Note the boutons on short stalks. (From Fyffe 1981.)

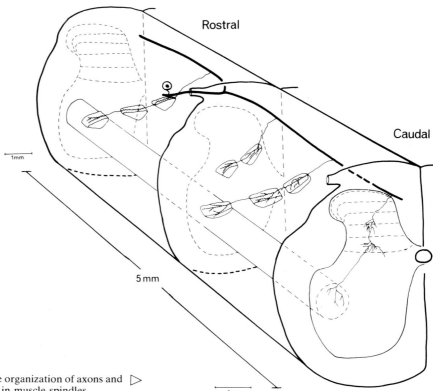

Fig. 13.6. Schematic diagram of the organization of axons and ▷ collaterals from secondary endings in muscle spindles.

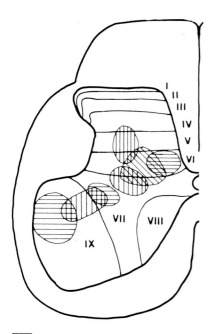

▤ Ia terminals

▨ Ib terminals

▥ II terminals

dorsal VII in the medial and central parts of the grey matter. Occasional Ib terminals are found in lamina IV. Both the Group Ia and the Group II axons generate three clear arborization regions. The Ia collaterals arborize in medial lamina VI, in lamina VII dorsal and dorso-medial to the motor nuclei, and in the motor nuclei (lamina IX) themselves. In contrast the Group II collaterals have terminations in laminae IV–VI, laminae VI and VII and in the ventral horn in lamina IX and dorsal to it. In the ventral horn there is overlap between the ventral Group II arborization and the lamina VII and lamina IX terminations of Group Ia axon collaterals. In the intermediate region overlap between the lamina VI arborization from Ia collaterals and the laminae VI–VII termination of Group II collaterals seems unlikely as the Group II region is usually lateral to the middle of the grey matter whereas the Ia region is

◁ **Fig. 13.7.** Diagrammatic representation of the areas of termination of muscle afferent fibres from lateral gastrocnemius/soleus near their point of entry into the spinal cord. The average areas of termination are shown.

usually medial to it. The areas occupied by the terminals of Group Ia and Ib collaterals in lamina VI overlap.

Obviously the information summarized in Fig. 13.7 provides only generalizations about regions of termination. However, it does suggest where neurones monosynaptically excited by the different inputs might be located. The presence of the dorsal Group II termination in lamina IV is of considerable interest as this part of the cord is dominated by cutaneous input from slowly adapting mechanoreceptors of hairy and glabrous skin and rapidly adapting mechanoreceptors of glabrous skin.

14 Relationships between Group Ia afferent fibres and motoneurones

In Chapter 11 the afferent fibres from the primary endings in muscle spindles (Group Ia axons) were discussed. It was shown that each Ia afferent fibre, near its entrance into the spinal cord, gives off collaterals at an average frequency of one every millimetre. The collaterals have three main areas of termination in the lumbosacral cord: in lamina VI, in lamina VII (to the region containing the Ia inhibitory interneurones) and in lamina IX (the motor nuclei).

Horseradish peroxidase injections into single Ia afferent fibres allowed some indirect estimates to be made about the organization of the monosynaptic reflex arc between axons from primary endings in muscle spindles and motoneurones. It was suggested that, on average, each collateral of a Ia afferent fibre from triceps surae supplies about 20–50 triceps surae motoneurones. Furthermore, in counterstained material, although some Ia boutons were observed in apparent contact with motoneuronal somata many were not, even though they were located within lamina IX. These boutons presumably contacted dendrites, as suggested by other evidence both electrophysiological and anatomical (see the review by Burke and Rudomin 1977).

In the present chapter the Ia–motoneuronal synaptic system will be considered in more detail. The morphology of the α-motoneurone will be described and new evidence presented on the geometry and extent of its dendritic tree. More quantitative data on the Ia–motoneuronal system will be discussed and direct evidence on the distribution of Ia synapses on motoneurones will be presented (see Brown and Fyffe 1981a).

A. α-Motoneurones

I. Anatomy

α-Motoneurones have their cell bodies within the motor cell columns of the ventral horn (Romanes 1951), that is, in Rexed's lamina IX. Their somata are amongst the largest in the central nervous system being 30–70 μm in diameter with a surface area of some 10^{-5}–10^{-3} cm^2 (Rall 1959; Aitken and Bridger 1961; Gelfan et al. 1970; Lux et al. 1970). This large soma undoubtedly provides one of the reasons for the popularity of motoneurones with electrophysiologists; it is possible to maintain intracellular microelectrode recordings from motoneurones for many hours and they will withstand many experimental manoeuvres such as current and ion injection etc.

The dendritic trees of motoneurones are extensive. It is instructive to consider the differences in dendritic tree morphology as revealed by different methods. Classically the silver staining methods have provided details of dendritic trees (see Ramon y Cajal 1909). Unfortunately most studies using these techniques have been carried out on very young animals (e.g. Scheibel and Scheibel 1969) and it is thought that considerable remodelling of dendritic trees may take place early in life (Conradi and Ronnevi 1975).

The first detailed study using Golgi-impregnated material in adult cats was that of Aitken and Bridger (1961). In a sample of large ventral horn neurones (presumed motoneurones) they observed between two and 14 primary dendrites per cell (mean seven). A similar result was obtained by Gelfan et al. (1970) for large neurones in the ventral horn of adult dogs. The geometrical length of the dendrites, from their origin at the soma to their termination, was up to about 1 mm in both studies. It is necessary to point out that single sections only were examined. This would lead to an under-representation of dendritic length.

The introduction of Procion dyes for intracellular staining (Stretton and Kravitz 1968) provided another method for studying motoneuronal morphology in adult animals. Barrett and Crill (1974a) described ten motoneurones from the cat's lumbosacral cord. Between eight and 22 primary dendrites per cell were observed but the total dendritic lengths were only 300–800 μm. That is, the Procion method demonstrated more dendrites than the Golgi method but the dendrites were shorter. However, Barrett and Crill (1974a) estimated the surface area of the soma plus dendrites at 79 000–250 000 μm^3, considerably more than estimates based on Golgi preparations (Aitken and Bridger 1961; Gelfan et al. 1970).

The two sets of results suggest that the Golgi method fails to demonstrate all the dendrites. Whether the Procion method stains all dendrites is open to question, but it certainly shows more than the Golgi method. But the Procion method certainly does not stain the total length of the dendrites: Golgi-stained dendrites are considerably longer.

An independent check on the two methods was provided by Lux et al. (1970) who injected tritiated glycine into single motoneurones. Their results were similar to Barrett and Crill's with regard to numbers of dendrites and to the results from silver staining with regard to dendritic length. A further major difference between the results of Lux et al. and Barrett and Crill was in the degree of dendritic tapering observed (see Sect. A.II below).

Horseradish peroxidase injection (Brown and Fyffe 1981a) demonstrates clearly that both the Golgi and Procion techniques are deficient in that they do not reveal the total extent of motoneuronal dendritic trees. Neither all the dendrites nor their complete lengths are demonstrated. Whether horseradish peroxidase reveals all the dendritic tree is a matter of some concern and a final answer will have to await reconstructions from serial electron micrographs. For the time being, however, the light microscope picture as revealed by this method is the most complete that is available.

Representative reconstructions of α-motoneurones from both transversely and longi-

tudinally cut sections of lumbosacral cord are shown in Fig. 14.1. Quantitative data from a sample of α-motoneurones are presented in Table 14.1. The most immediately striking thing about the reconstructions, especially in comparison with single silver-stained sections or Procion Yellow reconstructions, is the enormous total extent of the dendritic tree relative to the size of the soma (see also Fig. 1 in Cullheim and Kellerth 1976). Furthermore, it is obvious that motoneurones have a considerable number of primary dendrites (between 7 and 18 in our sample of reconstructed motoneurones; mean 11.6).

As pointed out by Sterling and Kuypers (1967b) and Scheibel and Scheibel (1969) the orientation of motoneuronal dendrites varies according to the location of the cell body. Motoneurones situated ventrally in the ventral horn have most of their dendrites running rostrally or caudally away from the cell body in the longitudinal direction. Those situated dorsally and laterally within the motor cell columns also have many longitudinally running dendrites but in addition have a greater development of 'radially' oriented dendrites, i.e. dendrites extending away from the soma in all directions.

Motoneurones with cell bodies situated close to the border of the grey and white matter usually have some dendrites that follow this border closely. But the dendrites of these cells and other motoneurones are not restricted to the grey matter. Most motoneurones have dendrites that extend into the white matter of the lateral and ventral columns (Fig. 14.1C, D, F).

The total geometric length of motoneuronal dendrites (from somatic origin to termination) is usually at least 1 mm and often 1.5 mm or so. The horseradish peroxidase method therefore demonstrates longer dendrites than have been shown by other methods. The total lengths of dendrites from motoneurones have been measured (Table 14.1) and these range up to 1.5 mm or even longer. The dendrites extend well beyond the confines of lamina IX into laminae VIII and VII and dorsally into lamina VI and even V.

The question immediately arises as to whether there are synapses on these very distal dendrites, particularly those out in the white matter. Furthermore, it is obvious that synaptic boutons of primary afferent fibres, descending axons or local interneurones do not have to be within lamina IX in order for them to contact motoneurones.

Table 14.1. Some geometrical and electrophysiological data for the six motoneurones shown in Fig. 14.1.

Motoneurone[a]	Soma diameter (μm)	Conduction velocity (m s^{-1})	No. of primary dendrites	Dendritic spread (μm)		
				Rostro-caudal	Medio-lateral	Dorso-ventral
A Lg-S	60 × 40	83	11	2131	2000	1938
B Mg	45 × 50	90	14	1969	1800	2063
C Lg-S	48 × 45	74	8	2600	1720	1915
D Lg-S	45 × 50	86	11	2600	1975	2185
E Mg	75 × 50	92	9	1100	1688	1625
F Mg	45 × 55	76	11	2100	1781	2371

[a] Lg-S, lateral gastrocnemius/soleus; Mg, medial gastrocnemius.

Boutons of Group Ia and Group II axons (from muscle spindle primary and secondary endings respectively) are found dorsal to the motor nuclei, as well as within them (Chapters 11, 13), and contacts onto motoneuronal dendrites could be made in these regions.

Horseradish peroxidase injections have also allowed the axon collateral systems of motoneurones to be reconstructed. However it is outside the scope of the present treatment to discuss this fascinating new information and interested readers should consult the original papers (Cullheim and Kellerth 1978a, b, c; Cullheim et al. 1977).

II. Electrophysiology

The electrophysiology of cat α-motoneurones has been reviewed many times. For the now classical picture see Eccles (1957, 1964) and for more modern interpretations Jack et al. (1975), Burke and Rudomin (1977) and Rall (1977). Although often considered as a 'model' vertebrate neurone, the motoneurone is, in fact, highly specialized for its functional role in the control of skeletal muscle. In the present context only those matters of special significance for an understanding of the Ia afferent fibre–motoneurone system will be touched upon.

Intracellular microelectrode recording from motoneurones has a history of about 30 years. In the early studies it was assumed that motoneuronal dendrites were, in electrical terms, rather long and this, coupled with an under-estimate of membrane resistivity (R_m), at about 500 Ω cm^2 rather than the presently accepted value of about 2500 Ω cm^2, led to an under-estimate of the dendritic contribution to input conductance measured at the soma. There was a corresponding neglect of the possible importance of synapses on distal dendrites (see Eccles 1964; Rall 1977).

It was pointed out by Rall (1959) that, for an intrasomatic microelectrode recording from a neurone with cell body and dendrites, membrane resistivity (R_m) was related to the ratio of current flow into the dendrites to that across the somatic membrane (the dendritic to soma conductance ratio, ρ) and that

$$R_N = R_m \, 1/(\rho + 1)A_s,$$

where R_N is the input resistance and A_s the area of isopotential 'somatic' membrane. For a class of dendritic trees that could be reduced to an equivalent cylinder (Rall 1962a, b, 1964) the electrotonic dendritic length (of the equivalent cylinder) could be estimated by injecting a short current pulse into the soma.

Electrophysiological studies (Rall et al. 1967; Nelson and Lux 1970; Jack et al. 1971) have shown that the electrotonic dendritic lengths of motoneurones are short, probably less than twice the length constant, λ, of the membrane. These conclusions have been supported by combined morphological and electrophysiological studies (Lux et al. 1970; Barrett and Crill 1974a). The results of Barrett and Crill (though not those of Lux et al.) indicated considerable dendritic tapering throughout the tree and this led them to reject the equivalent cylinder model. Even so they estimated dendritic lengths at between 1.1 and 1.5λ. According to Rall (1977) the deviations of actual motoneuronal morphology from the theoretical

Fig. 14.1. Reconstructions, from sagittal (**A** and **B**) and transverse (**C–F**) sections, of α-motoneurones innervating triceps surae. In **C–F** the surface of the spinal cord is shown as a *thick solid line* and the border of the ventral horn by a *dashed line*. Note the numerous dendrites in the white matter, some reaching to within 100 μm of the surface of the cord. The axons are also indicated by *broken lines*. (From Brown and Fyffe 1981a.)

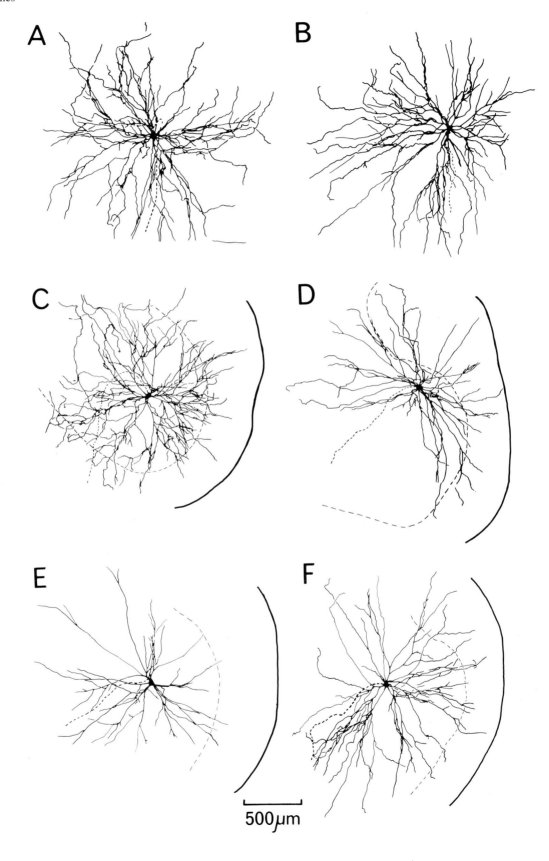

500μm

shape assumed by him do not upset the conclusions drawn from the equivalent cylinder model concerning electrotonic dendritic length. Furthermore, the fact that motoneuronal dendrites are geometrically much longer than previously thought (see above) emphasizes their electrotonic shortness.

Important points that have emerged from recent work, especially the modelling studies of Rall (see Rall 1977) and Redman and his associates (see Jack et al. 1975; Redman 1976) include the following. (1) Even distal dendrites have an important role to play in the integrative activity of motoneurones. (2) The dendritic to soma conductance ratio varies from about 2 to 25, with most values greater than 6 (Barrett and Crill 1974a; Iansek and Redman 1973a). (3) Synapses on distal dendrites may deliver more than one-half of the charge that can be injected by juxtasomatic terminals on the same cell (Iansek and Redman 1973b; Barrett and Crill 1974b) if all excitatory synapses produce the same conductance change. According to Redman (1976) somatic charge is almost independent of synaptic location and if any dependence exists it is such as to allow distal synapses to provide more somatic charge than proximal ones. This is an important point in dispelling the idea that distal dendrites are ineffective. (4) Because most of the motoneuronal dendritic tree is usually incapable of generating action potentials (see Rall 1964; Nelson and Frank 1964a, b) dendrites act as passive cables. When seen from the soma—the usual site for microelectrode penetration and the site of origin of action potentials at and near the initial segment—excitatory post-synaptic potentials generated far out on the dendrites have long rise times and long half-widths (durations) in comparison with those generated close to or on the soma. Therefore distal dendritic actions have more lasting effects on impulse generation in motoneurones than do proximal ones.

In order to test the validity of motoneuronal models and to determine whether synapses on distal dendrites are as effective as suggested it is necessary to have an experimental preparation in which monosynaptic excitatory connexions are made onto motoneurones, preferably with synapses spread rather widely over the dendritic tree. Ia afferent fibres from the primary endings of muscle spindles make such connexions and this system has been used to test the theory. It is also of considerable importance that the system should be studied in its own right as a basic spinal reflex mechanism.

B. Actions of Ia afferent fibres upon motoneurones

An introduction to the monosynaptic reflex was given in Chapter 11. Activity in afferent fibres from the primary endings in muscle spindles leads to the production of a depolarizing potential in motoneurones (the monosynaptic excitatory post-synaptic potential (EPSP) seen in motoneurones innervating the muscle containing the spindle and in its synergists: Coombs et al. 1955). These Ia EPSPs are made up of a hierarchy of smaller components designated by Burke and Rudomin (1977) as follows:

1) *Composite EPSP*, produced by impulses arriving more or less synchronously in two or more afferent fibres. It may be produced by electrical stimulation of muscle nerves (Coombs et al. 1955) or by sudden muscle stretch (Lundberg and Winsbury 1960a).

2) *Single fibre EPSP*, produced by activity in a single Ia afferent fibre (Mendell and Henneman 1971; see also Kuno 1964a).

3) *Single terminal EPSP*, produced by transmitter release from a single Ia terminal (i.e. at a single synapse).

4) *Quantal EPSP*, produced by liberation of a single quantum (package) of transmitter by analogy with quantal release at the neuromuscular junction (see Katz 1969).

It should be realized that this hierarchy is theoretical in part. Only the first two categories have been demonstrated unequivocally.

The composite EPSP was the one available for study to Eccles. Because it decays with a time course longer than that of the single exponential of membrane time constant (Curtis and Eccles 1959) it was thought that there was some sort of delayed transmitter action. It is now known, however, that the delayed decay is due to synaptic actions located on distal dendrites. The initial observations (see Eccles 1964) indicated that composite EPSPs may summate linearly with one another, thus suggesting that the synaptic sites were far enough apart to reduce any interaction to a minimum. But more recent studies (Burke 1967) have shown that some composite EPSPs evoked by activity in muscle nerves supplying synergists may add non-linearly, suggesting that synaptic sites are located close enough to each other (in electrotonic terms) to allow interaction of conductances, and therefore voltage, changes.

Studies of single fibre EPSPs have been of special importance in showing that Ia synapses are distributed on motoneuronal receptive surfaces from proximal to distal sites. Single fibre Ia EPSPs range from those with fast rise times and fast decays (indicative of proximal synaptic locations) to those with slow rise and decay times (indicative of distal locations), as shown for EPSPs in both flexor and extensor motoneurones in Fig. 14.2A. The data are plotted as EPSP half-width (duration at half maximal amplitude) against rise time (shape index of Rall 1967), which demonstrates the positive correlation between the two values and the wide range of shapes. Both of these findings suggest that Ia synapses are found at various spatial locations on motoneurones—provided all Ia synapses produce the same conductance change and provided motoneuronal membranes have the same properties from soma to dendritic distal termination. The histogram of Fig. 14.2B shows the estimated positions of the synapses producing the EPSPs of Fig. 14.2A; most contacts were estimated at between 0.2 and 0.6 length constants, that is about half way along the dendrites. A greater range of locations, 0 to 1.25λ, has been estimated by Iansek and Redman (1973b).

A single Ia afferent fibre can produce EPSPs with quite different shapes in different motoneurones, as shown in Fig. 14.2C. This suggests that a single Ia afferent fibre distributes its input to different motoneurones in different ways and that it does not always have synaptic boutons limited to the same part of the motoneuronal receptive surface.

Single fibre EPSPs, and the interpretation of results from experiments in which they are studied, are not quite as simple as they might appear at first sight. If all single Ia afferent fibres terminated on motoneurones with a single synaptic knob then the situation would be straightforward. But presumed Ia collaterals terminate with a number of boutons on motoneurones (see Conradi 1969; Réthelyi and Szentágothai 1973; Iles 1976) and identified Ia afferent fibres have been

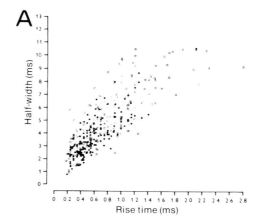

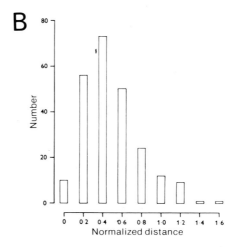

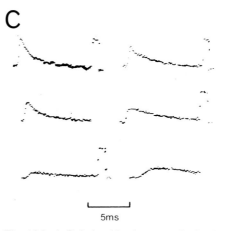

Fig. 14.2. A Relationships between the half-widths of single fibre Ia EPSPs and their rise times. **B** Histogram to show the estimated electronic positions of the synapses producing the EPSPs of **A**. (From Jack et al. 1971.) **C** EPSPs produced by a single Ia fibre in six different motoneurones. (Modified from Mendell and Henneman 1971.)

shown to have more than one bouton in close association with the somata and proximal dendrites of individual motoneurones (Brown and Fyffe 1978a; Ishizuka et al. 1979; Chapter 11). As will be described later in the present chapter, Ia afferent fibres terminate widely on motoneurones, with varying numbers of synaptic boutons in a variety of arrangements.

For convenience it is often assumed (see Jack et al. 1971; Iansek and Redman 1973b) that there is a single locus of action for single fibre EPSPs. Although single Ia fibres often terminate on different parts of a motoneurone's dendritic tree (Burke et al. 1979; Brown and Fyffe 1981a; see below) the assumption of a single *electrotonic* locus may not be far from the actual situation in most instances.

Electrophysiological data show the complexity of single fibre EPSPs. Such potentials elicited in single motoneurones may not add linearly even when their shapes are quite different (Kuno and Miyahara 1969a), suggesting that some of the synaptic sites are situated close together electronically, even though the majority may not be. Furthermore, single fibre EPSPs with slow rise and decay times, indicating distal locations, often have maximal amplitudes greater than expected (Burke 1967; Iansek and Redman 1973b). This suggests that distally located Ia synapses have a greater average membrane area per synaptic bouton or that the number of boutons per Ia fibre increases with distance from the soma. According to Redman (1976) the implication is that there is no spatial weighting attached to different fibres through the location of their synapses on the dendrites.

Electrophysiological examination of electrically evoked single fibre EPSPs (Kuno and Miyahara 1969b; Jack et al. 1971; Iansek and Redman 1973b), stretch-induced presumed single fibre EPSPs (Burke 1967) and the charge content of single fibre EPSPs (Edwards et al. 1976a) has shown that each single fibre Ia EPSP is composed of smaller unitary EPSPs. Between one and 15 unitary EPSPs make up a single fibre EPSP, the usual number being less than five. Early reports (Kuno 1964a, b; Kuno and Miyahara 1969a, b; Mendell and Weiner 1976) suggested that these quantal fluctuations followed Poisson statistics in a way similar to miniature end-plate potentials at the neuromuscular junction. More recent studies have indicated that other models may be more

appropriate (Zucker 1973; Edwards et al. 1976a, b). The anatomical situation at the Ia–motoneurone synapses lends itself to a number of interpretations of these results. At one extreme each component in the single fibre EPSP could reflect the release of a single package of transmitter, as at the neuromuscular junction. Alternatively it could reflect release from single boutons with failure occurring randomly. Another explanation would be action potential failure at branch points on the Ia axon collateral.

Satisfactory explanations of the variation in size of the single fibre EPSP will only be possible when a combined anatomical and electrophysiological analysis of pairs of Ia afferent fibres and motoneurones is undertaken. The rest of this chapter will be concerned with the morphology of the Ia–motoneurone system as revealed by horseradish peroxidase injections. Some of the data will provide answers to questions about this system, such as: Where are the synaptic contacts made? How many contacts are there between a single Ia fibre and a motoneurone? Are the contacts all made at similar distances out on the dendritic tree? Are the contacts limited to a single dendrite and its branches or are they on more than one dendritic system? Do synapses on distal dendrites have larger contact areas? Are there more synaptic boutons per Ia fibre when the contacts are made distally? In any one Ia–motoneurone pair do all synaptic boutons arise from a single terminal axon or from several terminal axons? What are the most reasonable estimates of the total numbers of boutons given by a single Ia fibre to motoneurones? How many Ia boutons does a single motoneurone receive?

C. Ia afferent fibre terminations upon motoneurones

I. Terminations upon motoneuronal somata and proximal dendrites

By combining horseradish peroxidase injection into identified Ia afferent fibres with counterstaining of the spinal cord sections to demonstrate motoneuronal somata and proximal dendrites it is possible to provide quantitative information about Ia contacts on the stained parts of the motoneurones (Ishizuka et al. 1979; Brown and Fyffe 1981a). The results of Ishizuka et al. and Brown and Fyffe are in close agreement, any differences probably being due to the greater lengths of proximal dendrite stained in the study of Ishizuka et al. compared with ours (up to 100 μm and 30 μm respectively).

Figure 14.3 shows micrographs of horseradish peroxidase stained Ia afferent fibres and counterstained motoneurones. Up to six boutons were seen on the soma and proximal 30 μm of dendrite (Fig. 14.3D), although two or three was a more common number. Ishizuka et al. (1979) observed up to ten boutons on a motoneurone in their material, with an average of 3.3. Boutons were of both the *en passant* (Fig. 14.3C) and *terminal* types, and could arise from different branches of the same collateral (Fig. 14.3D). But all boutons on any one motoneurone always arose from a branch or branches of the same collateral (see also Sect. C.II below).

Only a minority of Ia boutons within the confines of lamina IX were in close apposition to motoneuronal somata and proximal dendrites. Of 500 lamina IX boutons, from six collaterals from different Ia axons innervating lateral gastrocnemius/soleus, only 45 were shown in counterstained material to be upon motoneurones. That is, only 9% of the total were on somata and proximal dendrites and the remaining 91% must be assumed to contact more distal dendrites. Ishizuka et al. (1979) have provided similar figures: about 20% for medial gastrocnemius Ia afferent fibres, 10% for soleus, 20% for plantaris, 11% for flexor digitorum hallucis longus and 20% for hamstring muscles. About 10%–15% would seem to be appropriate figures for the proportion of lamina IX Ia boutons that end on motoneuronal somata and the most proximal parts of the dendrites (up to about 30 μm from the soma). Somatic contacts are obviously in a small minority.

In our sample of six Ia afferent fibre collaterals from lateral gastrocnemius, 22 motoneurones received the 45 contacts observed, with an average of 2.05 boutons per cell. In their mixed sample of afferent fibres, Ishizuka et al. (1979) report an average of 3.3 contacts per motoneurone with about 20% of 152 motoneurones receiving only a single contact. Again, the higher values reported by the Japanese workers are presumably due to

examination of longer lengths of dendrites. Finally, with six collaterals contacting 22 motoneurones each collateral terminated upon an average of 3.66 somata or proximal dendrites. As will be shown below (Sect. C.II; see also Chapter 11) each triceps collateral contacts, on average, about 40–50 motoneurones, so that between 70% and 90% of the motoneurones receive dendritic contacts exclusively.

II. Terminations upon dendritic trees

In order to determine the numbers and locations of dendritic terminations of Ia fibres upon motoneurones, we (Brown and Fyffe 1981a) stained both identified Ia afferents and identified α-motoneurones with horseradish peroxidase in the same cat. Ten Ia afferent fibre–motoneurone pairs with contacts between the two were stained. In a preliminary report Burke et al. (1979) have described similar results for three pairs.

There are certain difficulties in the interpretation of double-stained material such as this. When it is examined solely with the light microscope one cannot be sure whether apparent contacts between boutons and dendrites are in fact real contacts; only electron microscopical examination would reveal whether structural synapses were present. Furthermore, it is not necessarily the case that contacts have to involve a pre-synaptic enlargement (bouton) on the axon, since Bodian and Taylor (1963) and Waxman (1975) have shown that synaptic specializations can occur at nodes of Ranvier without any such axonal enlargement. But in the light microscope it is impossible to determine whether an axonal profile without a swelling but running apparently in contact with a dendritic profile represents a possible functional contact. For this reason we limited our identification of possible contact sites to those where an obvious bouton was in apparent contact with a dendrite. We may, therefore, have underestimated the number of contacts. Burke et al. (1979) did include apparent contacts without axonal swellings. On average they observed about one contact per cell more than we did but the two samples are so small that this is insignificant.

Figures 14.4–14.11 illustrate some of the material from eight of our stained pairs. In the reconstructions the motoneurones have not been drawn in full, and only those dendrites receiving contacts are complete. Most of the branches of the Ia

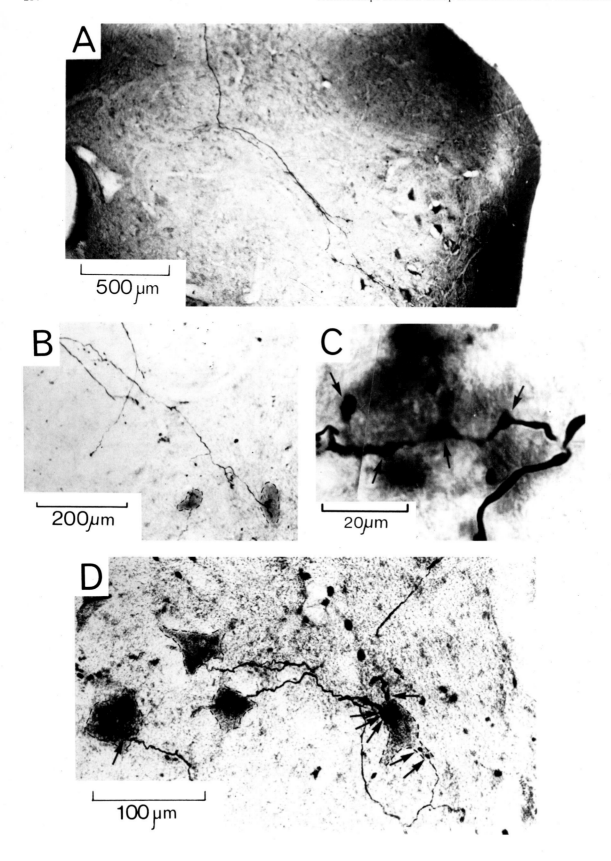

Fig. 14.3. Photomicrographs, from 100-μm transverse sections, of horseradish peroxidase-stained Ia afferent fibre collaterals terminating on counterstained motoneurones. **A** Low-power view showing a collateral running to the motor nuclei. **B–D** Synaptic boutons on motoneuronal somata and proximal dendrites. The *arrows* in **C** and **D** indicate sites of contact. (From Brown and Fyffe 1981a.)

collaterals are shown ventral to lamina VI, except in the drawings at higher magnifications, where only the pre-terminal parts are shown.

In Figs. 14.4–14.6 and Fig. 14.8 it will be seen that only a single Ia collateral is shown. This is because in all ten pairs (and in the three pairs of Burke et al. 1979) although two or three collaterals usually projected through the dendritic tree of the motoneurone contacts were only made by branches of one of them. This observation confirms suggestions made by Mendell and Henneman (1971) and Jack et al. (1971) from electrophysiological data: single fibre EPSPs evoked by Ia afferent usually have a simple time course which implies that all synapses are active almost

synchronously. Restriction of contacts to branches of a single collateral will reduce time dispersion of the input signals. Another possible functional result of this arrangement, suggested by Ishizuka et al. (1979), is that it might help to link inhibitory effects from lamina VI interneurones onto the motoneurones excited by the same Ia fibre that activates these interneurones. Some selective process must occur during development of the connexions between Ia axons and moto-

neurones to produce this striking result (see also Chapter 7). It is not known whether contacts are made from more than one collateral initially with subsequent withdrawal or whether there are always only terminals from a single collateral.

Figure 14.4 shows a reconstruction, from sagittal sections, of a lateral gastrocnemius/soleus Ia–motoneurone pair. The collateral intersected the caudally directed dendrites and four probable contact sites were identified at two widely separated locations on branches of two different primary dendrites. At A (see also Fig. 14.12E) there was a single contact made by a bouton *en passant* at about 765 μm from the soma on a dendrite of the third order. At B there was a series of three boutons *de passage* at about 360 μm from the soma on a second-order dendritic branch.

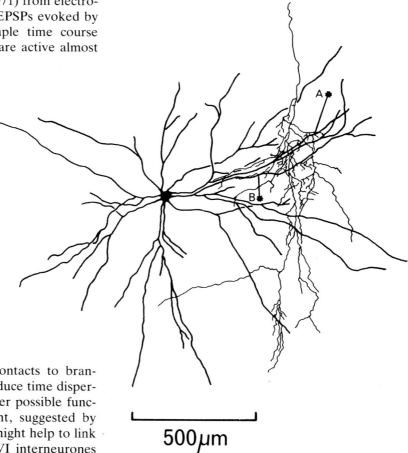

500μm

Fig. 14.4. Reconstructions, from sagittal sections, of a lateral gastrocnemius/soleus Ia–motoneurone pair. Four contact sites are present, one at A and three at B. For further description see the text. (From Brown and Fyffe 1981a.)

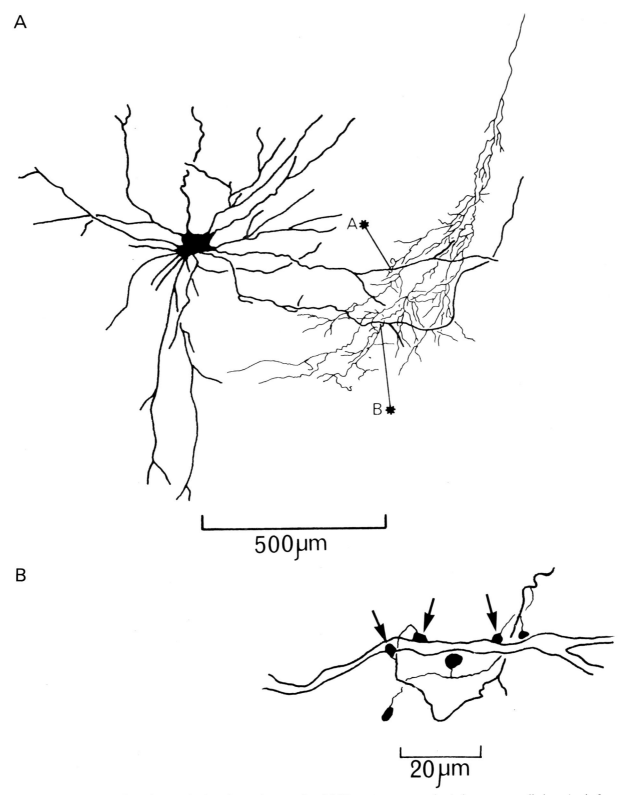

Fig. 14.5. Reconstructions, from sagittal sections, of a posterior tibial Ia-motoneurone pair. **A** shows an overall view. Again four contacts were present, one at A and three at B. **B** shows the contacts made at B in more detail. (From Brown and Fyffe 1981a.)

In Fig. 14.5 a pair with axons in the posterior tibial nerve is shown (see also Fig. 14.12F). Again contacts were at two main locations on branches of two primary dendrites: a single contact (*en passant*) at 500 μm on a second-order dendrite, and at about the same distance a more complex set of terminations involving three boutons on a third-order dendrite (Fig. 14.5B).

The reconstruction in Fig. 14.6 is from transverse sections of the cord and all of the Ia collateral is shown with its more dorsal arborizations as well as those in lamina IX. In this lateral gastrocnemius/soleus pair there were five contacts (Figs. 14.7, 14.12G): three at about 360 μm on a third-order dendrite and two single contacts at 190 and 250 μm on a second- and third-order

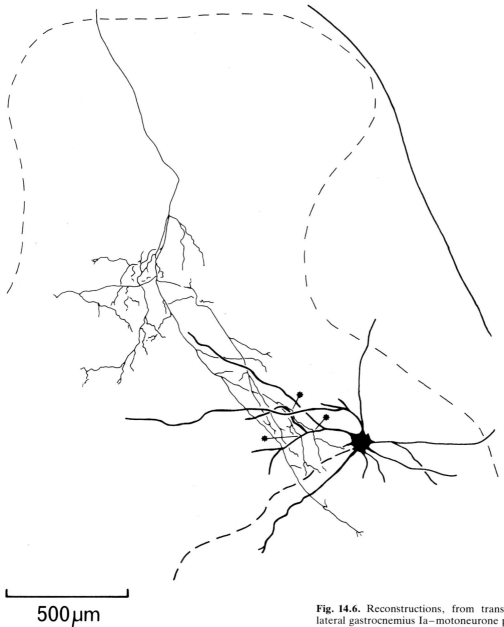

500μm

Fig. 14.6. Reconstructions, from transverse sections, of a lateral gastrocnemius Ia–motoneurone pair. Only part of the dendritic tree is shown but all of the collateral has been drawn. Five contacts were seen (see Fig. 14.7). (From Brown and Fyffe 1981a.)

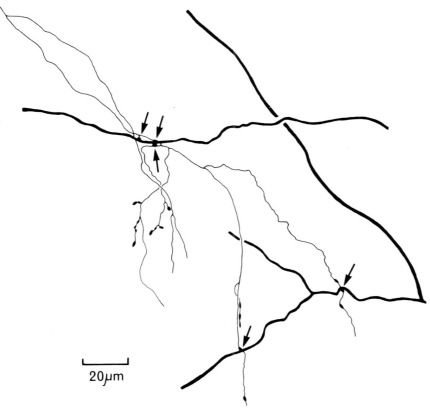

Fig. 14.7. Details of the contacts between the Ia fibre and motoneurone dendrite shown in Fig. 14.6. (From Brown and Fyffe 1981a.)

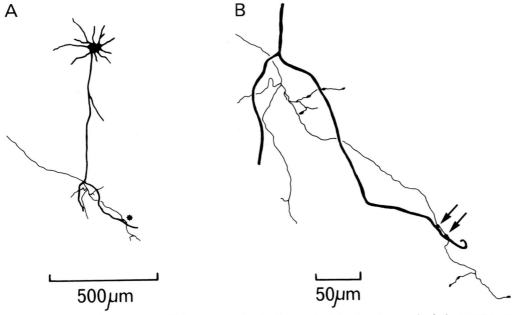

Fig. 14.8. Contacts between a medial gastrocnemius Ia fibre and a lateral gastrocnemius/soleus motoneurone. The contacts, shown in more detail in **B**, are on a ventral dendrite about 820 μm from the soma. (From Brown and Fyffe 1981a.)

branch respectively of another primary dendrite. More examples of distal contacts are shown in Figs. 14.8 and 14.9. In Fig. 14.8 a collateral of a medial gastrocnemius Ia axon intersects a ventral dendrite of a lateral gastrocnemius/soleus motoneurone and two contacts are made at about 820 μm from the soma on a third-order dendrite (see also Fig. 14.12I). Figure 14.9 shows photomicrographs of a single 100 μm thick transverse section of cord illustrating contacts made by a lateral gastrocnemius/soleus Ia collateral on a medial gastrocnemius motoneurone. Three contacts may be seen, all on branches of the same primary dendrite, all of the crossing-over type:

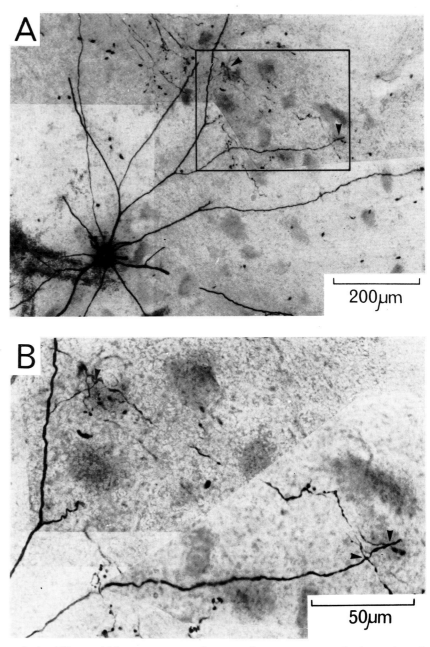

Fig. 14.9. Photomicrographs, from a single 100-μm thick transverse section, to show contacts made by a lateral gastrocnemius/soleus Ia fibre on a medial gastrocnemius motoneurone. **A** is a low-power view and **B** a high-power view. (From Brown and Fyffe 1981a.)

two are at about 620 μm on a third-order dendrite and one at about 520 μm on a fourth-order dendrite. This set of contacts is shown diagrammatically in Fig. 14.12H.

Contacts closer to the motoneuronal soma are shown in Figs. 14.10 and 14.11. Both examples of Fig. 14.10 are from Ia axons and motoneurones of the lateral gastrocnemius/soleus muscles. In Fig. 14.10A two *en passant* contacts are located on a primary dendrite near its bifurcation at about 20 μm and 30 μm from the soma (see also Fig. 14.12D). It is possible that more contacts were made as the axonal branch passed close to the soma but the intensity of staining of the latter precluded differentiation of the axon from the motoneurone. The example of Fig. 14.10B (also Fig. 14.12B) shows four contacts, all within 70 μm of the soma on second- and third-order dendrites. Finally, the photomicrographs of Fig. 14.11 show juxtasomatic contacts between a medial gastrocnemius Ia fibre and a medial gastrocnemius motoneurone (see Fig. 14.12A). Five contacts were observed, all within 40 μm of the soma on three different ventrally directed primary dendrites.

Diagrammatic summaries of the contacts made in the ten pairs of our sample are shown in Fig. 14.12, and similar diagrams from Burke et al. (1979) in Fig. 14.13. In the total of 13 pairs there are many points in common. Forty-seven contacts were identified, giving an average of 3.6 contacts per motoneurone (3.4 in our sample and 4.3 in that of Burke et al.). When all the anatomical information is taken into account, including that on somatic contacts detailed above, it can be concluded that Ia afferent fibres usually make less than five synaptic contacts with their target motoneurones, the average figure probably being between three and four; these values are in remarkably good agreement with suggestions from electrophysiological data (see Sect. B above). With two to four contacts per motoneurone a triceps surae Ia afferent fibre should distribute between about 1000 and 2000 contacts to the 450–500 of the 750 triceps motoneurones it excites monosynaptically (Boyd and Davey 1968; Mendell and Henneman 1971; Iles 1976; Scott and Mendell 1976; Munson and Sypert 1979b). Over the 10 mm or so length of the triceps motor cell column (Romanes 1951; Sprague and Ha 1964) a single Ia axon will give off ten collaterals on average (Brown and Fyffe 1978a; Ishizuka et al. 1979;

Munson and Sypert 1979a) and each should carry some 100–200 boutons for termination upon motoneurones. Ishizuka et al. (1979) report an average of 135 boutons per collateral in lamina IX and our own figures are in agreement with this value. Obviously the observed numbers of Ia boutons agree very closely with the estimated requirements for satisfying the demand, especially when it is realized (see below) that although motoneuronal dendrites may pass into the dorsal horn and out into white matter, all contacts made

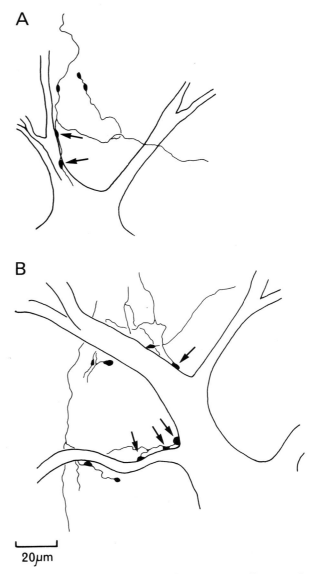

20μm

Fig. 14.10. Proximal contacts between Ia fibres and motoneurones. **A** and **B** are from different lateral gastrocnemius/soleus Ia–motoneurone pairs. (From Brown and Fyffe 1981a.)

by Ia fibres upon the motoneurones are made within or very close to the motor nuclei.

As shown in Figs. 14.12 and 14.13 contacts were made on the somata and dendrites of the motoneurones up to about 800 μm out on dendrites up to the fifth order. Most contacts, however, were within 600 μm of the soma and therefore in the proximal geometrical half of the dendritic tree—as predicted by electrophysiological results (Jack et al. 1971; Iansek and Redman 1973b). Since the Ia synapses are located on the proximal half of the dendritic tree, it may be assumed that the remaining, distal, half (including those dendrites in the white matter) receive inputs from

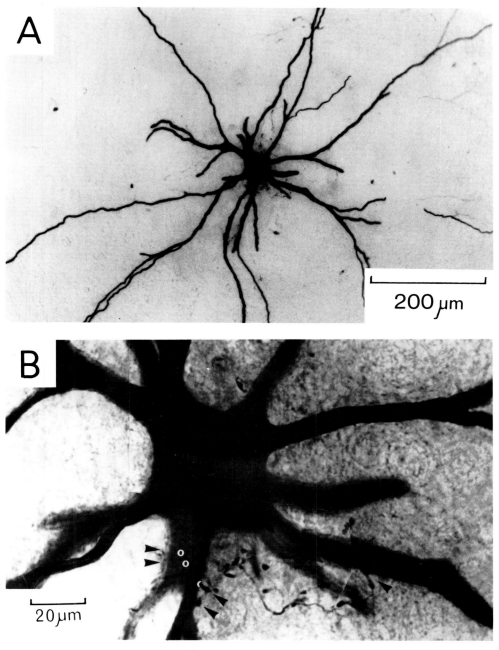

Fig. 14.11. Photomicrographs of contacts made by a medial gastrocnemius Ia fibre on proximal dendrites of a medial gastrocnemius motoneurone. In the high-power view (**B**) the contacts are indicated by *either arrows* or *white circles* and a *semicircle*. (From Brown and Fyffe 1981a.)

other sources. Rose and Richmond (1978) have shown that motoneurones in the cervical cord also send dendrites out into the lateral and ventral funiculi where they make synaptic contacts.

A striking feature of Figs. 14.12 and 14.13 is that with only a few isolated exceptions nearly all Ia synapses upon motoneurones are made at about the same geometrical distance even though they may be on different dendrite systems. This

restriction of synaptic location was suggested from anatomical data by Scheibel and Scheibel (1969) and from electrophysiological evidence by Kuno and Miyahara (1969a, b), Mendell and Henneman (1971) and Jack et al. (1971). When such clustering occurs on one dendritic branch the effect will be as though only a single synapse were involved (an assumption made in electrophysiological analyses), provided all boutons are active

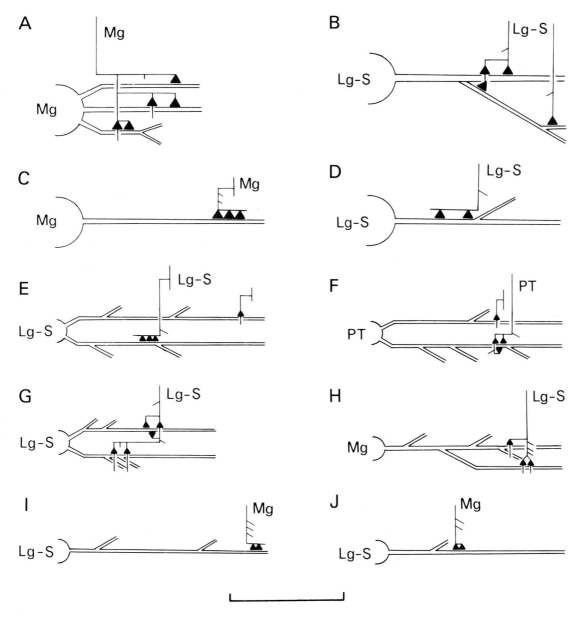

Fig. 14.12. Summary diagram of the locations of Ia synapses on motoneurones. The motoneurones and Ia fibres are identified: Mg, medial gastrocnemius; Lg–S, lateral gastrocnemius/soleus; PT, posterior tibial. The *scale bar* represents 50 μm in **A** and **B** and 500 μm in **C–J**. (From Brown and Fyffe 1981a.)

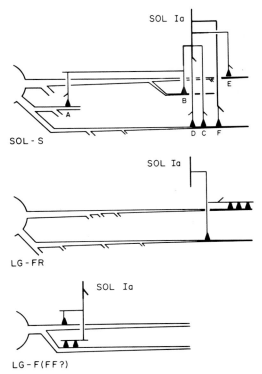

Fig. 14.13. Summary diagram of the locations of soleus Ia (SOL Ia) synapses on motoneurones. SOL-S, slow soleus motoneurone; LG-FR and LG-F(FF?), fast lateral gastrocnemius motoneurones. (From Burke et al. 1979.)

contacts with a mean of 2.8 contacts per motoneurone. Where the position was equivocal (five pairs) the number of contacts ranged from two to five with a mean of 4.4. The sample is very small but the results suggest further study would be worthwhile. Most electrophysiological observations (Kuno and Miyahara 1969a, b; Mendell and Henneman 1971; Jack et al. 1971) have provided no evidence for differences in amplitude, number of component parts (m values), shape index or distribution on the motoneurone between homonymous and heteronymous EPSPs produced by single Ia fibres. Recently, however, Munson and Sypert (1979b) have shown significant differences between single fibre homonymous and heteronymous EPSPs in their rise times but not their amplitudes or half-widths. They conclude that the differences are due to differences in the motoneurones and not in the Ia connectivities. Differences in single fibre EPSP amplitudes have also been reported, homonymous EPSPs being larger than heteronymous ones (Scott and Mendell 1976; Watt et al. 1976).

It has been suggested (Burke 1967; Iansek and Redman 1973b) that, because single fibre EPSPs with slow rise times and slow decay times often have amplitudes greater than expected, distally located synapses have either more contacts compared with proximally located ones or have greater contact area per bouton. In our material there were no obvious correlations between the size and numbers of contacts per motoneurone nor between bouton size and contact location. Where distal contacts were made the boutons were usually larger than the diameter of the dendrite but examination with the electron microscope is required to determine the area of the true contact site.

III. Conclusions

The data presented in this section provide answers to the questions posed at the end of Sect. B.

1) In the Ia–motoneurone system synaptic contacts are made on the motoneuronal somata and on the dendrites up to about 800 μm away from the soma. Most contacts are within 600 μm of the soma. Since motoneuronal dendrites are usually at least 1000 μm long, and can be up to 1600 μm, Ia synapses are therefore located within the proximal geometrical half of the dendritic tree. These anatomical data agree with the estimates that Ia

and failure of transmission at individual boutons does not occur. If failure does occur then the individual components would add non-linearly and could still be assigned a single locus. With distribution of terminals to different dendritic systems, but at similar electrotonic distances from the soma, linear or near-linear summation might be expected between EPSPs as a result of conductance changes in different dendrites. Where synaptic inputs are clearly separated (e.g. Figs. 14.12E, 14.13A) then EPSPs with dissociation of the rise time/half-width relation might be expected, as has been recorded (Rall et al. 1967; Jack et al. 1971; Iansek and Redman 1973b).

In the total of 13 sets of contacts reported so far, there were more contacts between homonymous pairs than heteronymous ones. Thus for three homonymous pairs (two medial gastrocnemius and one soleus) there were 14 contacts (mean 4.7) whereas for five heteronymous pairs (three involving medial gastrocnemius and either lateral gastrocnemius or soleus and two involving lateral gastrocnemius and soleus) there were 14 synapses are located in the proximal *electrotonic* half of the dendritic equivalent cylinder (Jack et al. 1971; Iansek and Redman 1973b).

2) In the studies of Burke et al. (1979), Ishizuka et al. (1979) and Brown and Fyffe (1981a), between one and ten contacts have been identified between single Ia fibres and α-motoneurones. The vast majority of Ia fibres gives less than five boutons to a single motoneurone, the average number being three to four, which again is in excellent agreement with electrophysiological data (Kuno and Miyahara 1969a, b; Burke 1967; Jack et al. 1971; Iansek and Redman 1973b; Edwards et al. 1976a).

3) The synapses made between a single Ia fibre and a motoneurone are usually clustered so that they all occur at about the same distance from the soma. In only two of the 13 sets of contacts analysed so far has there been any marked dispersion of contact sites. Again these data are in agreement with suggestions made from electrophysiological analyses (Kuno and Miyahara 1969a, b; Mendell and Henneman 1971; Jack et al. 1971) and also independent anatomical data (Scheibel and Scheibel 1969).

4) Contacts are not necessarily limited to a single dendritic system of a motoneurone. Often contacts are made on branches of different (up to four) primary dendrites even though they are usually always at about the same distance from the soma. This could account for linear summation of unitary EPSPs with similar shape indices evoked from the same Ia afferent fibre.

5) So far there is no evidence for synapses on distal dendrites having larger contact areas than those more proximally located, nor is there any evidence that when contacts are made distally there are more of them (Burke 1967; Iansek and Redman 1973b).

6) In any Ia–motoneurone pair all contacts identified so far have arisen from a single collateral of the Ia fibre. This, too, agrees with suggestions made from electrophysiological observations (Mendell and Henneman 1971; Jack et al. 1971).

7) At present the most reasonable estimate for the total number of boutons given by a Ia fibre to α-motoneurones (in the cat lumbosacral cord) is of the order of 1000–2000. This figure is derived from an average of about 135 boutons per collateral and about ten collaterals per axon (Brown and Fyffe 1978a; Ishizuka et al. 1979; Munson and Sypert 1979a) and applies mainly to Ia fibres belonging to muscles innervated by a few hundred motoneurones, such as members of the triceps surae group.

8) The probable number of Ia boutons received by a single motoneurone can be assessed from data on (i) the number of spindles in the homonymous and heteronymous muscles, (ii) the number of contacts made, on average, by each Ia afferent fibre, and (iii) the projection ratios for the homonymous and heteronymous pairs. For triceps surae the estimates are as follows. Triceps surae contains about 153 spindles (35 in lateral gastrocnemius, 62 in medial gastrocnemius and 56 in soleus: Chin et al. 1962) and each spindle may be assumed to be innervated by a single Ia fibre; projection ratios may be taken as 90% for homonymous and 60% for heteronymous connexions (Mendell and Henneman 1971; Scott and Mendell 1976; Munson and Sypert 1979b). Using values of two to four for the numbers of contacts made by each Ia afferent fibre upon its target motoneurones, then each triceps motoneurone will receive between 200 and 450 contacts from triceps Ia afferent fibres. Furthermore, with 450–500 triceps motoneurones receiving monosynaptic excitation from triceps Ia fibres (see above), and each fibre having about ten collaterals, each Ia collateral will terminate on 45–50 motoneurones. Only four or five of these motoneurones will receive somatic or proximal dendritic contacts.

Appendix 1   Methods

The decision to include details of the methods used in my laboratory was taken after some hesitation. Scientific methods in the biological sciences are generally very personal things. Furthermore, they are constantly changing even in the hands of a single investigator. The last thing I want to do is present our techniques as though they represent the only way to success. All methods should be adapted to suit both the experimenter and the problem being tackled and all methods should undergo constant assessment. Having stated that, I would also urge anyone who has made a technique work, after arduous learning and developmental stages, to hold on to it and not be easily side-tracked to another approach.

The electrophysiological techniques to be described all depend on satisfactory intracellular recording methods. It cannot be emphasized too strongly that in order to carry out these techniques the animal preparation must be in excellent condition and the part of the central nervous system containing the target neurones must be free from movement. These two aspects have received more consideration in my laboratory over the years than anything else. For in vivo work on mammalian preparations it is essential to monitor arterial blood pressure, end-tidal P_{CO_2} (blood gases or cerebrospinal fluid pH may be preferable) and body temperature as indicators of the state of the preparation. The only interferences that we allow to adjust these parameters are: small (up to 10 ml) injections of dextran solution; injections of glucose-saline; injections of 10 mmol l^{-1} sodium bicarbonate in Normal saline; alteration of the frequency and/or volume of respiration; alteration of the thermostat setting of the electric blanket keeping the preparation warm. No drugs are given to prevent or correct hypotension. In all preparations the bladder is kept empty via an indwelling catheter. The state of the pupils of the eyes is a sensitive indicator of the general condition, especially in paralysed preparations; pupillary dilation indicates some stress. Finally, visual examination (using an operating microscope) of the local blood flow at the surface of the region of interest provides some indication of local conditions.

Maximal mechanical stability must be achieved. We carry out the following procedures routinely: (1) paralysis with positive pressure ventilation; (2) bilateral pneumothoraces (dehydration of the preparation must be guarded against, either by closing the end of the pneumothorax tubes with thin-walled plastic or rubber balloons or by replacing lost water); (3) bladder catheterization to prevent surges in blood pressure due to a full bladder (this procedure also allows renal function to be assessed and helps to monitor the hydration of the preparation); (4) for investigation on the lumbosacral spinal cord the spinal column is stretched between pins on the iliac crests and a clamp on the dorsal processes of the first *and* second lumbar vertebrae.

A. Electrophysiological methods

I. Solutions for intracellular ionophoresis of horseradish peroxidase

The following solution is used routinely: 4–8% horseradish peroxidase (Type VI, Sigma Chemical Co., London) in 0.1 mol l^{-1} Tris/HCl buffer (pH 8.6) containing 0.2 mol l^{-1} KCl (see Snow et al. 1976). The lower enzyme concentrations are preferable for staining neurones where intracellular recordings can be maintained for 30 min or more. The higher concentrations, which predispose to electrode blocking, are more suitable for smaller neurones and axons.

II. Microelectrodes

1. Electrode blanks

Glass microelectrodes are pulled from 1.5–2.0 mm (o.d.) glass tubing containing a single glass capillary filament. The capillary filaments may be inserted and glued in place a few days prior to use or suitable filament-containing tubing may be purchased commercially. The geometry of the shank and taper of microelectrodes suitable for particular purposes varies and must be established by trial and error.

2. Filling the electrode

The use of filament-containing microelectrodes greatly facilitates filling; they can be filled just prior to use by inserting the tip into either Tris/HCl solution or the horseradish peroxidase solution. This fills the tip by capillarity. The remainder of the electrode is back-filled; the use of a very fine polyethylene cannula, inserted to below the surface of the solution in the tip, helps prevent air bubbles entering the electrode.

3. Breaking and bevelling

The final tip size of the microelectrode is determined by the target neurone. In most cases a compromise has to be reached between a large tip that allows currents of greater than 10 nA to be passed and a small tip that allows satisfactory neuronal membrane penetration.

For large neurones such as α-motoneurones and some cells in the spinal cord dorsal horn the electrodes may simply be broken to a tip resistance of 15–25 MΩ (original resistances range from 80 to 250 MΩ). This is done by touching the electrode tip onto a piece of tissue paper. For small neurones and axons the electrode is bevelled. We now use a Narishige Model EG-5 microgrinder (Narishige Scientific Instrument Laboratory, Japan) in which the grinding surface is 0.06 μm AlO$_2$ particles embedded in a polyurethane varnish coating on a flat glass disc. An advantage of this system is that continuous electrode resistance measurements can be made during bevelling by means of a conventional electrometer and a saline-soaked wick contacting the bevelling surface. Final resistances of 25–60 MΩ indicate tip sizes of the order of 2.0–0.5 μm.

III. Intracellular injection of horseradish peroxidase

1. Intracellular penetration and recording

The standard criteria for 'good' intracellular conditions should be used. Thus a stable membrane potential of at least 40 mV (preferably 60 mV or more) and overshooting action potentials are prerequisites for consistently satisfactory results. Any initial injury discharge should be over in a matter of a few seconds. Figure A.1 shows the quality of typical intrasomatic (A, B) and intra-axonal (C) recordings.

2. Current passing

Conventional recording and ionophoretic techniques are used. A satisfactory electrometer should allow continuous electrode resistance measurements and incorporate an internal bridge balancing current for simultaneous recording and current injection.

Horseradish peroxidase is injected by means of a 450-ms depolarizing rectangular current pulse repeated every 600 ms. Currents of 10–30 nA, usually around 15 nA, are used. Microelectrode resistance is continuously measured at the start of each oscilloscope sweep; blockage of the electrode tip is indicated by an increased resistance and an inability to balance current pulses of more than a few nanoamps. Occasionally a blocked electrode may be cleared by rapidly increasing the amount of capacity compensation applied to it ('ringing'). Examples of recording and current passing are shown in Fig. A.1 and illustrate the reduction in size of action potentials recorded when the applied current and membrane potential are balanced.

Successful enzyme injection usually requires upwards of 40 nA min of current. Experience will indicate the probable requirement; smaller cells require less. Even for the largest cells or axons 200–250 nA min will be sufficient.

At the end of the current-passing period the neurones should still show a membrane potential upon electrode withdrawal. Usually this is up to 40 mV and action potentials are still recordable from the neurone.

Microelectrodes are seldom used for more than one injection. In our experience the probability of electrode block is increased after an injection. The horseradish peroxidase solution can be removed from the electrode and used to fill another one.

It is usually convenient to mark injection sites by inserting a blank microelectrode at some known distance from the site. This greatly helps subsequent handling of the tissue during histological procedures.

3. Criteria for probable success

i) 'Good' intracellular penetration with membrane potential greater than 40 mV and overshooting action potentials.

ii) Microelectrode capable of passing more than 10 nA of current for pulses at least 450 ms in duration.

iii) Current and membrane potential balanced.

iv) No electrode blocking.

v) No injury discharge.

vi) Action potentials generated throughout injection.

vii) Membrane potential of several tens of millivolts after injection period.

viii) Total current passed of at least 40 nA min.

IV. Histological methods

1. Perfusion of the preparation

Solutions used are:

i) 0.9% NaCl containing 100 units heparin per ml.

ii) 0.9% NaCl.

iii) Modified Karnovsky's fixative: 1% paraformaldehyde; 2% glutaraldehyde in 0.05 mol l^{-1} phosphate buffer, pH 7.6.

iv) Ralston's fixative (Ralston 1979): 3.0% paraformaldehyde; 1.0% glutaraldehyde in 0.1 mol l^{-1} phosphate buffer, plus 4% sucrose, pH 7.4.

Method of perfusion is as follows:

Ten to 15 minutes prior to perfusion, 10 000–25 000 units of heparin are injected IV. Perfusion commences with 100–200 ml of warm (37 °C) saline or saline plus heparin at about 100 mm Hg pressure via a cannula in the descending aorta (for lumbosacral cord). The saline is followed by 500–1000 ml warm fixative at similar pressure initially and then a further 500–1000 ml at a slightly reduced pressure. This is followed by a further 500–1000 ml fixative at 4 °C. The appropriate blocks of tissue are excised and stored for 6–10 h in fixative at 4 °C. This method will produce satisfactory tissue for electron microscopy (Fig. A.2).

2. Preparation of sections

For frozen sections the tissue is rinsed in 0.1 mol l^{-1} phosphate buffer, pH 7.6, containing 10–30% sucrose. Frozen sections are cut at 50–100 μm and stored in phosphate buffer. Sections may also be cut on the vibratome after postfixation.

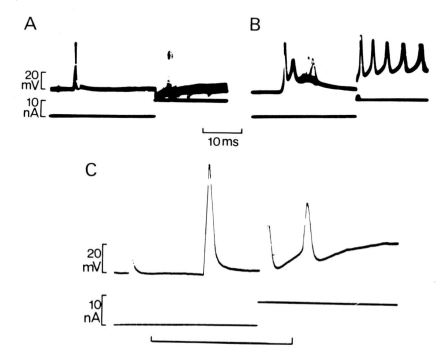

Fig. A.1. Injection of horseradish peroxidase. Each set of records shows the intracellular recording (*upper trace*) and the applied current pulse (*lower trace*). **A** and **B** are from dorsal horn neurones—a post-synaptic dorsal column neurone in **B**. Several sweeps are superimposed. **C** is from a Ia primary afferent fibre and shows a single sweep. Note the action potentials evoked by the onset of the current pulse and the reduction in size of action potentials during the passage of the current pulse.

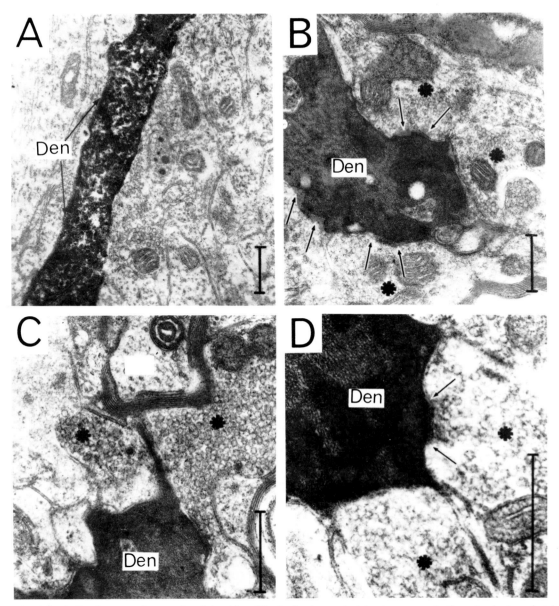

Fig. A.2. A–D, electron micrographs of dendrites (Den) of spinocervical tract neurones in the cat spinal cord stained with an intracellular injection of horseradish peroxidase. The *asterisks* indicate pre-synaptic terminals containing agranular, circular vesicles. Synaptic thickenings are shown between the *arrows*. Ax, an axon with a myelin sheath. (Micrographs prepared by Dr D. J. Maxwell.)

3. Histochemical demonstration of horseradish peroxidase

a) Diaminobenzidine method (see Graybiel and Devor 1974; Snow et al. 1976). Sections are incubated, with gentle agitation, at 25 °C for 20–30 min in the following medium: 0.33% diaminobenzidine tetrahydrochloride; 0.1% H_2O_2 dissolved in 0.05 mol l^{-1} Tris/HCl buffer, pH 7.4. The solution is prepared just before use and the

reaction terminated by transferring the sections into phosphate buffer.

Diaminobenzidine is carcinogenic. Full precautions for handling carcinogenic materials should be carried out during the above procedure. This method is no longer used in my laboratory, partly because of the danger but also because the following method gives better results.

b) Phenylenediamine–paracatechol method (see

Hanker et al. 1977). Sections are incubated for 10 min at 25 °C in: 0.033% *p*-phenylenediamine (PPD); 0.066% *p*-catechol (PC); 0.05% H_2O_2 in 0.1 mol l^{-1} Tris/HCl buffer, pH 7.6. The solution is prepared just before use by dissolving the PPD and PC in the buffer and then adding H_2O_2. The solution is then filtered once or twice. We also take full precautions to avoid contact with or inhalation of PPD and PC.

In both methods processed sections are rinsed in buffer, then distilled water and mounted on gelatin-coated slides. The slides are dried in air and placed in formalin vapour for 12–18 h. They are then dehydrated in an ascending series of alcohols (2 min in 50%; 4 min in 70%; 10 min in 90%; 5 min in absolute alcohol; 10 min in fresh absolute alcohol followed by 5–10 min in two changes of xylene). Sections may be counterstained, e.g. with methyl green.

Appendix 2 Nomenclature

At a very recent symposium on 'Sensory Processing in the Dorsal Horn' (see Brown 1981), held under the auspices of the Somatosensory Commission of the International Union of Physiological Sciences, the following recommendations were made.

A. Anatomy of the spinal grey matter

Rexed's cytoarchitectonic scheme should be used, based on the criteria laid down by Rexed (1952, 1954). The term *superficial dorsal horn* should refer to lamina I and lamina II together and the terms *marginal zone* and *substantia gelatinosa* should refer to lamina I and lamina II respectively. Lamina II may be divided into inner and outer parts (II_i, II_o) as described by Rexed. Deeper parts of the spinal grey matter should be described according to Rexed's cytoarchitectonic scheme for the time being, taking into account differences within and between species.

B. Nomenclature for somatosensory neurones

It was recommended that neurones be described in terms of their afferent input and their location, origin and axonal projection as far as possible.

I. Afferent input

Afferent input should be defined as *excitatory* or *inhibitory*. Neurones should be described accord-ing to their dominant input if this was recognizable as from a particular class of afferent fibres, e.g. *thermoreceptive*, *mechanoreceptive*, *chemoreceptive*, *nocireceptive*, with appropriate subdivisions such as *hair mechanoreceptive*. If input is from two or more of the above categories, neurones should be described as *multireceptive* and if possible further descriptive terms be applied, such as *mechano-noci-multireceptive* etc. This classification is meant to be flexible, to invite more rigorous receptor identification and to avoid ambiguous terms such as Class I, lamina IV type, wide dynamic range, etc.

II. Location of the neuronal soma

The location of the neuronal soma should be stated in terms of Rexed's scheme and whenever possible should be identified by intracellular dye injection. The origin and projection of the axon should be stated whenever possible. Thus, cells might be described as a lamina III spinomedullary (or post-synaptic dorsal column) neurone, a lamina IV spinocervical tract cell, etc. Cells with no recognized axonal projection should still be defined as having their soma in a particular location.

Thus, descriptions of neurones would be as follows: hair mechanoreceptive lamina IV spinocervical tract cell; nocireceptive lamina I spinothalamic tract cell; multireceptive lamina II cell. Obviously, for many purposes appropriate abbreviations will have to be used, but the use of such a system should overcome many of the problems discussed in Chapters 1 and 10.

References

Adams JC (1977) Technical considerations on the use of horseradish peroxidase as a neuronal marker. Neuroscience 2:141–145

Adrian ED (1931) The messages in sensory nerve fibres and their interpretation. Proc R Soc Lond [Biol] 109:1–18

Adrian ED, Umrath K (1929) The impulse discharge from the Pacinian corpuscle. J Physiol (Lond) 68:139–154

Adrian ED, Zotterman Y (1926) The impulses produced by sensory nerve endings. III. Impulses set up by touch and pressure. J Physiol (Lond) 61:465–483

Aitken JT, Bridger JE (1961) Neuron size and neuron population density in the lumbosacral region of the cat's spinal cord. J Anat 95:38–53

Albe-Fessard D, Levante A, Lamour Y (1974a) Origin of spinothalamic tract in monkeys. Brain Res 65:503–509

Albe-Fessard D, Levante A, Lamour Y (1974b) Origin of spinothalamic and spinoreticular pathways in cats and monkeys. In: Bonica JJ (ed) International Symposium on Pain. Adv Neurol 4:157–166. Raven Press, New York

Alnaes E (1967) Static and dynamic properties of Golgi tendon organs in the anterior tibial and soleus muscle of the cat. Acta Physiol Scand 70:176–187

Anden N-E, Jukes MGM, Lundberg A, Vyklicky L (1966) The effect of DOPA on the spinal cord. I. Influences on transmission from primary afferents. Acta Physiol Scand 67:373–386

Andersen P, Eccles JC, Sears TA (1962) Presynaptic inhibitory action of cerebral cortex on spinal cord. Nature 194:740–743

Andersen P, Eccles JC, Sears TA (1964) Cortically evoked depolarization of primary afferent fibres in the spinal cord. J Neurophysiol 27:63–77

Andres KH, Von During M (1973) Morphology of cutaneous receptors. In: Iggo A (ed) Handbook of sensory physiology: vol II, Somatosensory system. Springer, Berlin Heidelberg New York, pp 3–28

Angaut-Petit D (1975a) The dorsal column system. I. Existence of long ascending postsynaptic fibres in the cat's fasciculus gracilis. Exp Brain Res 22:457–470

Angaut-Petit D (1975b) The dorsal column system. II. Functional properties and bulbar relay of the postsynaptic fibres of the cat's fasciculus gracilis. Exp Brain Res 22:471–493

Aoyama M, Hongo T, Kudo N (1973) An uncrossed ascending tract originating from below Clarke's column and conveying group I impulses from the hindlimb muscles in the cat. Brain Res 62:237–241

Applebaum ML, Clifton GL, Coggeshall RE, Coulter JD, Vance WH, Willis WD (1976) Unmyelinated fibres in the sacral 3 and caudal 1 ventral roots of the cat. J Physiol (Lond) 256:557–572

Armett CJ, Gray JAB, Hunsperger RW, Lal S (1962) The transmission of information in primary receptor neurones and second order neurones of a phasic system. J Physiol (Lond) 164:395–421

Armett CJ, Gray JAB, Palmer JF (1961) A group of neurones in the dorsal horn associated with cutaneous mechanoreceptors. J Physiol (Lond) 156:611–622

Armett CJ, Hunsperger RW (1961) Excitation of receptors in the pad of the cat by single and double mechanical pulses. J Physiol (Lond) 158:15–38

Armstrong DM, Eccles JC, Harvey RJ, Matthews PBC (1968) Responses in the dorsal accessory olive of the cat to stimulation of hind limb afferents. J Physiol (Lond) 194:125–145

Armstrong R, Blesovsky L, Corsiglia R, Gordon G (1979) Descending projections from the cat's dorsal column nuclei. J Physiol (Lond) 296:43P

Barilari MG, Kuypers HGJM (1969) Propriospinal fibers interconnecting the spinal enlargements in the cat. Brain Res 14:321–330

Barker D (1974) The morphology of muscle receptors. In: Hunt CC (ed) Handbook of sensory physiology: vol III/2, Muscle receptors. Springer, Berlin Heidelberg New York, pp 1–190

Barnes CD, Pompeiano O (1970a) Presynaptic inhibition of extensor monosynaptic reflex by Ia afferents from flexors. Brain Res 18:380–383

Barnes CD, Pompeiano O (1970b) Inhibition of monosynaptic extensor reflex attributable to presynaptic depolarization of the group Ia afferent fibres produced by vibration of flexor muscle. Arch Ital Biol 108:233–258

Barrett JN, Crill WE (1971) Specific membrane resistivity of dye-injected cat motoneurons. Brain Res 20:556–561

Barrett JN, Crill WE (1974a) Specific membrane properties of cat motoneurones. J Physiol (Lond) 239:301–324

Barrett JN, Crill WE (1974b) Influence of dendritic location and membrane properties on the effectiveness of synapses on cat motoneurones. J Physiol (Lond) 239:325–345

Barrett JN, Graubard K (1970) Fluorescent staining of cat motoneurons in vivo with beveled micropipettes. Brain Res 18:565–568

Basbaum AI, Clanton CH, Fields HL (1976) Opiate and stimulus-produced analgesia: Functional anatomy of a medullospinal pathway. Proc Natl Acad Sci USA 73:4685–4688

Basbaum AI, Clanton CH, Fields HL (1978) Three bulbospinal pathways from the rostral medulla of the cat: An autoradiographic study of pain modulating systems. J Comp Neurol 178:209–224

Basbaum AI, Fields HL (1977) The dorsolateral funiculus of the spinal cord: A major route for descending brainstem control. Neurosci Abs 3:499

Basbaum AI, Wall PD (1976) Chronic changes in the response of cells in adult cat dorsal horn following partial deafferentation: The appearance of responding cells in a previously non-responsive region. Brain Res 116:181–204

Beal JA, Cooper MH (1978) The neurons in the gelatinosal complex (laminae II and III) of the monkey (*Macaca mulatta*): A Golgi study. J Comp Neurol 179:89–122

Beall JE, Martin RF, Applebaum AE, Willis WD (1976)

Inhibition of primate spinothalamic tract neurons by stimulation in the region of the nucleus raphe magnus. Brain Res 114:328–333

Bennett GJ, Hayashi H, Abdelmoumene M, Dubner R (1979) Physiological properties of stalked cells of the substantia gelatinosa intracellularly stained with horseradish peroxidase. Brain Res 164:285–289

Besson JM, Guilbaud G, Le Bars D (1975) Descending inhibitory influences excited by the brain stem upon the activities of dorsal horn lamina V cells induced by intra-arterial injection of bradykinin into the limbs. J Physiol (Lond) 248:725–739

Bessou P, Laporte Y (1960) Activation des fibres afférentes myelinisées de petit calibre d'origine musculaire (fibres du Group III). CR Soc Biol (Paris) 154:1093–1096

Bessou P, Laporte Y (1961) Some observations on receptors of the soleus muscle innervated by Group III afferent fibres. J Physiol (Lond) 155:19P

Bianconi R, Van der Meulen JP (1963) The response to vibration of the end organs of mammalian muscle spindles. J Neurophysiol 26:177–190

Bodian D, Taylor N (1965) Synapse arising at a central node of Ranvier, and a note on fixation in the central nervous system. Science 139:330–332

Boivie JJG, Perl ER (1975) Neural substrates of somatic sensation. In: Hunt CC (ed) MTP international review of science: Physiology, series I, vol 3, Neurophysiology. Butterworth, London; University Park Press, Baltimore, pp 303–411

Boyd IA, Davey MR (1968) Composition of peripheral nerves. Livingstone, Edinburgh London

Boyd IA, Roberts TDM (1953) Proprioceptive discharges from stretch-receptors in the knee-joint of the cat. J Physiol (Lond) 122:38–58

Bradley K, Eccles JC (1953) Analysis of the fast afferent impulses from thigh muscles. J Physiol (Lond) 122:462–473

Brock LG, Coombs JS, Eccles JC (1952) The recording of potentials from motoneurones with an intracellular electrode. J Physiol (Lond) 117:431–460

Brock LG, Eccles JC, Rall W (1951) Experimental investigations on the afferent fibres in muscle nerves. Proc R Soc Lond [Biol] 138:453–475

Brodal A, Angaut P (1967) The termination of spinovestibular fibres in the cat. Brain Res 5:494–500

Brodal A, Taber E, Walberg T (1960) The raphe nuclei of the brain stem in the cat. II. Efferent connections. J Comp Neurol 114:239–260

Brown AG (1968) Cutaneous afferent fibre collaterals in the dorsal columns of the cat. Exp Brain Res 5:293–305

Brown AG (1971) Effects of descending impulses on transmission through the spinocervical tract. J Physiol (Lond) 219:103–125

Brown AG (1973) Ascending and long spinal pathways: Dorsal columns, spinocervical tract and spinothalamic tract. In: Iggo A (ed) Handbook of sensory physiology: vol II, Somatosensory system. Springer Verlag, Berlin Heidelberg New York, pp 315–338

Brown AG (1976) The spinocervical tract: Organization and neuronal morphology. In: Zotterman Y (ed) Sensory functions of the skin in primates, with special reference to man. Pergamon Press, Oxford New York, pp 91–102

Brown AG (ed) (1981) Spinal cord sensation: sensory processing in the dorsal horn. Scottish Academic Press, Edinburgh

Brown AG, Franz DN (1969) Responses of spinocervical tract neurones to natural stimulation of identified cutaneous receptors. Exp Brain Res 7:231–249

Brown AG, Franz DN (1970) Patterns of response in spinocervical tract neurones to different stimuli of long duration. Brain Res 17:156–160

Brown AG, Fyffe REW (1978a) Morphology of Group Ia afferent fibre collaterals in the spinal cord of the cat. J Physiol (Lond) 274:111–127

Brown AG, Fyffe REW (1978b) The morphology of Group Ib muscle afferent fibre collaterals. J Physiol (Lond) 277:44–45P

Brown AG, Fyffe REW (1979) The morphology of Group Ib afferent fibre collaterals in the spinal cord of the cat. J Physiol (Lond) 296:215–228

Brown AG, Fyffe REW (1981a) Direct observations on the contacts made between Ia afferent fibres and α-motoneurones in the cat's lumbosacral spinal cord. J Physiol (Lond) (in press)

Brown AG, Fyffe REW (1981b) Form and function of spinal neurones with axons ascending the dorsal columns in the cat. J Physiol (Lond) (in press)

Brown AG, Gordon G (1977) Subcortical mechanisms concerned in somatic sensation. Br Med Bull 33:121–128

Brown AG, Hayden RE (1971) The distribution of cutaneous receptors in the rabbit's hind limb and differential electrical stimulation of their axons. J Physiol (Lond) 213:495–506

Brown AG, Iggo A (1967) A quantitative study of cutaneous receptors and afferent fibres in the cat and rabbit. J Physiol (Lond) 193:707–733

Brown AG, Martin HF (1973) Activation of descending control of the spinocervical tract by impulses ascending the dorsal column and relaying through the dorsal column nuclei. J Physiol (Lond) 235:535–550

Brown AG, Noble R (1979) Connexions between hair follicle afferent fibres and spinocervical tract neurones in the cat: the synthesis of receptive fields. J Physiol (Lond) 296:38–39P

Brown AG, Noble R (1981) Connexions between hair follicle afferent fibres and spinocervical tract neurones in the cat. (In press)

Brown AG, Short AD (1974) Effects from the somatic sensory cortex on transmission through the spinocervical tract. Brain Res 74:338–341

Brown AG, Kirk EJ, Martin HF (1973) Descending and segmental inhibition of transmission through the spinocervical tract. J Physiol (Lond) 230:689–705

Brown AG, Gordon G, Kay RH (1974) A study of single axons in the cat's medial lemniscus. J Physiol (Lond) 236:225–246

Brown AG, Hamann WC, Martin HF (1975) Effects of activity in non-myelinated afferent fibres on the spinocervical tract. Brain Res 98:243–259

Brown AG, House CR, Rose PK, Snow PJ (1976) The morphology of spinocervical tract neurones in the cat. J Physiol (Lond) 260:719–738

Brown AG, Coulter JD, Rose PK, Short AD, Snow PJ (1977a) Inhibition of spinocervical tract discharges from localized areas of the sensorimotor cortex in the cat. J Physiol (Lond) 264:1–16

Brown AG, Rose PK, Snow PJ (1977b) The morphology of spinocervical tract neurones revealed by intracellular injection of horseradish peroxidase. J Physiol (Lond) 270:747–764

Brown AG, Rose PK, Snow PJ (1977c) The morphology of hair follicle afferent fibre collaterals in the spinal cord of the cat. J Physiol (Lond) 272:779–797

Brown AG, Rose PK, Snow PJ (1978) Morphology and organization of axon collaterals from afferent fibres of slowly adapting Type I units in cat spinal cord. J Physiol (Lond) 277:15–27

Brown AG, Fyffe REW, Heavner JE, Noble R (1979) The morphology of collaterals from axons innervating Pacinian corpuscles. J Physiol (Lond) 292:24–25P

Brown AG, Fyffe REW, Noble R, Rose PK, Snow PJ (1980a) The density, distribution and topographical organization of spinocervical tract neurones in the cat. J Physiol (Lond) 300:409–428

Brown AG, Rose PK, Snow PJ (1980b) Dendritic trees and cutaneous receptive fields of adjacent spinocervical tract neurones in the cat. J Physiol (Lond) 300:429–440

Brown AG, Fyffe REW, Noble R (1980c) Projections from Pacinian corpuscles and rapidly adapting mechanoreceptors of glabrous skin to the cat's spinal cord. J Physiol (Lond) 307:385–400

Brown AG, Fyffe REW Rose PK, Snow PJ (1981) Spinal cord collaterals from axons of Type II slowly adapting units in the cat. (In press)

Brown MC, Engberg I, Matthews PBC (1967) The relative sensitivity to vibration of muscle receptors of the cat. J Physiol (Lond) 192:773–800

Brown PB, Culberson JL (1981) Dorsal horn projections of the cutaneous component of hindlimb dorsal roots. J Neurophysiol (in press)

Brown PB, Fuchs JL (1975) Somatotopic representation of hindlimb skin in cat dorsal horn. J Neurophysiol 38:1–19

Brown PB, Moraff H, Tapper DN (1973) Functional organization of the cat's dorsal horn: Spontaneous activity and central cell responses to single impulses in single Type I fibers. J Neurophysiol 36:827–839

Brown PB, Fuchs JL, Tapper DN (1975) Parametric studies of dorsal horn neurons responding to tactile stimulation. J Neurophysiol 38:19–25

Bryan RN, Trevino KL, Coulter JD, Willis WD (1973) Location and somatotopic organization of the cells of origin of the spino-cervical tract. Exp Brain Res 17:177–189

Burgess PR, Howe JF, Lessler MJ, Whitehorn D (1974) Cutaneous receptors supplied by myelinated fibers in the cat. II. Numbers of mechanoreceptors excited by local stimulus. J Neurophysiol 37:1373–1386

Burgess PR, Petit D, Warren RM (1968) Receptor types in cat hairy skin supplied by myelinated fibers. J Neurophysiol 31:833–848

Burgess PR, Perl ER (1973) Cutaneous mechanoreceptors and nociceptors. In: Iggo A (ed) Handbook of sensory physiology: vol II, Somatosensory system. Springer, Berlin Heidelberg New York, pp 29–78

Burke RE (1967) Composite nature of the monosynaptic excitatory postsynaptic potential. J Neurophysiol 30:1114–1136

Burke RE, Rudomin P (1977) Spinal neurons and synapses. In: Kandel ER (ed) Handbook of physiology: sect 1, vol I, The nervous system: the cellular biology of neurons. American Physiological Society, Washington, pp 877–944

Burke RE, Levine DN, Zajac FE, Tsairis P, Engel WK (1971a) Mammalian motor units: physiological–histochemical correlation in three types in cat gastrocnemius. Science 174:709–712

Burke RE, Lundberg A, Weight F (1971) Spinal border cell origin of the ventral spinocerebellar tract. Exp Brain Res 12:283–294

Burke RE, Levine DN, Zajac FE (1973) Physiological types and histochemical profiles in motor units of the cat gastrocnemius. J Physiol 234:723–748

Burke RE, Levine DN, Salcman M, Tsairis P (1974) Motor unit types in cat soleus muscle: Physiological, histochemical and morphological characteristics. J Physiol 238:503–514

Burke RE, Walmsley B, Hodgson JA (1979) HRP anatomy of group Ia afferent contacts on alpha motoneurons. Brain Res 160:347–352

Burke RE, Walmsley B, Hodgson JA (1980) Structural–functional relations in monosynaptic action on spinal motoneurons. (In press)

Burton H, Loewy AD (1976) Descending projections from the marginal cell layer and other regions of the monkey spinal cord. Brain Res 116:485–491

Burton H, Loewy, AD (1977) Projections to the spinal cord from medullary somatosensory relay nuclei. J Comp Neurol 173:773–792

Busch HFM (1961) An anatomical analysis of the white matter in the brain stem of the cat. van Gorcum, Leiden (Doctoral thesis)

Cangliano A, Lutzemberger L (1972) The action of selectively activated group II muscle afferent fibers on extensor motoneurons. Brain Res 41:475–478

Carpenter D, Lundberg A, Norrsell U (1962) Effects from the pyramidal tract on primary afferents and on spinal reflex actions to primary afferents. Experientia 18:337–338

Carpenter D, Lundberg A, Norrsell U (1963a) Decerebrate control of reflexes to primary afferents. Acta Physiol Scand 59:424–437

Carpenter D, Lundberg A, Norrsell U (1963b) Primary afferent depolarization evoked from the sensorimotor cortex. Acta Physiol Scand 59:126–142

Carstens E, Trevino DL (1978a) Laminar origins of spinothalamic projection in the cat as determined by the retrograde transport of horseradish peroxidase. J Comp Neurol 182:151–166

Carstens E, Trevino DL (1978b) Anatomical and physiological properties of ipsilaterally projecting spinothalamic neurons in the second cervical segment of the cat's spinal cord. J Comp Neurol 182:167–184

Cervero F, Iggo A (1978) Reciprocal sensory interaction in the spinal cord. J Physiol (Lond) 284:84–85P

Cervero F, Iggo A, Ogawa H (1976) Nociceptor-driven dorsal horn neurones in the lumbar spinal cord of the cat. Pain 2:5–24

Cervero F, Iggo A, Molony V (1977) Responses of spinocervical tract neurones to noxious stimulation of the skin. J Physiol (Lond) 267:537–558

Cervero F, Iggo A, Molony V (1979a) Ascending projections of nociceptor-driven lamina I neurones in the cat. Exp Brain Res 35:135–149

Cervero F, Iggo A, Molony V (1979b) An electrophysiological study of neurones in the substantia gelatinosa Rolandi of the cat's spinal cord. Q L Exp Physiol 64:297–314

Chambers MR (1969) The properties of a slowly-adapting mechanoreceptor in the skin of the cat. MSc thesis, University of Edinburgh

Chambers MR, Iggo A (1967) Slowly-adapting cutaneous mechanoreceptors. J Physiol (Lond) 192:26–27

Chambers MR, Andres KH, Von Duering M, Iggo A (1972) The structure and function of the slowly adapting Type II mechanoreceptor in hairy skin. Q J Exp Physiol 57:417–445

Chan-Palay V, Palay SL (1977) Ultrastructural identification of substance P cells and their processes in rat sensory ganglia and their terminals in spinal cord by immunocytochemistry. Proc Natl Acad Sci USA 74:4050–4054

Chin NK, Cope M, Pang M (1962) Number and distribution of spindle capsules in seven hind-limb muscles of the cat. In: Barker D (ed) Symposium on muscle receptors. University Press, Hong Kong, pp 24–28

Christensen BN, Perl ER (1970) Spinal neurons specifically excited by noxious or thermal stimuli: The marginal zone of the dorsal horn. J Neurophysiol 33:293–307

Clarke J (1851) Researches into the structure of the spinal cord Phil Trans R Soc Lond [Biol] 1:607–621

Clarke J (1859) Further researches on the gray substance of the spinal cord. Phil Trans R Soc Lond [Biol] 149:437–467

Clifton GL, Coggeshall RE, Vance WH, Willis WD (1976) Receptive fields of unmyelinated ventral root afferent fibres in the cat. J Physiol (Lond) 256:573–600

Clifton GL, Vance WH, Applebaum KL, Coggeshall RE,

Willis WD (1974) Responses of unmyelinated afferents in the mammalian ventral root. Brain Res 82:163–167

Coggeshall RE, Coulter JD, Willis WD (1973) Unmyelinated fibers in the ventral root. Brain Res 57:229–233

Coggeshall RE, Coulter JD, Willis WD (1974) Unmyelinated axons in the ventral roots of the cat lumbosacral enlargement. J Comp Neurol 153:39–58

Coimbra A, Sodre-Borges BP, Magelhaes MM (1974) The substantia gelatinosa Rolandi of the rat. Fine structure, cytochemistry (acid phosphatase) and changes after dorsal root section. J Neurocytol 3:199–217

Conradi S (1969) On motoneuron synaptology in adult cats. Acta Physiol Scand 78: [Suppl 332] 1–115

Conradi S, Ronnevi L-O (1975) Spontaneous elimination of synapses on cat spinal motoneurones after birth: Do half the synapses on the cell bodies disappear? Brain Res 92:505–510

Cook WA, Neilson DR, Brookhart JM (1965) Primary afferent depolarization and monosynaptic reflex depression following succinylcholine administration. J Neurophysiol 28:290–311

Cook WA, Cangiano A, Pompeiano O (1969a) Dorsal root potentials in the lumbar cord evoked from the vestibular system. Arch Ital Biol 107:275–295

Cook WA, Cangiano A, Pompeiano O (1969b) Vestibular control of transmission in primary afferents to the lumbar spinal cord. Arch Ital Biol 107:296–320

Coombs JS, Curtis DR, Landgren S (1956) Spinal cord potentials generated by impulses in muscle and cutaneous afferent fibres. J Neurophysiol 19:452–467

Coombs JS, Eccles JC, Fatt P (1955) Excitatory synaptic action on motoneurones. J Physiol (Lond) 130:374–395

Cooper S (1961) The responses of the primary and secondary endings of muscle spindles with intact motor innervation during applied stretch. Q J Exp Physiol 46:389–398

Cooper S, Sherrington CS (1940) Gower's tract and spinal border cells. Brain 63:123–134

Coppin CML, Jack JJB, Mcintyre AK (1969) Properties of group I afferent fibres from semitendinosus muscle in the cat. J Physiol (Lond) 203:45–46P

Coulter JD, Foreman RD, Beall JE, Willis WD (1976) Cerebral cortical modulation of primate spinothalamic neurons. In: Bonica JJ, Albe-Fessard D (eds) Advances in pain research and therapy, vol 1. Raven Press, New York, pp 271–277

Coulter JD, Jones EG (1977) Differential distribution of corticospinal projections from individual cytoarchitectonic fields in the monkey. Brain Res 129:335–340

Coulter JD, Maunz RA, Willis WD (1974) Effects of stimulation of sensorimotor cortex on primate spinothalamic neurons. Brain Res 66:351–356

Craig AD (1976) Spinocervical tract cells in cat and dog, labelled by the retrograde transport of horseradish peroxidase. Neurosci Lett 3:173–177

Craig AD (1978) Spinal and medullary input to the lateral cervical nucleus. J Comp Neurol 18:729–744

Crowe A, Matthews PBC (1964) Further studies of static and dynamic fusimotor fibres. J Physiol (Lond) 174:132–151

Cullheim S, Kellerth J-O (1976) Combined light and electron microscope tracing of neurons including axons and synaptic terminals, after intracellular injection of horseradish peroxidase. Neurosci Lett 2:307–313

Cullheim S, Kellerth J-O (1978a) A morphological study of the axons and recurrent axon collaterals of cat sciatic α-motoneurons after intracellular staining with horseradish peroxidase. J Comp Neurol 178:537–558

Cullheim S, Kellerth J-O (1978b) A morphological study of the axons and recurrent axon collaterals of cat α-motoneurones supplying different hind-limb muscles. J Physiol (Lond) 281:285–299

Cullheim S, Kellerth J-O (1978c) A morphological study of the axons and recurrent axon collaterals of cat α-motoneurones supplying different functional types of muscle unit. J Physiol (Lond) 281:301–313

Cullheim S, Kellerth J-O, Conradi S (1977) Evidence for direct synaptic interconnections between cat spinal α-motoneurones via the recurrent axon collaterals: A morphological study using intracellular injection of horseradish peroxidase. Brain Res 132:1–10

Curtis DR, Eccles JC (1959) The time courses of excitatory and inhibitory synaptic actions. J Physiol (Lond) 145:529–546

Czarkowska J, Jankowska E, Sybirska E (1976) Axonal projections of spinal interneurones excited by group I afferents in the cat, revealed by intracellular staining with horseradish peroxidase. Brain Res 118:115–118

Dahlström A, Fuxe K (1965) Evidence for the existence of monoamine neurons in the central nervous system. Acta Physiol Scand 64: [Suppl 247] 1–36

Danforth CH (1925) Studies on hair. Arch Dermat Syphilol 11:637–653

Darian-Smith I, Phillips G, Ryan RD (1963) Functional organization in the trigeminal main sensory and rostral spinal nuclei of the cat. J Physiol (Lond) 168:129–146

Dart AM (1971) Cells of the dorsal column nuclei projecting down into the spinal cord. J Physiol (Lond) 219:29–30

Dart AM, Gordon G (1973) Some properties of spinal connections of the cat's dorsal column nuclei which do not involve the dorsal columns. Brain Res 48:61–68

Devor M, Merrill EG, Wall PD (1977) Dorsal horn cells that respond to stimulation of distant dorsal roots. J Physiol (Lond) 270:519–531

Devor M, Wall PD (1978) Reorganization of spinal cord sensory map after peripheral nerve injury. Nature 267:75–76

Dilly PN, Wall PD, Webster KE (1968) Cells of origin of the spinothalamic tract in the cat and rat. Exp Neurol 21:550–562

Dogiel AS (1903) Über die Nervenendapparate in der Haut des Menschen. Z wiss Zool 65:46

Douglas AS, Barr KL (1950) The course of the pyramidal tract in rodents. Rev Can Biol 9:118–122

Eccles JC (1953) The neurophysiological basis of mind: the principles of neurophysiology. Clarendon Press, Oxford

Eccles JC (1957) The physiology of nerve cells. Johns Hopkins Press, Baltimore

Eccles JC (1962) Central connexions of muscle afferents. In: Barker D (ed) Symposium on muscle receptors. University Press, Hong Kong, pp 81–101

Eccles JC (1964) The physiology of synapses. Springer, Berlin Heidelberg New York

Eccles JC, Pritchard JJ (1937) The action potential of motoneurones. J Physiol (Lond) 89:43–45P

Eccles JC, Rall W (1951) Repetitive monosynaptic activation of motoneurones. Proc R Soc Lond [Biol] 138:475–498

Eccles JC, Fatt P, Koketsu K (1954b) Cholinergic and inhibitory synapses in a pathway from motor axon collaterals to motoneurones. J Physiol (Lond) 126:524–562

Eccles JC, Fatt P, Landgren S (1954c) The 'direct' inhibitory pathway in the spinal cord. Aust J Sci Res 16:130–134

Eccles JC, Fatt P, Landgren S, Winsbury GJ (1954a) Spinal cord potentials generated by volleys in the large muscle afferents. J Physiol (Lond) 125:590–606

Eccles JC, Fatt P, Landgren S (1956) Central pathway for direct inhibitory action of impulses in largest afferent nerve fibres to muscle. J Neurophysiol 19:75–98

Eccles JC, Eccles RM, Lundberg A (1957a) Synaptic actions on motoneurones in relation to the two components of the group I muscle afferent volley. J Physiol (Lond) 136:527–546

Eccles JC, Eccles RM, Lundberg A (1957b) The convergence of monosynaptic excitatory afferents on to many different species of alpha motoneurones. J Physiol (Lond) 137:22–50

Eccles JC, Eccles RM, Lundberg A (1957c) Synaptic actions on motoneurones caused by impulses in Golgi tendon organ afferents. J Physiol (Lond) 138:227–252

Eccles JC, Eccles RM, Lundberg A (1960) Types of neurone in and around the intermediate nucleus of the lumbosacral cord. J Physiol (Lond) 154:89–114

Eccles JC, Eccles RM, Magni F (1961a) Central inhibitory action attributable to presynaptic depolarization produced by muscle afferent volleys. J Physiol (Lond) 159:147–166

Eccles JC, Hubbard JI, Oscarsson O (1961b) Intracellular recording from cells of the ventral spino-cerebellar tract. J Physiol (Lond) 158:486–516

Eccles JC, Kozak W, Magni F (1961c) Dorsal root reflexes of muscle Group I afferent fibres. J Physiol (Lond) 159:128–146

Eccles JC, Oscarsson O, Willis WD (1961d) Synaptic action of Group I and II afferent fibres of muscle on the cells of the dorsal spino-cerebellar tract. J Physiol (Lond) 158:517–543

Eccles JC, Magni F, Willis WD (1962) Depolarization of central terminals of Group I afferent fibres from muscle. J Physiol (Lond) 160:62–93

Eccles JC, Schmidt RF, Willis WD (1963) The location and mode of action of the presynaptic inhibitory pathways on the Group I afferent fibers from muscle. J Neurophysiol 26:506–522

Eccles RM (1965) Interneurons activated by higher threshold group I muscle afferents. In: Curtis DR, McIntyre AK (eds) Studies in physiology, Springer, Berlin Heidelberg New York, pp 59–64

Eccles RM, Lundberg A (1958a) Integrative patterns of Ia synaptic actions in motoneurones in hip and knee muscles. J Physiol (Lond) 144:271–298

Eccles RM, Lundberg A (1958b) The synaptic linkage of 'direct' inhibition. Acta Physiol Scand 43:204–215

Eccles RM, Lundberg A (1959a) Supraspinal control of interneurones mediating spinal reflexes. J Physiol (Lond) 147:565–584

Eccles RM, Lundberg A (1959b) Synaptic actions in motoneurones by afferents which may evoke the flexion reflex. Arch Ital Biol 97:199–221

Edinger L (1889) Vergleichend-entwicklungsgeschichtliche und anatomische Studien im Bereiche des Zentralnervensystems. II. Über die Fortsetzung der hinteren Rückenmarkswurzeln zum Gehirn. Anat Anz 4:121–128

Edward FR, Redman SJ, Walmsley B (1976a) Non-quantal fluctuations and transmission failures in charge transfer at Ia synapses on spinal motoneurones. J Physiol (Lond) 259:689–704

Edwards FR, Redman SJ, Walmsley B (1976b) The effect of polarizing currents on unitary Ia excitatory post-synaptic potentials evoked in spinal motoneurones. J Physiol (Lond) 259:705–723

Egger DM, Wall PD (1971) The plantar cushion reflex circuit: An oligosynaptic cutaneous reflex. J Physiol (Lond) 216:483–501

Eldred E, Granit R, Merton PA (1953) Supraspinal control of the muscle spindle and its significance. J Physiol (Lond) 122:498–523

Engberg I, Ryall RW (1966) The inhibitory action of noradrenaline and other monoamines on spinal neurones. J Physiol (Lond) 185:298–322

Engberg I, Lundberg A, Ryall RW (1968a) The effect of reserpine on transmission in the spinal cord. Acta Physiol Scand 72:115–122

Engberg I, Lundberg A, Ryall RW (1968b) Is the tonic decerebrate inhibition of reflex paths mediated by monoaminergic pathways? Acta Physiol Scand 72:123–133

Engberg I, Lundberg A, Ryall RW (1968c) Reticulospinal inhibition of transmission in reflex pathways. J Physiol (Lond) 194:201–223

Engberg I, Lundberg A, Ryall RW (1968d) Reticulospinal inhibition of interneurones. J Physiol (Lond) 194:225–236

Erulkar SD, Nichols CW, Popp MB, Koelle GB (1968) Renshaw elements: Localization and acetylcholinesterase content. J Histochem Cytochem 16:128–135

Erulkar SD, Sprague JM, Whitsel BL, Dogan S, Janetta PJ (1966) Organization of vestibular projection to the spinal cord of the cat. J Neurophysiol 29:626–664

Fedina L, Gordon G, Lundberg A (1968) The source and mechanisms of inhibition in the lateral cervical nucleus of the cat. Brain Res 11:694–696

Fetz EE (1968) Pyramidal tract effects on interneurons in the cat lumbar dorsal horn. J Neurophysiol 31:69–80

Fields HL, Basbaum AI, Clanton CH, Anderson, SD (1977) Nucleus raphe magnus inhibition of spinal cord dorsal horn neurons. Brain Res 126:441–453

Fitzgerald OJ (1940) Discharges from the sensory organ of the cat's vibrissae and the modifications in their activity by ions. J Physiol (Lond) 98:163–178

Frankenhaeuser B (1949) Impulses from a cutaneous receptor with slow adaption and low mechanical threshold. Acta Physiol Scand 18:68–74

Fu TC, Schomburg ED (1974) Electrophysiological investigation of the projection of secondary muscle spindle afferents in the cat spinal cord. Acta Physiol Scand 91:314–329

Fu TC, Santini M, Schomburg ED (1974) Characteristics and distribution of spinal focal synaptic potentials generated by group II muscle afferents. Acta Physiol Scand 91:298–313

Fuller DRG, Gray JAG (1966) The relation between mechanical displacements applied to a cat's pad and the resultant impulse patterns. J Physiol (Lond) 182:465–483

Fyffe REW (1979) The morphology of Group II muscle afferent fibre collaterals. J Physiol (Lond) 296:39–40

Fyffe REW (1981) Spinal cord terminations of afferent fibres from cat hind limb muscles. PhD thesis, University of Edinburgh

Gelfan S, Kao G, Ruchkin DS (1970) The dendritic tree of spinal neurons. J Comp Neurol 139:385–412

Gobel S (1974) Synaptic organization of the substantia gelatinosa glomeruli in the spinal trigeminal nucleus of adult cat. J Neurocytol 3:219–243

Gobel S (1975a) Golgi studies of the substantia gelatinosa neurons in the spinal trigeminal nucleus. J Comp Neurol 162:397–416

Gobel S (1976) Dendroaxonic synapses in the substantia gelatinosa glomeruli of the spinal trigeminal nucleus of the adult cat. J Comp Neurol 167:165-176

Gobel S (1978a) Golgi studies of the neurons in layer I of the dorsal horn of the medulla (Trigeminal Nucleus Caudalis). J Comp Neruol 180:375–393

Gobel S (1978b) Golgi studies of the neurons in layer II of the dorsal horn of the medulla (Trigeminal Nucleus Caudalis). J Comp Neurol 180:395–413

Gobel S, Falls WM, Hockfield S (1977) The division of the dorsal and ventral horn of the mammalian caudal medulla into eight layers using anatomical criteria. In: Anderson DJ, Matthews BM (eds) Pain in the trigeminal region. Elsevier/North Holland Biomedical Press, Amsterdam, pp 443–453

Goglia G, Sklenska A (1969) Ricerche ultrastrutturali sopra i corpuscoli di Ruffini della capsule articolari nel coniglio. Quad Anat Prat 25:14–27

Goode GE (1976) The ultrastructural identification of primary and suprasegmental afferents in the marginal and gelatinous layers of lumbar spinal cord following central and peripheral lesions. Neurosci Abstr 2:975

Gordon G, Grant G (1972) Afferents to the dorsal column nuclei from the dorsolateral funiculus of the spinal cord. Acta Physiol Scand 84:30–31A

Gordon G, Jukes MGM (1964) Dual organization of the exteroceptive components of the cat's gracile nucleus. J Physiol (Lond) 173:263–290

Gordon G, Miller R (1969) Identification of cortical cells projecting to the dorsal column nuclei of the cat. Q J Exp Physiol 54:85–98

Gottschaldt K-M, Iggo A, Young DW (1973) Functional characteristics of mechanoreceptors in sinus hair follicles of the cat. J Physiol (Lond) 235:287–315

Granit R (1950) Reflex self-regulation of muscle contraction and autogenetic inhibition. J Neurophysiol 13:351–372

Granit R, Henatsch HD (1956) Gamma control of dynamic properties of muscle spindles. J Neurophysiol 19:356–366

Grant G, Ygge J (1978) Transganglionic degeneration used for studying the projection of the body segment on the dorsal horn. Neurosci Lett [Suppl] 1:95

Grant G, Arvidsson J, Robertson B, Ygge J (1979) Transganglionic transport of horseradish peroxidase in primary sensory neurons. Neurosci Lett 21:23–28

Gray JAB, Lal S (1965) Effects of mechanical and thermal stimulation of cat's pad on the excitability of dorsal horn neurones. J Physiol (Lond) 179:154–162

Gray JAB, Matthews PBC (1951) A comparison of the adaptation of the Pacinian corpuscle with accommodation of its own axon. J Physiol (Lond) 114:454–464

Graybiel AM, Devor M (1974) A micro-electrophoretic delivery technique for use with horseradish peroxidase. Brain Res 68:167–173

Gregor M, Zimmermann M (1972) Characteristics of spinal neurones responding to cutaneous myelinated and unmyelinated fibres. J Physiol (Lond) 221:555–576

Grillner S (1970) Is the tonic stretch reflex dependent upon Group II excitation? Acta Physiol Scand 78:431–432

Guilbaud G, Oliveras JL, Giesler G, Besson J-M (1977) Effects induced by stimulation of the centralis inferior nucleus of the raphe on dorsal horn interneurons in cat's spinal cord. Brain Res 126:355–360

Ha H, Liu C-N (1968) Cell origin of the ventral spinocerebellar tract. J Comp Neurol 133:185–206

Hagbarth KE, Jerr DIB (1954) Central influences on spinal afferent conduction. J Neurophysiol 17:295–307

Handwerker HO, Iggo A, Zimmermann M (1975) Segmental and supraspinal actions on dorsal horn neurons responding to noxious and non-noxious skin stimuli. Pain 1:147–165,

Hanker JS, Yates PE, Metz CB, Rustioni A (1977) A new, specific, sensitive and non-carcinogenic reagent for the demonstration of horseradish peroxidase. Histochem J 9:789–792

Harrington T, Merzenich MM (1970) Neural coding in the sense of touch: Human sensations of skin indentation compared with the responses of slowly adapting mechanoreceptive afferents innervating the hairy skin of monkeys. Exp Brain Res 10:251–264

Harvey R, Matthews PBC (1961) The response of the de-efferented muscle spindle ending in the cat's soleus to slow extension of the muscle. J Physiol (Lond) 157:370–392

Heath JP (1978) The cutaneous sensory input to the spinocervical tract of the cat and the corticofugal modulation of transmission from the forelimb component. PhD thesis, University of Edinburgh

Hentall I (1977) A novel class of unit in the substantia gelatinosa of the spinal cat. Exp Neurol 57:792–806

Hokfelt T, Kellerth J-O, Nilsson G, Pernow B (1975) Experimental immuno-histochemical studies on the localization and distribution of substance P in cat primary sensory neurons. Brain Res 100:235–252

Holmqvist B, Lundberg A (1959) On the organization of the supraspinal inhibitory control of interneurones of various spinal reflex arcs. Arch Ital Biol 97:340–356

Holmqvist B, Lundberg A (1961) Differential supraspinal control of synaptic actions evoked by volleys in the flexion reflex afferents in alpha motoneurones. Acta Physiol Scand 54:[Suppl 186] 1–51

Holmqvist B, Lundberg A, Oscarsson O (1960) Supraspinal inhibitory control of transmission to three ascending spinal paths influenced by the flexion reflex afferents. Arch Ital Biol 98:60–80

Hongo T, Jankowska E (1967) Effects from the sensorimotor cortex on the spinal cord in cats with transected pyramids. Exp Brain Res 3:117–134

Hongo T, Koike H (1975) Some aspects of synaptic organization in the spinocervical tract cell in the cat. In: Kornhuber HH (ed) The somatosensory system. Thieme, Stuttgart, pp 218–226

Hongo T, Jankowska E, Lundberg A (1966) Convergence of excitatory and inhibitory action on interneurones in the lumbosacral cord. Exp Brain Res 1:338–358

Hongo T, Jankowska E, Lundberg A (1968) Post-synaptic excitation and inhibition from primary afferents in neurones of the spinocervical tract. J Physiol (Lond) 199:569–592

Hongo T, Jankowska E, Lundberg A (1969) The rubrospinal tract. II. Facilitation of interneuronal transmission in reflex paths to motoneurones. Exp Brain Res 7:365–391

Hongo T, Ishizuka N, Mannen H, Sasaki S (1978) Axonal trajectory of single Group Ia and Ib fibres in the cat spinal cord. Neurosci Lett 8:321–328

Horch KW, Tuckett RP, Burgess PR (1977) A key to the classification of cutaneous mechanoreceptors. J Invest Dermatol 69:75–82

Houk J, Henneman E (1967) Responses of Golgi tendon organs to active contractions of the soleus muscle of the cat. J Neurophysiol 30:1482–1493

Hubbard JI, Oscarsson O (1962) Localization of the cell bodies of the ventral spinocerebellar tract in lumbar segments of the cat. J Comp Neurol 118:199–204

Hubbard SJ (1958) A study of rapid mechanical events in a mechanoreceptor. J Physiol (Lond) 141:198–218

Hultborn H, Jankowska E, Lindström S (1971a) Recurrent inhibition from motor axon collaterals of transmission in the Ia inhibitory pathway to motoneurones. J Physiol (Lond) 215:591–612

Hultborn H, Jankowska E, Lindström S (1971b) Recurrent inhibition of interneurones monosynaptically activated from Group Ia afferents. J Physiol (Lond) 215:613–636

Hultbor H, Jankowska E, Lindström S (1971c) Relative contribution from different nerves to recurrent depression of Ia IPSP's in motoneurones. J Physiol (Lond) 215:637–664

Hunt CC (1952) The effect of stretch receptors from muscle on the discharge of motoneurones. J Physiol (Lond) 117:359–379

Hunt CC (1954) Relation of function to diameter in afferent fibres of muscle nerves. J Gen Physiol 38:111–131

Hunt CC (1961) On the nature of vibration receptors in the hind limb of the cat. J Physiol (Lond) 155:175–186

Hunt CC (1974) The physiology of muscle receptors. In: Hunt CC (ed) Handbook of sensory physiology, vol III/2, Muscle receptors. Springer, Berlin Heidelberg New York, pp 191–234

Hunt CC, Kuffler SW (1951) Stretch receptor discharges during muscle contraction. J Physiol (Lond) 113:298–315

Hunt CC, McIntyre AK (1960a) Characteristics of responses from receptors from the flexor longus digitorum muscle and adjoining interosseous region of the cat. J Physiol (Lond) 153:74–87

Hunt CC, McIntyre AK (1960b) Properties of cutaneous touch receptors in cat. J Physiol (Lond) 53:88–98

Hunt CC, McIntyre AK (1960c) An analysis of fibre diameter and receptor characteristics of myelinated cutaneous afferent fibres in cat. J Physiol (Lond) 153:99–112

Hunt CC, Ottoson D (1973) Receptor potentials and impulse activity in isolated mammalian spindles. J Physiol (Lond) 230:49–50P

Hursh JB (1939) Conduction velocity and diameter of nerve fibers. Am J Physiol 127:131–139

Hyvärinen J, Poranen A (1978) Receptive field integration and submodality convergence in the hand area of the postcentral gyrus of the alert monkey. J Physiol (Lond) 283:539–556

Iansek R, Redman SJ (1973a) An analysis of the cable properties of spinal motoneurones using a brief intracellular current pulse. J Physiol (Lond) 234:613–636

Iansek R, Redman SJ (1973b) The amplitude, time course and charge of unitary excitatory post-synaptic potentials evoked in spinal motoneurone dendrites. J Physiol (Lond) 234:665–688

Iggo A (1963a) New specific sensory structures in hairy skin. Acta Neurovegetativa 24:175–180

Iggo A (1963b) An electrophysiological analysis of afferent fibres in primate skin. Acta Neurovegetativa 24:225–240

Iggo A (1966) Cutaneous receptors with a high sensitivity to mechanical displacement. In: de Reuck EVS, Knight J (eds) Ciba foundation symposium on touch, heat and pain. Churchill, London, pp 237–256

Iggo A (1968) Electrophysiological and histological studies of cutaneous mechanoreceptors. In: Kenshalo DR (ed) The skin senses. Thomas, Springfield, pp 84–106

Iggo A (1969) Cutaneous thermoreceptors in primates and sub-primates. J Physiol (Lond) 200:403–430

Iggo A (ed) (1973) Handbook of sensory physiology: vol 2, Somatosensory system. Springer, Berlin Heidelberg New York

Iggo A (1974) Activation of cutaneous nociceptors and their actions on dorsal horn neurons. In: Bonica JJ (ed) International symposium on pain. Raven Press, New York (Advances in neurology, vol 4, pp 1–9)

Iggo A, Muir AR (1969) The structure and function of a slowly adapting touch corpuscle in hairy skin. J Physiol (Lond) 200:763–796

Iggo A, Ogawa H (1977) Correlative physiological and morphological studies of rapidly adapting mechanoreceptors in cat's glabrous skin. J Physiol (Lond) 266:275–296

Iggo A, Ramsey RL (1976) Thermosensory mechanisms in the spinal cord of monkeys. In: Zotterman Y (ed) Sensory functions of the skin in primates, with special reference to man. Pergamon Press, New York Oxford, pp 285–306

Iles JF (1976) Central terminations of muscle afferents on motoneurones in the cat spinal cord. J Physiol (Lond) 262:91–117

Illert M, Lundberg A, Tanaka R (1976) Integration in descending motor pathways controlling the forelimb in the cat. II. Convergence on neurones mediating disynaptic corticomotoneuronal excitation. Exp Brain Res 26:521–540

Illis L (1967) The relative densities of monosynaptic pathways to the cell bodies and dendrites of the cat ventral horn. J Neurol Sci 4:259–270

Imai Y, Kusama T (1969) Distribution of the dorsal root fibers in the cat. An experimental study with the Nauta method. Brain Res 13:338–359

Ishizuka N, Mannen H, Hongo T, Sasaki S (1979) Trajectory of Group Ia afferent fibres stained with horseradish peroxidase in the lumbosacral spinal cord of the cat: Three dimensional reconstructions from serial sections. J Comp Neurol 186:189–212

Jack JJB, MacLennan CR (1971) The lack of an electrical threshold discrimination between group Ia and group Ib fibres in the nerve to the cat peroneus longus muscle. J Physiol (Lond) 212:35–36

Jack JJB, Noble D, Tsien RW (1975) Electric current flow in excitable cells. Clarendon Press, Oxford

Jack JJB, Redman SJ (1971) An electrical description of the motoneurone and its application to the analysis of synaptic potentials. J Physiol (Lond) 215:321–352

Jack JJB, Miller S, Porter R, Redman S (1971) The time course of minimal excitatory post-synaptic potentials evoked in spinal motoneurones by group Ia afferent fibres. J Physiol (Lond) 215:353–380

Jänig W (1971a) The afferent innervation of the central pad of the cat's hind foot. Brain Res 28:203–216

Jänig W (1971b) Morphology of rapidly and slowly adapting mechanoreceptors in the hairless skin of the cat's hind foot. Brain Res 28:217–231

Jänig W, Spilok N (1978) Functional organization of the sympathetic innervation supplying the hairless skin of the hindpaw in chronic spinal cats. Pflügers Arch 377:25–31

Jänig W, Schmidt RF, Zimmermann M (1968a) Single unit responses and the total afferent outflow from the cat's foot pad upon mechanical stimulation. Brain Res 6:100–115

Jänig W, Schmidt RF, Zimmermann M (1968b) Two specific feedback pathways to the central afferent terminals of phasic and tonic mechanoreceptors. Exp Brain Res 6:116–129

Jankowska E, Lindström S (1970) Morphological identification of physiologically defined neurons in the cat spinal cord. Brain Res 20:323–326

Jankowska E, Lindström S (1971) Morphological identification of Renshaw cells. Acta Physiol Scand 81:428–430

Jankowska E, Lindström S (1972) Morphology of interneurones mediating Ia reciprocal inhibition of motoneurones in the spinal cord of the cat. J Physiol (Lond) 226:805–823

Jankowska E, Lindström S (1973) Procion Yellow staining of functionally identified interneurons in the spinal cord of the cat. In: Kator SB, Nicholson C (eds) Intracellular staining in neurobiology. Springer, Berlin Heidelberg New York, pp 199–209

Jankowska E, Roberts WJ (1972a) An electrophysiological demonstration of the axonal projections of single spinal interneurones in the cat. J Physiol (Lond) 222:597–622

Jankowska E, Roberts WJ (1972b) Synaptic actions of single interneurones mediating reciprocal Ia inhibition of motoneurones. J Physiol (Lond) 222:623–642

Jankowska E, Lund S, Lundberg A, Pompeiano O (1968) Inhibitory effects evoked through ventral reticulospinal pathways. Arch Ital Biol 106:124–140

Jankowska E, Rastad J, Westman J (1976) Intracellular application of horseradish peroxidase and its light and electron microscopical appearance in spinocervical tract cells. Brain Res 105:557–562

Jankowska E, Rastad J, Zarzecki P (1979) Segmental and supraspinal input to cells of origin of non-primary fibres in the feline dorsal column. J Physiol (Lond) 290:185–200

Jansen JKS, Rudjord T (1964) On the silent period and Golgi tendon organs of the soleus muscle of the cat. Acta Physiol Scand 62:364–379

Jansen JKS, Rudjord T (1965) Dorsal spinocerebellar tract: Response pattern of nerve fibers to muscle stretch. Science 149:1109–1111

Johansson RS (1978) Tactile sensibility in the human hand: Receptive field characteristics of mechanoreceptive units in the glabrous skin area. J Physiol (Lond) 281:101–123

Kahler O (1882) Faserverlauf in den Hintersträngen des Rückenmarks. Berl Klin Wochenschr: 640–641

Katz B (1969) The release of neuronal transmitter substance. University Press, Liverpool

Kennard MA (1954) The course of ascending fibers in the spinal cord of the cat essential to the recognition of painful stimuli. J Comp Neurol 100: 511–524

Kenton B, Kruger L, Woo M (1971) Two classes of slowly adapting mechanoreceptor fibres in reptile cutaneous nerve. J Physiol (Lond) 212: 21–44

Kerr FWL (1975a) Neuroanatomical substrates of nociception in the spinal cord. Pain 1: 325–356

Kerr FWL (1975b) Pain, a new central inhibitory balance theory. Mayo Clin Proc 50: 685–690

King JL (1910) The corticospinal tract of the rat. Anat Rec 4: 245–252

Kirkwood PA, Sears TA (1974) Monosynaptic excitation of motoneurones from secondary endings of muscle spindles. Nature 252: 242–244

Knibestöl M (1975) Stimulus–response functions of slowly adapting mechanoreceptors in the human glabrous skin area. J Physiol (Lond) 245: 63–80

Knibestöl M, Vallbo AB (1970) Single unit analysis of mechanoreceptor activity from the human glabrous skin. Acta Physiol Scand 80: 178–195

Koll W, Haase J, Schütz R-M, Muhlberg B (1961) Reflexentladungen der tiefspinalen Katze durch afferente Impulse aus Hochschwelligen nociceptiven A-Fasern (Post δ-Fasern) und aus nociceptiven C-Fasern Cutaner Nerven. Pflügers Arch 272: 270–289

Kolmodin GM (1957) Integrative processes in single spinal interneurones with proprioceptive connections. Acta Physiol Scand 40: [Suppl 139] 1–89

Kolmodin GM, Skoglund CR (1960) Analysis of spinal interneurons activated by tactile and nociceptive stimulation. Acta Physiol Scand 50: 337–355

Krause W (1860) Die terminalen Körperchen der einfachen sensiblen Nerven. Hahn'sche Hofbuchhandlung, Hannover

Kuffler SW, Hunt CC, Quilliam JP (1951) Function of medullated small nerve fibres in mammalian ventral roots: Efferent muscle spindle innervation. J Neurophysiol 14: 29–54

Kumazawa T, Perl ER (1978) Excitation of marginal and substantia gelatinosa neurons in the primate spinal cord: Indications of their place in dorsal horn organization. J Comp Neurol 177: 417–434

Kumazawa T, Perl ER, Burgess PR, Whitehorn D (1975) Ascending projections from marginal zone (lamina I) neurons of the spinal dorsal horn. J Comp Neurol 162: 1–11

Kuno M (1964a) Quantal components of excitatory synaptic potentials in spinal motoneurones. J Physiol (Lond) 175: 81–99

Kuno M (1964b) Mechanism of facilitation and depression of the excitatory synaptic potential in spinal motoneurones. J Physiol (Lond) 175: 100–112

Kuno M, Miyahara JT (1969a) Non-linear summation of unit synaptic potentials in spinal motoneurones of the cat. J Physiol (Lond) 201: 465–477

Kuno M, Miyahara JT (1969b) Analysis of synaptic efficacy in spinal motoneurones from 'quantum' aspects. J Physiol 201: 479–493

Kuypers HGJM, Tuerk JD (1964) The distribution of the cortical fibres within the nuclei cuneatus and gracilis in the cat. J Anat 98: 143–162

Lamotte C (1977) Distribution of the tract of Lissauer and the dorsal root fibers in the primate spinal cord. J Comp Neurol 172: 529–562

Laporte Y, Bessou P (1957) Etude des sous-groupes lent et rapide du groupe I (fibres afferentes d'origine musculaire de grand diametre) chez le chat. J Physiol (Paris) 49: 1025–1037

Laporte Y, Lloyd DPC (1952) Nature and significance of the reflex connections established by large afferent fibers of muscular origin. Am J Physiol 169: 609–621

Laporte Y, Lundberg A, Oscarsson O (1956) Functional organization of the dorsal spino-cerebellar tract in the cat. II. Single fibre recording in Fleschig's fasciculus on electrical stimulation of various peripheral nerves. Acta Physiol Scand 36: 188–203

Leontovich TA, Zhukova GP (1963) The specificity of the neuronal structure and topography of the reticular formation in the brain and spinal cord of carnivores. J Comp Neurol 121: 347–379

Light AR, Perl ER (1977a) Differential termination of large-diameter and small-diameter primary afferent fibers in the spinal dorsal gray matter as indicated by labelling with horseradish peroxidase. Neurosci Lett 6: 59–63

Light AR, Perl ER (1977b) Central termination of identified cutaneous afferent units with fine myelinated fibers. Neurosci Abs 3: 486

Light AR, Perl ER (1979a) Reexamination of the dorsal root projection to the spinal dorsal horn including observations on the differential termination of coarse and fine fibers. J Comp Neurol 186: 117–132

Light AR, Perl ER (1979b) Spinal termination of functionally identified primary afferent neurons with slowly conducting myelinated fibers. J Comp Neurol 186: 133–150

Light AR, Trevino DL, Perl ER (1979) Morphological features of functionally defined neurons in the marginal zone and substantia gelatinosa of the spinal dorsal horn. J Comp Neurol 186: 151–172

Lindblom U, Lund L (1966) The discharge from vibration sensitive receptors in the monkey foot. Exp Neurol 15: 401–417

Lindblom U, Tapper DN (1967) Terminal properties of vibrotactile sensor. Exp Neurol 17: 1–15

Lindström S, Takata M (1971) Cited in Oscarsson O (1973) Functional organization of spinocerebellar paths. In: Iggo A (ed) Handbook of sensory physiology: Vol 2, Somatosensory system. Springer, Berlin Heidelberg New York, pp 340–380

Liu CN, Chambers WW (1964) An experimental study of the cortico-spinal system in the monkey (Macacca mulatta). The spinal pathways and preterminal distribution of the degenerating fibres following discrete lesions of the pre- and postcentral gyri and bulbar pyramid. J Comp Neurol 123: 257–284

Lloyd DPC (1943a) Reflex action in relation to pattern and peripheral source of afferent stimulation. J Neurophysiol 6: 111–120

Lloyd DPC (1943b) Neuron patterns controlling transmission of ipsilateral hind limb reflexes in cat. J Neurophysiol 6: 293–315

Lloyd DPC (1946) Integrative pattern of excitation and inhibition in two-neuron reflex arcs. J Neurophysiol 9: 439–444

Lloyd DPC (1952) On reflex actions of muscular origin. Res Publ Assoc Res Nerv Ment Dis 30: 48–67

Loewenstein WR, Mendelson M (1963) Components of receptor adaptation in a Pacinian corpuscle. J Physiol (Lond) 177: 377–397

Lucas ME, Willis WD (1974) Identification of muscle afferents which activate interneurons in the intermediate nucleus. J Neurophysiol 37: 282–293

Lundberg A (1964a) Ascending spinal hindlimb pathways in the cat. In: Eccles JC, Schadé JP (eds) Progress in brain research: vol 12, Physiology of spinal neurons. Elsevier, Amsterdam London New York, pp 135–163

Lundberg A (1964b) Supraspinal control of transmission in

reflex paths motoneurones and primary afferents. In: Eccles JC, Schadé JP (eds) Progress in brain research: vol 12, Physiology of spinal neurons. Elsevier, Amsterdam London New York, pp 197–221

Lundberg A (1971) Function of the ventral spinocerebellar tract: A new hypothesis. Exp Brain Res 12:317–330

Lundberg A, Malmgren K, Schomberg ED (1977) Cutaneous facilitation of transmission in reflex pathways from Ib afferents to motoneurones. J Physiol (Lond) 265:763–780

Lundberg A, Malmgren K, Schomberg ED (1978) Role of joint afferents in motor control exemplified by effects on reflex pathways from Ib afferents. J Physiol (Lond) 284:327–343

Lundberg A, Oscarsson O (1960) Functional organization of the dorsal spino-cerebellar tract in the cat. VII. Identification of units by antidromic activation from the cerebellar cortex with recognition of five functional subdivisions. Acta Physiol Scand 50:356–374

Lundberg A, Oscarsson O (1961) Three ascending spinal pathways in the dorsal part of the lateral funiculus. Acta Physiol Scand 51:1–16

Lundberg A, Weight F (1971) Functional organization of connexions to the ventral spinocerebellar tract. Exp Brain Res 12:295–316

Lundberg A, Winsbury G (1960a) Selective adequate activation of large afferents from muscle spindles and Golgi tendon organs. Acta Physiol Scand 49:155–164

Lundberg A, Winsbury G (1960b) Functional organization of the dorsal spino-cerebellar tract in the cat. VI. Further experiments on excitation from tendon organ and muscle spindle afferents. Acta Physiol Scand 49:165–170

Lux HD, Schubert P, Kreutzberg GW (1970) Direct matching of morphological and electrophysiological data in cat spinal motoneurones. In: Andersen P, Jansen JKKS (eds) Excitatory synaptic mechanisms. Universitetsförlaget, Oslo, pp 189–198

Lynn B (1969) The nature and location of certain phasic mechanoreceptors in the cat's foot. J Physiol (Lond) 201:765–773

Lynn B (1971) The form and distribution of the receptive fields of Pacinian corpuscles found in and around the cat's large foot pad. J Physiol (Lond) 217:755–771

Magoun HW, Rhines R (1946) An inhibitory mechanism in the bulbar reticular formation. J Neurophysiol 9:165–171

Maillard MC, Besson JM, Conseiller C, Aleonard P (1971) Effets provoqués par la stimulation du cortex orbitaire sur les cellules des couches IV et V de la corne dorsale de la moelle chez le chat. CR Acad Sci [D] (Paris) 272:729–732

Malinovsky L (1966) Variability of sensory nerve endings in foot pads of a domestic cat (Felis ocreata L., F. domestica). Acta Anat (Basel) 64:82–106

Mann MD (1971) Axons of dorsal spinocerebellar tract which respond to activity in cutaneous receptors. J Neurophysiol 34:1035–1050

Mann MD, Kasprzak H, Tapper DN (1971) Ascending dorsolateral pathways relaying Type I afferent activity. Brain Res 27:176–178

Mannen H (1975) Reconstruction of axonal trajectory of individual neurons in the spinal cord using Golgi-stained serial sections. J Comp Neurol 159:357–374

Mannen H, Sugiura Y (1976) Construction of neurons of dorsal horn proper using Golgi-stained serial sections. J Comp Neurol 168:303–312

Mark RF (1970) Chemospecific synaptic repression as a possible memory store. Nature 225:178–179

Mark RF (1974a) Selective innervation of muscle. Br Med Bull 30:122–125

Mark RF (1974b) Memory and nerve cell connections. Clarendon Press, Oxford

Martin HF, Manning JW (1972) Responses of A fibers of peripheral nerve to warming of cutaneous fields. Brain Res 43:653–656

Maruhashi J, Mizuguchi K, Tasaki I (1952) Action currents in single afferent fibres elicited by stimulation of the skin of the toad and the cat. J Physiol (Lond) 117:129–151

Matsushita M (1969) Some aspects of the interneuronal connections in cat's spinal gray matter. J Comp Neurol 136:57–80

Matsushita M (1970) The axonal pathways of spinal neurons in the cat. J Comp Neruol 138:391–417

Matthews BHC (1933) Nerve endings in mammalian muscles. J Physiol (Lond) 18:1–53

Matthews PBC (1963) The response of de-efferented muscle spindle receptors to stretching at different velocities. J Physiol (Lond) 168:660–678

Matthews PBC (1969) Evidence that the secondary as well as the primary endings of the muscle spindles may be responsible for the tonic stretch reflex of the decerebrate cat. J Physiol (Lond) 204:365–393

Matthews PBC (1972) Mammalian muscle spindles and their central actions. Arnold, London

McIntyre AK (1974) Central actions of impulse in muscle afferent fibres. In: Hunt CC (ed) Handbook of sensory physiology: vol III/2, Muscle receptors. Springer, Berlin Heidelberg New York, pp 235–288

McIntyre AK, Mark RF (1960) Synaptic linkage between afferent fibres of the cat's hind liimb and ascending fibres in the dorsolateral funiculus. J Physiol (Lond) 153:306–330

McLaughlin BJ (1972a) The fine structure of neurones and synapses in the motor nuclei of the cat spinal cord. J Comp Neurol 144:429–460

McLaughlin BJ (1972b) Dorsal root projections to the motor nuclei in the cat spinal cord. J Comp Neurol 144:461–474

MacLennan CR (1971) Studies on the selective activation of muscle receptor afferents. D Phil thesis, Oxford University

MacLennan CR (1972) The behaviour of receptors of extramuscular and muscular origin with afferent fibres contributing to the group I and the group II of the cat tibialis anterior muscle nerve. J Physiol (Lond) 222:90–91P

Melzack R, Wall PD (1965) Pain mechanisms: A new theory. Science 150:971–979

Mendell LM, Henneman E (1971) Terminals of Ia fibers: Location, density and distribution within a pool of 300 homonymous motoneurons. J Neurophysiol 34:171–187

Mendell LM, Sassoon EM, Wall PD (1978) Properties of synaptic linkage from long ranging afferents onto dorsal horn neurones in normal and deafferented cats. J Physiol (Lond) 285:299–310

Mendell LM, Weiner R ((1976) Analysis of pairs of individual Ia-e.p.s.p.s in single motoneurones. J Physiol (Lond) 255:81–104

Menetrey D, Giesler GJ, Besson JM (1977) An analysis of response properties of spinal cord dorsal horn neurones to non-noxious and noxious stimuli in the spinal rat. Exp Brain Res 27:15–33

Merkel F (1875) Tastzellen und Tastkörperchen bei den Haustieren und beim Menschen. Arch mikrosk Anat EntwMech 11:636–652

Merrill EG, Wall PD (1972) Factors forming the edge of a receptive field: The presence of relatively ineffective afferent terminals. J Physiol (Lond) 226:825–846

Merton PA (1953) Slowly conducting muscle spindle afferents. Acta Physiol Scand 29:87–88

Merzenich MM, Harrington T (1969) The sense of flutter-vibration evoked by stimulation of the hairy skin of primates: Comparison of human sensory capacity with the responses of mechanoreceptive afferents innervating the hairy skin of monkeys. Exp Brain Res 9:236–260

Mitchell D, Hellon RF (1977) Neuronal and behavioural responses in rats during noxious stimulation of the tail. Proc R Soc Lond [Biol] 197:169–194

Molenaar I, Kuypers HGJM (1978) Cells of origin of propriospinal fibers and of fibers ascending to supraspinal levels. A HRP study in cat and rhesus monkey. Brain Res 152:429–450

Morest DK (1967) Experimental study of the projections of the nucleus of the tractus solitarius and the area postrema in the cat. J Comp Neurol 130:277–299

Morin F (1955) A new spinal pathway for cutaneous impulses. Am J Physiol 183:245–252

Mountcastle VB, Talbot WH, Sakata H, Hyvärinen J (1969) Cortical neuronal mechanisms in flutter vibration studied in unanaesthetized monkeys. Neuronal periodicity and frequency discrimination. J Neurophysiol 32:452–484

Munger B, Pubols LM (1972) The sensory neuronal organization of the digital skin of the raccoon. Brain Behav Evol 5:367–393

Munson JB, Sypert GW (1979a) Properties of single central Ia afferent fibres projecting to motoneurones. J Physiol (Lond) 296:315–327

Munson JB, Sypert GW (1979b) Properties of single fibre excitatory post-synaptic potentials in triceps surae motoneurones. J Physiol (Lond) 296:329–342

Münzer E, Wiener H (1910) Experimentelle Beiträge zur Lehre von endogenen Fasersystemen des Rückenmarkes. Monatsschr Psychiatr Neurol 28:1–25

Necker R, Hellon RF (1978) Noxious thermal input from the rat tail: Modulation by descending inhibition influences. Pain 4:231–242

Nelson PG, Frank K (1964a) Extracellular potential fields of single spinal motoneurons. J Neurophysiol 27:913–927

Nelson PG, Frank K (1964b) Orthodromically produced changes in motoneuronal extracellular fields. J Neurophysiol 27:928–941

Nelson PG, Lux HD (1970) Some electrical measurements of motoneuron parameters. Biophys J 10:55–73

Nilsson BY (1969a) Structure and function of the tactile hair receptors on the cat's foreleg. Acta Physiol Scand 77:396–416

Nilsson BY (1969b) Hair discs and Pacinian corpuscles functionally associated with the carpal tactile hairs in the cat. Acta Physiol Scand 77:417–428

Nilsson BY, Skoglund CR (1965) The tactile hairs on the cat's foreleg. Acta Physiol Scand 65:364–369

Nyberg-Hansen R (1965) Sites and mode of termination of reticulo-spinal fibers in the cat. J Comp Neurol 124:71–100

Nyberg-Hansen R, Brodal A (1963) Sites of termination of corticospinal fibers in the cat. An experimental study with silver impregnation methods. J Comp Neurol 120:369–391

Ormea F, Goglia G (1969) Ultrastructural researches on the Krause's nerve endings (cylindrische Endkolben und küglige Endkolben). Ital Gen Rev Dermatol 9:9–30

Oscarsson O (1968) Termination and functional organization of the ventral spino-olivocerebellar path. J Physiol (Lond) 196:453–478

Oscarsson O (1973) Functional organization of spinocerebellar paths. In: Iggo A (ed) Handbook of sensory physiology: vol II, Somatosensory system. Springer, Berlin Heidelberg New York, pp 340–380

Ozeki M, Sato M (1965) Changes in the membrane potential and the membrane conductance associated with a sustained compression of the non-myelinated nerve terminal in Pacinian corpuscles. J Physiol (Lond) 180:186–208

Paintal AS (1960) Functional analysis of group II afferent fibres of mammalian muscles. J Physiol (Lond) 152:250–270

Perl ER (1968) Myelinated afferent fibres innervating primate skin and their responses to noxious stimuli. J Physiol (Lond) 197:593–615

Perl ER, Whitlock DG, Gentry JR (1962) Cutaneous projection to second order neurons of the dorsal column system. J Neurophysiol 25:337–358

Petit D (1971) Données nouvelles sur l'organisation des messages d'origine cutanée, à la périphérie et dans le système des colonnes dorsales. Thèse de Doctorat d'Etat, Paris

Petit D, Burgess PR (1968) Dorsal column projection of receptors in cat hairy skin supplied by myelinated fibers. J Neurophysiol 31:849–855

Petit D, Lackner D, Burgess PR (1969) Mise en évidence de fibres à activité postsynaptique au niveau des colonnes dorsales chez le chat. J Physiol (Paris) 61:372–373

Petras JM (1967) Cortical, rectal and tegmental fiber connections in the spinal cord of the cat. Brain Res 6:275–324

Phillips CG, Porter R (1977) Corticospinal neurones: Their role in movement. Academic Press, London New York San Francisco

Pickel VM, Reis DJ, Leeman SE (1977) Ultrastructural localization of substance P in neurons of rat spinal cord. Brain Res 122:534–540

Pinkus F (1904) Über Hautsinnesorgane neben dem menschlichen Haar (Haarscheiben) udd ihre vergeichend anatomische Bedeutung. Arch mikrosk Anat EntwMech 65:121–179

Poggio GF, Mountcastle VB (1960) A study of the functional contributions of the lemniscal and spinothalamic system to somatic sensibility. Bull Johns Hopkins Hosp 106:266–316

Poggio GF, Mountcastle VB (1963) The functional properties of ventrobasal thalamic neurons studied in unanaesthetized monkeys. J Neurophysiol 26:775–806

Polacek P, Halata Z (1970) Development of simple encapsulated corpuscles in the nasolabial region of the cat. Ultrastructural study. Folia Morphol (Praha) 18:359–368

Pomeranz B, Wall PD, Weber WV (1968) Cord cells responding to fine myelinated afferents from viscera, muscle and skin. J Physiol (Lond) 199:511–532

Pompeiano O, Brodal A (1957) Spino-vestibular fibers in the cat. An experimental study. J Comp Neurol 108:353–381

Price DD, Hayashi H, Dubner R, Ruda MA (1979) Functional relationships between neurons of the marginal and substantia gelatinosa layers of the primate dorsal horn. J Neurophysiol 42:1590–1608

Proshansky E, Egger MD (1977) Dendritic spread of dorsal horn neurons in cats. Exp Brain Res 28:153–166

Proudfit HK, Anderson EG (1974) New long latency bulbospinal evoked potentials blocked by serotonin antagonists. Brain Res 65:542–546

Rall W (1959) Branching dendritic trees and motoneuron membrane resistivity. Exp Neurol 1:491–527

Rall W (1962a) Theory of physiological properties of dendrites. Ann NY Acad Sci 96:1071–1092

Rall W (1962b) Electrophysiology of a dendritic neuron model. Biophys J 2:145–167

Rall W (1964) Theoretical significance of dendritic trees for neuronal input–output relations. In: Reiss R (ed) Neural theory and modeling. University Press, Stamford, pp 73–97

Rall W (1967) Distinguishing theoretical synaptic potentials computed for different soma-dendritic distributions of synaptic input. J Neurophysiol 30:1138–1168

Rall W (1977) Core conductor theory and cable properties of neurons. In: Kandel ER (ed) Handbook of physiology: Sect 1, vol 1, The nervous system: The cellular biology of neurons. American Physiological Society, Washington, pp 39–97

Rall W, Smith TG, Frank K, Burke RE, Nelson PG (1967) Dendritic location of synapses and possible mechanisms for the monosynaptic EPSP in motoneurons. J Neurophysiol 30:1169–1193

Ralston HJ (1965) The organization of the substantia gelatinosa Rolandi in the cat lumbosacral spinal cord. Z Zellforsch mikrosk Anat 67:1–23

Ralston HJ (1968a) The fine structure of neurons in the dorsal horn of the cat spinal cord. J Comp Neurol 132:275–302

Ralston HJ (1968b) Dorsal root projections to dorsal horn neurons in the cat spinal cord. J Comp Neurol 132:303–330

Ralston HJ (1971) Evidence for presynaptic dendrites and a proposal for mechanism of action. Nature 230:585–587

Ralston HJ (1979) The fine structure of laminae I, II and III of the macaque spinal cord. J Comp Neurol 184:619–642

Ralston HJ, Ralston DD (1979) The distribution of dorsal root axons in laminae I, II and III of the macaque spinal cord: A quantitative electron microscope study. J Comp Neurol 184:643–644

Ramon-Moliner E (1962) An attempt at classifying nerve cells on the basis of their dendritic patterns. J Comp Neurol 119:211–227

Ramon-Moliner E, Nauta WJH (1966) The isodendritic core of the brain stem. J Comp Neurol 126:311–336

Ramon Y Cajal S (1909) Histologie du système nerveux de l'homme et des vertébrés, vol 1. Maloine, Paris

Randic M, Yu HH (1978) Effects of 5-hydroxytryptamine and bradykinin in cat dorsal horn neurones activated by noxious stimuli. Brain Res 111:197–203

Ranson SW (1913a) The course within the spinal cord of the non-medullated fibres of the dorsal roots. A study of Lissauer's tract in the cat. J Comp Neurol 23:259–281

Ranson SW (1913b) The fasciculus cerebro-spinalis in the albino rat. Am J Anat 14:411–424

Ranson SW (1914a) The tract of Lissauer and the substantia gelatinosa Rolandi. Am J Anat 16:97–126

Ranson SW (1914b) A note on the degeneration of the fasciculus cerebro-spinalis in the albino rat. J Comp Neurol 24:503–507

Ranson SW, Billingsley PR (1916) The conduction of painful impulses in the spinal nerves. Am J Physiol 40:571–589

Ranson SW, Hess CLV (1915) The conduction within the spinal cord of afferent impulses producing pain and the vasomotor reflexes. Am J Physiol 38:129–152

Redman SJ (1976) A quantitative approach to integrative function of dendrites. In: Porter R (ed) International review of physiology: vol 10, Neurophysiology II. University Park Press, Baltimore, London Tokyo, pp 1–35

Renshaw B (1940) Activity in the simplest spinal reflex pathways. J Neurophysiol 3:373–387

Réthelyi M (1968) The Golgi architecture of Clarke's column. Acta Morphol Acad Sci Hung 16:311–330

Réthelyi M (1970) Ultrastructural synaptology of Clarke's column. Exp Brain Res 11:159–174

Réthelyi M (1976) Central core in the spinal grey matter. Acta Morphol Acad Sci Hung 24:63–70

Réthelyi M (1977) Preterminal and terminal axon arborizations in the substantia gelatinosa of cat's spinal cord. J Comp Neurol 172:511–528

Réthelyi M, Szentágothai J (1969) The large synaptic complexes of the substantia gelatinosa. Exp Brain Res 7:258–274

Réthelyi M, Szentagothai J (1973) Distribution and connections of afferent fibres in the spinal cord. In: Iggo A (ed) Handbook of sensory physiology: vol II, Somatosensory system. Springer, Berlin Heidelberg New York, pp 207–252

Reveley IL (1915) The pyramidal tract of the guinea pig (Cavia aperea). Anat Rec 9:297–305

Rexed B (1952) The cytoarchitectonic organization of the spinal cord in the cat. J Comp Neurol 96:415–495

Rexed B (1954) A cytoarchitectonic atlas of the spinal cord in the cat. J Comp Neurol 100:297–379

Rolando L (1824) Ricerche anatomiche sulla struttura del midollo spinale, p 60. Torino (1824). Cited by Ramon Y Cajal, S (1909), p 409

Romanes GJ (1951) The motor cell columns of the lumbosacral cord of the cat. J Comp Neurol 94:313–364

Rose PK, Richmond FJR (1978) Dendrites in white matter of the upper cervical cord of the adult cat. Neurosci Abs 4:567

Rothmann M (1899) Ueber die secundären Degenerationen nach Ausschaltung des Sacral- und Lendenmarkgrav durch Rückenmarksembolie beim Hunde. Arch Anat Physiol (Leipzig) pp 120–157

Rufini A (1894) Sur un nouvel organe nerveux terminal et sur la présence des corpuscules Golgi-Mazzoni dans le conjonctif sous-cutané de la pulpe des doigts de l'homme. Arch Ital Biol 21:249–265

Rustioni A (1973) Non-primary afferents to the nucleus gracilis from the lumbar cord of the cat. Brain Res 51:81–95

Rustioni A (1974) Non-primary afferents to the cuneate nucleus in the brachial dorsal funiculus of the cat. Brain Res 75:247–259

Rustioni A (1977) Spinal cord neurons projecting to the dorsal column nuclei of rhesus monkey. Science 196:656–658

Rustioni A, Kaufman AB (1977) Identification of cells of origin of non-primary afferents to the dorsal column nuclei of the cat. Exp Brain Res 27:1–14

Rustioni A, Molenaar I (1975) Dorsal column nuclear afferents in the lateral funiculus of the cat: Distribution pattern and absence of sprouting after chronic deafferentation. Exp Brain Res 23:1–12

Sato M (1961) Responses of Pacinian corpuscles to sinusoidal vibration. J Physiol (Lond) 159:391–409

Scheibel ME, Scheibel AB (1966a) Spinal motoneurons, interneurons and Renshaw cells. A Golgi study. Arch Ital Biol 104:328–353

Scheibel ME, Scheibel AB (1966b) Terminal axonal patterns in cat spinal cord. I. The lateral corticospinal tract. Brain Res 2:333–350

Scheibel ME, Scheibel AB (1966b) Terminal axonal patterns in cat spinal cord. II. The dorsal horn. Brain Res 9:32–58

Scheibel ME, Scheibel AB (1969) Terminal patterns in cat spinal cord. III. Primary afferent collaterals. Brain Res 13:417–443

Schmidt RF (1973) Control of the access of afferent activity to somatosensory pathways. In: Iggo A (ed) Handbook of sensory physiology: vol II, Somatosensory system. Springer, Berlin Heidelberg New York, pp 151–206

Scott JG, Mendell LM (1976) Individual EPSPs produced by single triceps surae Ia afferent fibers in homonymous and heteronymous motoneurons. J Neurophysiol 39:679–692

Sherrington CS (1906) The integrative action of the nervous system. Yale University Press, New Haven

Sherrington CS (1909) On plastic tonus and proprioceptive reflexes. Q J Exp Physiol 2:109–156

Simpson S (1914) The pyramidal tract in the red squirrel (Sciurus gudsonius) and chipmunk (Tamius striatus lipteris). J Comp Neurol 24:137–160

Simpson S (1915a) The motor areas and pyramidal tract in the Canadian porcupine (Erethrizon dorsatus Linn.). Q J Exp Physiol 8:79–102

Simpson S (1915b) The pyramidal tract in the striped gopher. Q J Exp Physiol 8:383–390

Skoglund S (1956) Anatomical and physiological studies of knee joint innervation in the cat. Acta Physiol Scand 36: [Suppl 124] 1–101

Smith KR (Jr) (1967) The structure and function of *Haar-scheibe*. J Comp Neurol 13:459–474

Smith KR (Jr) (1970) The ultrastructure of the human *Haar-scheibe* and Merkel cell. J Invest Dermatol 54:150–159

Snow PJ, Rose PK, Brown AG (1976) Tracing axons and axon collaterals of spinal neurons using intracellular injection of horseradish peroxidase. Science 191:312–313

Sprague JM (1958) The distribution of dorsal root fibres on motor cells in the lumbosacral spinal cord of the cat, and the site of excitatory and inhibitory terminals in monosynaptic pathways. Proc R Soc Lond [Biol] 140:534–556

Sprague JM, Ha H (1964) The terminal fields of dorsal root fibers in the lumbosacral spinal cord of the cat, and the dendritic organization of the motor nuclei. In: Eccles JC, Schadé JP (eds) Progress in brain research: vol. 11, Organization of the spinal cord, Elsevier, Amsterdam, London, New York, pp 120–152

Stauffer EK, Watt DGD, Taylor A, Reinking RM, Stuart DG (1976) Analysis of muscle receptor connections by spike-triggered averaging. II. Spindle Group II afferents. J Neurophysiol 39:1393–1402

Sterling P, Kuypers HGJM (1967a) Anatomical organization of the brachial spinal cord of the cat. I. The distribution of dorsal root fibers. Brain Res 4:1–15

Sterling P, Kuypers HGJM (1967b) Anatomical organization of the brachial spinal cord of the cat. II. The motoneuron plexus. Brain Res 4:16–32

Straile WE (1958) Atypical guard hair follicles in the skin of the rabbit. Nature 181:1604–1605

Straile WE (1960) Sensory hair follicles in mammalian skin: The tylotrich follicle. Am J Anat 106:133–147

Straile WE (1961) The morphology of tylotrich follicles in the skin of the rabbit. Am J Anat 109:1–13

Stretton AOW, Kravitz EQ (1968) Neuronal geometry: Determination with a technique of intracellular dye injection. Science 162:132–134

Sugiura Y (1975) Three dimensional analysis of neurons in the substantia gelatinosa Roland. Proc Jap Acad 51:336–341

Sumner AJ (1961) Properties of IA and IB afferent fibres serving stretch receptors of cat's medial gastrocnemius muscle. Proc Univ Otago Medical School 39:3–5

Szentágothai J (1958) The anatomical basis of synaptic transmission of excitation and inhibition in motor neurons. Acta Morphol Acad Sci Hung 8:287–309

Szentágothai J (1964) Neuronal and synaptic arrangement in the substantia gelatinosa Rolandi. J Comp Neurol 122:219–240 (1964.)

Szentágothai J (1967a) Synaptic architecture of the spinal motoneuron pool. In: Widen L (ed) Recent advances in clinical neurophysiology. EEG Clin Neurophysiol, Suppl 25. Elsevier, Amsterdam, pp 4–19

Szentágothai J (1967b) The anatomy of complex integrative units in the nervous system. In: Lissak K (ed) Results in neuroanatomy, neurohistology, neuromorphology and neurophysiology. Academic Publishers, Budapest, pp 9–45

Takahashi T, Otsuka M (1975) Regional distribution of substance P in the spinal cord and nerve roots of the cat and the effects of dorsal root section. Brain Res 87:1–11

Talbot WH, Darian-Smith I, Kornhuber HH, Mountcastle VB (1968) The sense of flutter-vibration: comparison of the human capacity with response patterns of mechanoreceptive afferents from the monkey hand. J Neurophysiol 31:301–334

Tapper DN (1963) The cutaneous slowly-adapting mechanoreceptor of the cat. Physiologist 6:288

Tapper DN (1964) Input–output relationships in a skin tactile sensory unit of the cat. Trans N Y Acad Sci 26:697–701

Tapper DN (1965) Stimulus–response relationships in the cutaneous slowly-adapting mechanoreceptor in hairy skin of the cat. Exp Neurol 13:364–385

Tapper DN, Brown PB Muraff H (1973) Functional organization of the cat's dorsal horn: Connectivity of myelinated fiber systems of hairy skin. J Neurophysiol 36:817–826

Tapper DN, Mann MD, Brown PB, Cogdell B (1975) Cells of origin of the cutaneous subdivision of the dorsal spinocerebellar tract. Brain Res 85:59–63

Taub A (1964) Local, segmental and supraspinal interactions with a dorsolateral spinal cutaneous afferent system. Exp Neurol 10:357:374

Taub A, Bishop PO (1965) The spinocervical tract: Dorsal column linkage, conduction velocity, primary afferent spectrum. Exp Neurol 13:1–21

Terzuolo CA, Llinás R (1966) Distribution of synaptic inputs in the spinal motoneurone and its functional significance. In: Granit R (ed) Muscle afferents and motor control. Almqvist & Wiksell, Stockholm; Wiley, New York London Sydney, pp 373–384

Thomas RC, Wilson VJ (1965) Precise localization of Renshaw cells with a new marking technique. Nature 206:211–213

Trevino DL, (1976) The origin and projection of a spinal nociceptive and thermoreceptive pathway. In Y. Zotterman (ed) Sensory functions of the skin in primates with special reference to man. New York, Pergamon Press, pp 367–376

Trevino DL, Carstens E (1975) Confirmation of the location of spinothalamic neurons in the cat and monkey by the retrograde transport of horseradish peroxidase. Brain Res 98:177–182

Trevino DL, Coulter JD, Maunz RN, Willis WD (1974) Location and functional properties of spinothalamic cells in the monky. In: Bonica JJ (ed) International symposium on pain, Adv Neurol 4:167–170

Trevino DL, Maunz RA, Bryan RN, Willis WD (1972) Location of cells of origin of the spinothalamic tract in the lumbar enlargement of the cat. Exp Neurol 34:64–77

Trevino DL, Coulter JD, Willis WD (1973) Location of cells of origin of spinothalamic tract in lumbar enlargement of the monkey. J Neurophysiol 36:750–761

Uddenberg N (1968a) Differential organization in dorsal funiculi of fibres originating from different receptors. Exp Brain Res 4:367–376

Uddenberg N (1968b) Functional organization of long, second-order afferents in the dorsal funiculi. Exp Brain Res 4:377–382

Van Beusekom GT (1955) Fibre analysis of the anterior and lateral funiculi of the cord in the cat. (Doctoral thesis) E. Ijdo, Leiden

Vierck CJ (1973) Alteration of spatio-tactile discrimination after lesion of primate spinal cord. Brain Res 58:69–79

Voorhoeve PE, Verhey BA (1963) Pre- and postsynaptic effects on fusimotor and alpha motoneurones of the cat upon activation of muscle spindle afferents by succinylcholine. Acta Physiol Pharmacol Neerland 12:12–22

Waldeyer H (1888) Das Gorilla-Rückenmark. Abhandlungen der Preussichen Akademie der Wissenschaft en zu Berlin 3:1–147

Wall PD (1960) Cord cells responding to touch, damage and temperature of skin. J Neurophysiol 23:197–210

Wall PD (1967) The laminar organization of dorsal horn and effects of descending impulses. J Physiol (Lond) 188:403–424

Wall PD (1970) The sensory and motor role of impulses travelling in the dorsal column towards cerebral cortex. Brain 93:505–524

Wall PD (1973) Dorsal horn electrophysiology. In: Iggo A (ed) Handbook of sensory physiology, vol II, Somatosensory system. Springer, Berlin Heidelberg New York, pp 253–270

References

233

Wall Pd (1977) The presence of ineffective synapses and the circumstances which unmask them. Phil Trans R Soc Lond [Biol] 278:361–372

Wall PD, Werman R (1976) The physiology and anatomy of long ranging afferent fibres within the spinal cord. J Physiol (Lond) 255:321–334

Wall PD, Merrill EG, Yaksh TL (1979) Responses of single units in laminae 2 and 3 of cat spinal cord. Brain Res 160:245–260

Watt DGD, Stauffer EK, Taylor A, Reinking RM, Stuart DG (1976) Analysis of muscle receptor connections by spike triggered averaging. I. Spindle primary and tendon organ afferents. J Neurophysiol 39:1375–1392

Waxman SG (1975) Integrative properties and design principles of axons. Int Rev Neurobiol 18:1–39

Werner G, Mountcastle VB (1965) Neural activity in mechanoreceptive cutaneous afferents: Stimulus–response relations, Weber functions, and information transmission. J Neurophysiol 28:359–397

Werner G, Whitsel BL (1967) The topology of dermatomal projection in the medial lemniscal system. J Physiol (Lond) 192:123–144

Werner G, Whitsel BL (1968) Topology of the body representation in somatosensory area I of primates. J Neurophysiol 31:856–869

Westbury DR (1972) A study of stretch and vibration reflexes of the cat by intracellular recording from motoneurones. J Physiol (Lond) 226:37–56

Westbury DR (1979) The morphology of four gamma motoneurones of the cat examined by horseradish peroxidase histochemistry. J Physiol (Lond) 292:25–26P

Whitehorn D, Howe JF, Lessler MJ, Burgess PR (1974) Cutaneous receptors supplied by myelinated fibers in the cat. I. Number of receptors innervated by a single nerve. J Neurophysiol 37:1361–1372

Willis WD, Coggeshall RE (1978) Sensory mechanism of the spinal cord. Plenum Press, New York London

Willis WD, Haber LH, Martin RF (1977) Inhibition of spinothalamic tract cells and interneurons by brain stem stimulation in the monkey. J Neurophysiol 40:968–981

Willis WD, Leonard RB, Kenshalo DR (1978) Spinothalamic tract neurons in the substantia gelatinosa. Science 202:986–988

Willis WD, Trevino DL, Coulter JD, Maunz RN (1974) Responses of primate spinothalamic tract neurons to natural stimulation of hindlimb. J Neurophysiol 37:358–372

Willis WD, Weir MA, Skinner RD, Bryan RN (1973) Differential distribution of spinal cord field potentials. Exp Brain Res 17:169–176

Wilson VJ, Kato M (1965) Excitation of extensor motoneurons by group II afferent fibres in ipsilateral muscle nerves. J Neurophysiol 28:545–554

Winkelmann RK (1958) The sensory endings in the skin of the cat. J Comp Neurol 109:221–232

Witt I, Hensel H (1959) Afferent Impulse aus der Extremitätenhaut der Katze bei thermischer und mechanischer Reizung. Pflügers Arch 268:582–596

Zotterman Y (1939) Touch, pain and tickling: An electrophysiological investigation on cutaneous sensory nerves. J Physiol (Lond) 95:1–28

Zucker RS (1973) Changes in the statistics of transmitter release during facilitation. J Physiol (Lond) 229:787–810

Subject Index

The index should be used in conjunction with the Table of Contents. Entries in *italic* type refer to pages containing Figures but no text reference.

Afferent and Intrinsic Organization of Laminated Structures in the Brain

Editor: O. Creutzfeldt
1976. 127 figures. XXIII, 579 pages
(Experimental Brain Research, Supplementum 1)
ISBN 3-540-07923-8

Biological Order and Brain Organization

Selected Works of W. R. Hess
Editor: K. Akert
Translated from the German by K. Akert, M. Bornstein, V. Bucher, R. M. Hess, S. Hess, P. Levin, G. P. Michel
1981. 1 portrait, 91 figures. XII, 347 pages
ISBN 3-540-10551-4

H. Braak
Architectonics of the Human Telencephalic Cortex

1980. 43 figures, 1 table. X, 147 pages
(Studies of Brain Function, Volume 4)
ISBN 3-540-10312-0

V. Chan-Palay
Cerebellar Dentate Nucleus

Organization, Cytology and Transmitters

1977. 293 figures including 79 plates, some in color. XXI, 548 pages
ISBN 3-540-07958-0

The Cranial Nerves

Anatomy – Pathology – Pathophysiology – Diagnosis – Treatment

Editors: M. Samii, P. J. Jannetta
1981. Approx. 400 figures. Approx. 610 pages
ISBN 3-540-10620-0

Neurosecretion – The Final Neuroendocrine Pathway

6th International Symposium on Neurosecretion, London 1973
Editors: F. Knowles, L. Vollrath
1974. 92 figures. X, 345 pages
ISBN 3-540-06821-X

Neurosecretion and Neuroendocrine Activity. Evolution, Structure and Function

Proceedings of the VII. International Symposium on Neurosecretion, Leningrad, August 15–21, 1976
Editors: W. Bargmann, A. Oksche, A. Polenov, B. Scharrer
1978. 168 figures, 11 tables. XVI, 411 pages
ISBN 3-540-08637-4

The Pineal Gland

Proceedings of the International Symposium, Jerusalem, November 14–17, 1977
Editor: I. Nir, R. J. Reiter, R. J. Wurtman
1978. 79 figures, 39 tables. VIII, 408 pages
(Journal of Neural Transmission, Supplementum 13)
Wien–New York: Springer-Verlag
ISBN 3-211-81489-2

W. Precht
Neural Operations in the Vestibular System

1978. 105 figures, 3 tables. VIII, 226 pages
(Studies of Brain Function, Volume 2)
ISBN 3-540-08549-1

Springer-Verlag
Berlin
Heidelberg
NewYork

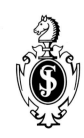

Advances in Anatomy, Embryology and Cell Biology

Volume 57
K. Niimi, H. Matsuoka

Thalamocortical Organization of the Auditory System in the Cat Studied by Retrograde Axonal Transport of Horseradish Peroxidase

1979. 30 figures, 1 table. IX, 56 pages
ISBN 3-540-09449-0

Volume 58
C. D. A. Verwoerd, C. G. van Oostrom

Cephalic Neural Crest and Placodes

1979. 41 figures. V, 75 pages
ISBN 3-540-09608-6

Volume 59
T. Bär

The Vascular System of the Cerebral Cortex

1980. 33 figures, 8 tables. VI, 62 pages
ISBN 3-540-09652-3

Volume 61
H. Korr

Proliferation of Different Cell Types in the Brain

1980. 21 figures, 1 table. VII, 72 pages
ISBN 3-540-09899-2

Volume 62
B. Brown Gould

Organization of Afferents from the Brain Stem Nuclei to the Cerebellar Cortex in the Cat

1980. 10 figures, 2 tables. VIII, 90 pages
ISBN 3-540-09960-3

Volume 64
A. Brodal, K. Kawamura

Olivocerebellar Projection: A Review

1980. 45 figures. VII, 140 pages
ISBN 3-540-10305-8

Volume 65
E. Pannese

The Satellite Cells of the Sensory Ganglia

1981. 30 figures. IX, 111 pages
ISBN 3-540-10219-1

Volume 67
H. Wolburg

Axonal Transport, Degeneration, and Regeneration in the Visual System of the Goldfish

1981. 28 figures. IX, 94 pages
ISBN 3-540-10336-8

Springer-Verlag
Berlin
Heidelberg
New York

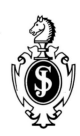